Nutrition for a Healthy Pregnancy

Nutrition for a Healthy Pregnancy

Editor: Jena Lin

AMERICAN
MEDICAL PUBLISHERS
www.americanmedicalpublishers.com

AMERICAN
MEDICAL PUBLISHERS
www.americanmedicalpublishers.com

Cataloging-in-Publication Data

Nutrition for a healthy pregnancy / edited by Jena Lin.
p. cm.
Includes bibliographical references and index.
ISBN 978-1-63927-761-2
1. Pregnancy--Nutritional aspects. 2. Prenatal care. 3. Pregnancy.
4. Nutrition--Requirements. I. Lin, Jena.
RG559 .N88 2023
618.24--dc23

American Medical Publishers,
41 Flatbush Avenue,
1st Floor, New York,
NY 11217, USA

ISBN 978-1-63927-761-2 (Hardback)

Contents

Preface

Pregnancy refers to a time where one or more offspring grows inside the womb of woman. A multiple pregnancy comprises more than one offspring, such as twins. Pregnancy generally occurs through sexual intercourse. It can also occur through assisted reproductive technology procedures. Nutrition is crucial while a woman is pregnant to maintain healthy development of the fetus. Nutrition at the time of pregnancy differs from the non-pregnant state. There is a need of specific micronutrients as well as increased energy. Sometimes, pregnant women might need to consult a doctor, if they have food allergies, specific religious/ethical beliefs and other medical conditions. During pregnancy, women should consume ample amount of healthy fats, lean protein, whole grains, vegetables and fruits. Foods rich in nutrients such as iron, vitamin D, folate and folic acid, protein and calcium should also be consumed. This book covers in detail some existent theories and innovative concepts revolving around nutrition and its role during pregnancy. It will serve as a reference to a broad spectrum of readers.

Various studies have approached the subject by analyzing it with a single perspective, but the present book provides diverse methodologies and techniques to address this field. This book contains theories and applications needed for understanding the subject from different perspectives. The aim is to keep the readers informed about the progresses in the field; therefore, the contributions were carefully examined to compile novel researches by specialists from across the globe.

Indeed, the job of the editor is the most crucial and challenging in compiling all chapters into a single book. In the end, I would extend my sincere thanks to the chapter authors for their profound work. I am also thankful for the support provided by my family and colleagues during the compilation of this book.

Editor

1

Maternal Omega-3 Nutrition, Placental Transfer and Fetal Brain Development in Gestational Diabetes and Preeclampsia

Prasad P. Devarshi *, Ryan W. Grant, Chioma J. Ikonte and Susan Hazels Mitmesser

Science and Technology, Pharmavite, LLC, West Hills, CA 91304, USA; rgrant@pharmavite.net (R.W.G.); cikonte@pharmavite.net (C.J.I.); smitmesser@pharmavite.net (S.H.M.)

* Correspondence: pdevarshi@pharmavite.net

Abstract: Omega-3 fatty acids, particularly docosahexaenoic fatty acid (DHA), are widely recognized to impact fetal and infant neurodevelopment. The impact of DHA on brain development, and its inefficient synthesis from the essential alpha-linolenic acid (ALA), has led to recommended DHA intakes of 250–375 mg eicosapentaenoic acid + DHA/day for pregnant and lactating women by the Dietary Guidelines for Americans. Despite these recommendations, the intake of omega-3s in women of child-bearing age in the US remains very low. The low maternal status of DHA prior to pregnancy could impair fetal neurodevelopment. This review focuses on maternal omega-3 status in conditions of gestational diabetes mellitus (GDM) and preeclampsia, and the subsequent impact on placental transfer and cord blood concentration of omega-3s. Both GDM and preeclampsia are associated with altered maternal omega-3 status, altered placental omega-3 metabolism, reduced cord blood omega-3 levels and have an impact on neurodevelopment in the infant and on brain health later in life. These findings indicate lower DHA exposure of the developing baby may be driven by lower placental transfer in both conditions. Thus, determining approaches which facilitate increased delivery of DHA during pregnancy and early development might positively impact brain development in infants born to mothers with these diseases.

Keywords: DHA; gestational diabetes; preeclampsia; placental transport

---

1. Introduction

Eicosapentaenoic acid (EPA, C20:5) and docosahexaenoic acid (DHA, C22:6) are omega-3 polyunsaturated fatty acids that are well-studied in humans [1–3]. Because they can be synthesized in the body from their precursor, alpha-linolenic acid (ALA, C18:3), EPA and DHA are not considered essential fatty acids. However, inefficient conversion of ALA to EPA and DHA [4,5] has led to recommendations to include food and dietary supplements as sources of EPA and DHA.

Wide recognition of the importance of EPA and DHA in infant development has led to recommendations for pregnant and lactating women from many regulatory bodies [6–10] and medical/scientific societies [11–17]. In the US, the American Academy of Pediatrics, American College of Obstetricians and Gynecologists, and March of Dimes recommend an intake of fish or omega-3 fatty acids resulting in ~200 mg DHA/day, and the Dietary Guidelines for Americans (DGA) recommends ~250–375 mg EPA + DHA/day. Despite these recommendations to promote the intake of omega-3 fatty acids, consumption of omega-3 fatty acids remains low across the US population [18], specifically in child-bearing-age, pregnant and lactating women [19]. Up to 95% of child-bearing-age and pregnant women do not meet the DGA recommendations for EPA + DHA intake [19]. Because of the impact DHA has on fetal development, the gap between the recommended and the actual DHA intake is concerning.

It is well established that DHA is an important structural component of the human brain and retina [20]. In the retina, DHA represents ~80% of all polyunsaturated fatty acids, while 60% of the dry weight of the brain is fatty acids, of which DHA is the major omega-3 fatty acid [21,22]. Omega-3 fatty acid deficiency leads to low levels of DHA in the cerebral cortex of the offspring and affects learning ability in animal models [23,24]. During fetal and infant development, membranes of the retina and brain grey matter become enriched with DHA [20]. During the third trimester, DHA selectively accumulates in the brain at a higher rate than other fatty acids [25]. This incorporation of DHA continues at these high rates until age 2 [26]. The first two years of life are an essential period of neurodevelopment for infants [27]. In the brain, DHA plays many important roles, including cell signaling, regulation of gene expression and neurotransmission [28–30]. In 60-day old rats, a diet deficient in omega-3 fatty acids led to altered physiology of neurotransmitters such as serotonin and dopamine, which are important for brain function [31]. Additionally, DHA deficiency led to decreased neuron size in various areas of the brain such as the hypothalamus and the hippocampus in animal models [32]. Normal neuron size is essential for their function in the brain [32]. Moreover, it was shown that maternal omega-3 deficiency not only affects neuronal size, but also neurogenesis in animals [33]. A lower rate of neurogenesis may affect cognitive function later in life [33]. Human studies have demonstrated that maternal omega-3 fatty acid supplementation increases maternal as well as fetal levels of DHA. DHA supplementation (200 mg/day) starting at the 21st week of gestation through lactation showed an increase in maternal red blood cells (RBCs) DHA at 37 weeks gestation and 3 months post birth. Additionally, this led to increased DHA in human milk and RBC DHA in the infant [34]. The benefits of omega-3 fatty acid supplementation during pregnancy have been well documented in the infant. After 1500 mg/week supplementation of DHA (as a functional food) during pregnancy, 9-month-old infants had improved performance on problem-solving tasks compared to the non-supplemented group [35]. Fish oil supplementation (2200 mg DHA and 1100 mg EPA per day) starting at 20 weeks gestation until birth showed an improvement in hand and eye coordination in the children at two and half years of age [36]. Additionally, hand and eye coordination scores positively correlated with omega-3 fatty acid levels in cord blood RBCs [36]. Supplementation of 600 mg/day of DHA from 14.5 weeks of gestation until birth, led to high levels of sustained attention in infants at 4, 6 and 9 month of age, while sustained attention declined in the control group during this period [37], suggesting the importance of omega-3 fatty acids in fetal brain development and function.

Despite the importance of omega-3 fatty acid intake on fetal brain development [38], most pregnant and child-bearing age women in the US are consuming less than the recommended amount [19]. While it is known that socioeconomic status influences infant cognitive development and nutrition [39,40], this review focuses on the effect of low placental omega-3 transfer in gestational diabetes mellitus (GDM) and preeclampsia on neurodevelopment. In addition to the low omega-3 fatty acid intake among pregnant women, in women with GDM and preeclampsia the transfer of DHA through the placenta to the fetus is compromised [41,42]. GDM is defined as impaired glucose tolerance first detected during pregnancy and is associated with various implications for fetal growth [43,44]. Preeclampsia is defined as systolic blood pressure of ≥140 mm Hg or diastolic blood pressure ≥90 mm Hg on two occasions at least 4 h apart, along with proteinuria, thrombocytopenia, renal insufficiency, impaired liver function, pulmonary edema, or cerebral or visual symptoms after 20 weeks of gestation [45]. Both GDM and preeclampsia are pregnancy disorders that have effects on fetal growth and development [43,44,46]. Due to the importance of omega-3 fatty acids in fetal brain development, it is important to understand the underlying mechanisms likely responsible for the reduced transfer of DHA to the fetus in GDM and preeclampsia. Here, we review the association of GDM and preeclampsia with maternal omega-3 fatty acid status, the impact of these disorders on the transfer of omega-3 fatty acids to the fetus, and subsequent effects on fetal brain development.

2. Gestational Diabetes

2.1. Maternal and Fetal Effects

In the course of gestation in all pregnancies, including normal pregnancies, insulin resistance increases progressively and is highest in the third trimester [47]. In normal pregnancies, the pancreatic beta cells produce higher levels of insulin which prevents hyperglycemia, whereas, in GDM, the response of these beta cells is inadequate, leading to hyperglycemia [47]. GDM is defined as impaired glucose tolerance first detected during pregnancy and is associated with various implications for fetal growth [43,44]. According to the 2014 analysis by the Centers for Disease Control and Prevention, GDM affects 9.2% of all pregnancies in the US [48]. Mechanisms involving progesterone and glucocorticoids and their effect on insulin sensitivity have been suggested to be responsible for the increase of insulin resistance during gestation [49,50]. Progesterone secretion increases during pregnancy and it has been shown to decrease the ability of insulin to suppress synthesis of glucose in the liver [49]. Cortisol is a glucocorticoid that increases during pregnancy and has have been shown to affect skeletal muscle insulin signaling [50,51]. Glucocorticoids reduce phosphorylation of the insulin receptor and reduce the content of insulin receptor substrate-1, which is involved in insulin signaling, in the skeletal muscle [50]. Women with GDM have higher levels of insulin resistance compared to normal pregnancy controls [52]. The combination of elevated insulin resistance and inadequate beta cells response both likely contribute to hyperglycemia in GDM [47,52,53]. GDM has a complicated etiology involving numerous metabolic and genetic factors with many underlying mechanisms [54]. A large prospective cohort study found that aging, obesity, non-white ethnicity, family history of diabetes and smoking increases the risk for developing GDM [55]. In addition, the development of GDM during pregnancy increases the risk of GDM in future pregnancies [56].The etiology of GDM is complex and comprises lifestyle and genetic risk factors, with many potential mechanisms.

GDM leads to adverse long-term effects including a higher risk of developing metabolic diseases in the mother and the child [57,58]. In addition to these adverse effects, the presence of diabetes during pregnancy is associated with impaired neurodevelopment [59–64]. Infants of mothers with GDM showed lower mental and psychomotor development indexes compared to infants of non-GDM mothers at 6 months of age [59]. Similarly, children below 9 years of age, of mothers with GDM, had lower verbal IQ scores than children of non-GDM mothers [60]. These children also scored low compared to children of non-GDM mothers in the Pollack tapper test, which is used to detect learning disabilities [60]. GDM also affects language development during childhood [61]. Children (18 and 30 months) of GDM mothers had lower expressive vocabulary and grammar scores compared to children of non-GDM mothers [61]. These children were at a 2.2-fold higher risk of having impaired language development [61]. In children of GDM mothers at 8 years of age, a trend towards lower IQ scores compared to children of non-GDM mothers was seen [64]. As DHA is an important nutrient for fetal brain development [38], it has been suggested that the effects on neurodevelopment may be as a result of low cord blood levels of DHA seen in GDM [59]. Additionally, in animal models, it has been suggested that inflammation due to GDM can lead to adverse effects on neurodevelopment in the offspring [65]. In totality, these studies demonstrate the influence of GDM on neurodevelopment.

2.2. Placental Transfer of Omega-3 Fatty Acids in GDM

The negative neurodevelopment effects observed in children of mothers with GDM could be a result of lower omega-3 fatty acid transfer from the mother to the fetus [66]. Maternal DHA is the primary source of DHA for the fetus as it cannot be synthesized in the fetus or the placenta [41]. The placenta preferentially absorbs DHA for transfer to the fetus during pregnancy and this is demonstrated by higher cord vein DHA levels compared to maternal blood DHA levels [67]. In GDM pregnancies, cord vein blood levels of DHA are lower than the levels in normal pregnancies [59,66,68]. Specifically, maternal DHA levels have been shown to be 11–44% higher in GDM, while cord blood levels were lower compared to normal pregnancies, indicating a possibility of reduced placental transfer of DHA to the fetus in GDM [69]. Thomas et al. similarly found that cord vein DHA was lower in GDM versus normal pregnancy [68]. Wijendran et al. observed that GDM mothers had a higher intake of omega-3 fatty acids during the third trimester of pregnancy compared to normal pregnancy controls [66]. Due to higher dietary intake, GDM mothers also had significantly higher maternal DHA erythrocyte content [66]. However, in spite of higher DHA intake and maternal DHA erythrocyte levels, DHA in cord vein erythrocytes was significantly lower (37% lower) than in normal pregnancy controls [66]. In this study, maternal plasma DHA positively correlated with DHA in fetal erythrocytes in the normal pregnancy control group, however this correlation was not present in GDM mothers [66]. Moreover, maternal hemoglobin A1c (HbA1C) levels were inversely related to fetal erythrocyte DHA content in GDM mothers, which suggests a relation between GDM and transfer of DHA to the fetus [66].

Several mechanisms have been proposed for the reduction in placental transfer of DHA in GDM. Peroxisome proliferator-activated receptor (PPAR)-alpha and PPAR-gamma belong to the family of nuclear receptors that control various fatty acid metabolism related genes, including genes related to fatty acid transport [70]. PPAR-alpha mainly controls fatty acid oxidation related genes and PPAR-gamma controls adipogenesis related genes [70]. PPAR-alpha was downregulated in GDM placentae compared to uncomplicated term placentae [71]. Also, PPAR-gamma had lower gene and protein expression in GDM placenta [71]. Lipoprotein lipase (LPL), which is expressed in the microvillous plasma membrane of the placenta, is needed to release free fatty acids from triglycerides in circulating lipoproteins, leading to uptake by the placenta [72]. In pregnancies complicated by type-1 diabetes, LPL activity in the microvillous plasma membrane of the placenta was increased by 39% compared to the normal pregnancy control, but no difference was seen in GDM pregnancies indicating that LPL is not involved in mechanisms related to reduced placental transfer of DHA in GDM [72,73]. The transport of fatty acid through the placenta is orchestrated by a number of proteins, including: Fatty acid transfer proteins such as fatty acid transport protein (FATP)-1-6, cluster of differentiation 36 (CD-36), fatty-acid-binding protein (FABP)-pm, placental-FABP-pm in the plasma membrane and FABP-1, 3, 4, 5, 7 [74]. In GDM placenta, it was seen that expression of FATP-1 and FATP-4 were decreased, while expression of CD-36 and FATP-6 were increased compared to normal pregnancy controls [75]. The major facilitator superfamily domain-containing protein 2A (MFSD2A) was identified as a brain choline and DHA transporter [76]. It was seen that MFSD2A was significantly reduced in GDM placentae [77]. DHA percentage in the cord vein blood correlated with levels of MFSD2A, suggesting a possible role in placental transfer of DHA to the fetus [77]. These alterations could be possibly responsible for reduced DHA transfer across the placenta.

Some studies have investigated the effect of omega-3 fatty acid supplementation during pregnancy on GDM [78–80]. Zhou et al. investigated the effect of DHA supplementation on the incidence of GDM [81]. DHA intake of 800 mg/day did not affect risk of developing GDM [81]. In GDM women, 800 mg/day of DHA supplementation starting at 17–33 weeks of gestation, increased DHA in maternal plasma and RBCs, but failed to increase DHA in cord vein plasma and RBCs. More studies investigating the effects of early DHA supplementation on placental expression of fatty acid metabolism-related genes and fetal outcomes are needed.

3. Preeclampsia

3.1. Maternal and Fetal Effects

Preeclampsia occurs in ~3% of pregnancies and negatively impacts both maternal and fetal health outcomes [45]. The American College of Obstetricians and Gynecologists defines preeclampsia as a systolic blood pressure of ≥140 mm Hg or diastolic blood pressure ≥90 mm Hg on two occasions at least 4 h apart, which co-occurs with proteinuria, thrombocytopenia, renal insufficiency, impaired liver function, pulmonary edema, or cerebral or visual symptoms after 20 weeks of gestation [45]. Although preeclampsia typically develops during the second trimester of pregnancy, its disease pathogenesis likely begins in the first trimester during implantation. Delivery of nutrients from the mother to the fetus depends on placental vasculature. Placental vascular development requires remodeling of the uterine spiral arteries from narrow vessels to wider, low resistance vessels [82]. Impairment of vascular remodeling during early gestation is thought to result in the later development of preeclampsia. Proposed mechanisms leading to preeclampsia include impairment of endothelial function and a maternal immune response to the invading trophoblast cells that remodel the spiral arteries [82]. During pregnancy, the maternal immune system develops tolerance to cells of the fetus [83]. Defects in the development of tolerance and activation of a pro-inflammatory response may be contributing factors to the development of preeclampsia [83].

Impairment of placental vascularization during preeclampsia limits efficient delivery of nutrients and oxygen to the fetus. Low oxygen levels lead to increased rates of neuronal apoptosis in experimental models of preeclampsia and perinatal asphyxia [84]. In addition to the sensitivity of neurons to low oxygen levels, hypoxia can drive tissue inflammatory responses. Preeclampsia upregulates placental expression of proinflammatory cytokines (tumor necrosis factor-α, Interleukin-1 (IL-1), and IL-18) and downregulates the anti-inflammatory cytokine IL-10 [85]. Indeed, human term placental explants exposed to low oxygen levels had increased production of tumor necrosis factor-α, IL-1α and β [86]. In ischemic brain injury, there is upregulation of both IL-1β and IL-18. Mice that lack production of IL-18 or were treated with an intracerebroventricular injection of an IL-1 receptor antagonist have reduced ischemic brain injury [87,88]. Hypoxia additionally promotes the production of reactive oxygen species and the development of oxidative stress, which can also contribute to neuronal apoptosis [89]. The impact of hypoxia on neuronal apoptosis, inflammation and oxidative stress likely function together to negatively impact brain development. In children, prenatal hypoxia is a known contributor to impaired cognitive development [90]. Specifically, preeclampsia negatively impacts several aspects of cognitive function including verbal reasoning and executive function during early childhood [91]. Preeclampsia may also impact brain health later in life. Children from mothers with preeclampsia had higher depression symptoms during adulthood [91]. These findings suggest that preeclampsia may impact the brain across the lifespan. To establish a link between preeclampsia and brain function, some studies have analyzed brain structure. Initial studies have demonstrated that children from preeclamptic pregnancies exhibit differences in the structure and connectivity of limbic system components, an area of the brain linked with mood, behavior and cognition [91]. Although the underlying factors that drive preeclampsia are not completely understood, evidence indicates that preeclampsia impacts maternal and fetal health, as well as long-term development.

3.2. *Placental Transfer of Omega-3 Fatty Acids in Preeclampsia*

Omega-3 fatty acids, and particularly DHA, are critical to the structure and function of developing nervous system cells. Several factors influence the availability of DHA and EPA to fetal tissues, including: Dietary intake, endogenous synthesis from alpha-linolenic acid, transport within the blood for delivery to placental tissues, placental tissue uptake and transfer to cord blood. Several case-controlled studies have demonstrated that during the third trimester or postpartum, blood levels of omega-3 fatty acids are reduced in mothers with preeclampsia compared to normal pregnancy. An initial study of postpartum mothers indicated that women in the lowest tertile of erythrocyte omega-3 fatty acid content were 7.6 times more likely to have preeclampsia compared with those in the highest tertile [92]. Kulkarni et al. found that at delivery, plasma DHA levels were reduced in preeclamptic vs. normotensive pregnancy, and this difference was also reflected in infant cord blood samples [93]. An additional study found that third trimester levels of omega-3 fatty acids were reduced in mothers with preeclampsia or intrauterine growth restriction (IUGR) compared to normal pregnancy [94]. Cord blood taken from these subjects also indicates a reduction in total omega-3 fatty acids and DHA compared to normal pregnancy [94]. Although differences in maternal omega-3 fatty acids during the third trimester are apparent, they don't account for exposure across the duration of pregnancy. A more recent study examined longitudinal changes of serum fatty acid proportions in normotensive and preeclamptic pregnant women. This study demonstrated reduced circulation of total omega-3 fatty acids, DHA and arachidonic acid at 16–20 weeks but not at 26–30 weeks or at delivery in preeclamptic pregnant women [95]. This study did confirm lower cord blood levels of both DHA and total omega-3 fatty acids at delivery with preeclampsia, which were similar to the differences found by Kulkarni et al. [95]. This study also revealed significant correlation of maternal plasma DHA with cord plasma DHA across all three time points [95], highlighting reduced maternal omega-3 fatty acids during preeclampsia.

Given that maternal blood levels of omega-3 fatty acids are low during preeclampsia, a key question is whether the placenta can compensate by upregulating the trafficking, synthesis and/or transfer of omega-3 fatty acids. The fatty acid composition of placentas from mothers with preeclampsia is different from those with normal pregnancies. Wang et al. demonstrated that placentas from preeclamptic women have reduced total non-esterified polyunsaturated fatty acids, including lower total omega-3 fatty acids and DHA compared to placenta from normal pregnant women [96]. The observation of reduced placental DHA has been confirmed by other studies [95,97,98]. An initial study comparing omega-3 fatty acid composition in different areas of the placenta indicates regional differences between normotensive controls, term pregnancy with preeclampsia and preterm pregnancy with preeclampsia. DHA and total omega-3 fatty acid concentrations were consistently lower in the central fetal and maternal areas of the placenta in mothers with preeclampsia and preterm delivery [97]. Additionally, in the central fetal area there were higher concentrations of ALA with preterm delivery and preeclampsia, indicating a possibility of inefficient conversion of ALA to DHA [97]. Because there were no matched normotensive preterm controls, it is unclear whether these changes are driven by gestational time or the severity of disease.

The placenta transports omega-3 fatty acids and expresses enzymes which contribute to the metabolism of ALA into EPA and DHA. Thus far, studies do not indicate increased capability for EPA + DHA synthesis or transport in preeclampsia. The expression of genes responsible for placental lipid transport (FATP 1 and 4) and fatty acid elongation (fatty acid desaturase 1) were reduced with preeclampsia, while others (fatty acid desaturase 2 and FABP-3) were not altered [95]. This indicates that during preeclampsia there may be a down regulation of the capacity to transport lipid in the placenta, and potentially a reduced capacity to synthesize DHA from ALA in placental tissue. Placental mRNA expression of MFSD2A, a DHA transporter in the brain, is reduced during severe preeclampsia compared to normotensive pregnancy [99]. However, it is unknown what the impact of this reduction is on fetal development. Collectively, these observations indicated altered transport and metabolism of omega-3 fatty acids during preeclampsia. These results are supported by reduced omega-3 fatty acids in placental tissue and cord blood from mothers with preeclampsia versus normal pregnancy. It is currently unknown whether cord blood DHA levels are responsive to increased dietary intake during preeclampsia.

A number of intervention trials were conducted to understand if supplemental omega-3 fatty acids from fish oil could impact maternal outcomes associated with preeclampsia. These studies have been largely ineffective [100] and vary widely in dose and composition of omega-3 fatty acids, as well as gestational age at the onset of the intervention [101]. Although studies have focused on the mother, this does not preclude impact on the baby. It was noted by Kulkarni et al. that cord blood DHA levels were correlated with serum DHA levels in mothers with preeclampsia. This raises the possibility that increasing maternal omega-3 fatty acid status may increase omega-3 fatty acid exposure of the developing baby. Future studies are needed to determine whether increased maternal prenatal omega-3 fatty acid intake can improve cord blood DHA and developmental outcomes in babies born to mothers with preeclampsia.

4. Conclusions

Despite the recommendations from various authorities, 95% of pregnant and child-bearing-age women do not consume enough omega-3 fatty acids [19,38]. Transfer of omega-3 fatty acids through the placenta to the cord blood and fetus is impaired in GDM and preeclampsia [41,42,75,77,95]. This is reflected in both conditions by lower cord vein DHA levels compared to normal pregnancies [66,93]. Given the role DHA plays in fetal neurodevelopment, lower DHA transfer to the fetus may contribute to impaired neurodevelopment.

Although it is apparent that GDM and preeclampsia are associated with lower cord blood levels of DHA, the impact of DHA and omega-3 fatty acid supplementation on fetal neurodevelopment in this population remains unclear. In GDM, increasing DHA intake later in pregnancy did not increase cord blood levels, possibly due to impaired DHA placental transfer [102]. Future studies in both GDM and preeclampsia need to focus on very early interventions. Such studies could elucidate the time course of serum fatty acids during pregnancy and the impact of DHA supplementation on maternal blood, placental and cord vein DHA levels. Additionally, there is a need to further link infant neurodevelopmental outcomes to omega-3 fatty acid intake. One factor that may influence the effects of omega-3 fatty acids on neurodevelopment may be socioeconomic status. Most of the studies discussed did not evaluate the impact of socioeconomic status on offspring neurodevelopment. This is a limitation, as socioeconomic status has been suggested to affect neurodevelopment and omega-3 nutrition [39,40]. Future studies are needed to determine the effect of socioeconomic status on maternal nutritional interventions and offspring neurodevelopment. While DHA intake prior to and during pregnancy is important, postnatal DHA intake could be an impactful opportunity to increase delivery of DHA to the breast-fed new born baby. Interventions supporting increased DHA consumption might positively impact neurodevelopmental outcomes associated with GDM and preeclampsia.

Author Contributions: Conceptualization, P.P.D. and R.W.G.; writing—original draft preparation, P.P.D. and R.W.G.; and writing—review and editing, C.J.I. and S.H.M.

References

1. Mozaffarian, D.; Wu, J.H.Y. Omega-3 Fatty Acids and Cardiovascular Disease. *J. Am. Coll. Cardiol.* **2011**, *58*, 2047. [CrossRef] [PubMed]
2. Lorente-Cebrián, S.; Costa, A.G.V.; Navas-Carretero, S.; Zabala, M.; Martínez, J.A.; Moreno-Aliaga, M.J. Role of omega-3 fatty acids in obesity, metabolic syndrome, and cardiovascular diseases: A review of the evidence. *J. Physiol. Biochem.* **2013**, *69*, 633–651. [CrossRef]
3. Ruxton, C.H.S.; Reed, S.C.; Simpson, M.J.A.; Millington, K.J. The health benefits of omega-3 polyunsaturated fatty acids: A review of the evidence. *J. Hum. Nutr. Diet.* **2004**, *17*, 449–459. [CrossRef] [PubMed]
4. Goyens, P.L.; Spilker, M.E.; Zock, P.L.; Katan, M.B.; Mensink, R.P. Compartmental modeling to quantify alpha-linolenic acid conversion after longer term intake of multiple tracer boluses. *J. Lipid Res.* **2005**, *46*, 1474–1483. [CrossRef] [PubMed]
5. Hussein, N.; Ah-Sing, E.; Wilkinson, P.; Leach, C.; Griffin, B.A.; Millward, D.J. Long-chain conversion of [13C]linoleic acid and alpha-linolenic acid in response to marked changes in their dietary intake in men. *J. Lipid Res.* **2005**, *46*, 269–280. [CrossRef] [PubMed]
6. Fats and fatty acids in human nutrition. Report of an expert consultation. *FAO Food Nutr. Pap.* **2010**, *91*, 1–166.
7. Koletzko, B.; Lien, E.; Agostoni, C.; Bohles, H.; Campoy, C.; Cetin, I.; Decsi, T.; Dudenhausen, J.W.; Dupont, C.; Forsyth, S.; et al. The roles of long-chain polyunsaturated fatty acids in pregnancy, lactation and infancy: Review of current knowledge and consensus recommendations. *J. Perinat. Med.* **2008**, *36*, 5–14. [CrossRef]
8. Koletzko, B.; Cetin, I.; Brenna, J.T.; Perinatal Lipid Intake Working Group; Child Health Foundation; Diabetic Pregnancy Study Group; European Association of Perinatal Medicine; European Society for Clinical Nutrition and Metabolism; European Society for Paediatric Gastroenterology, Hepatology and Nutrition; Committee on Nutrition; et al. Dietary fat intakes for pregnant and lactating women. *Br. J. Nutr.* **2007**, *98*, 873–877. [CrossRef]

9. Scientific Opinion on Dietary Reference Values for fats, including saturated fatty acids, polyunsaturated fatty acids, monounsaturated fatty acids, trans fatty acids, and cholesterol. *EFSA J.* **2010**, *8*, 1461. [CrossRef]
10. Simopoulos, A.P.; Leaf, A.; Salem, N., Jr. Workshop on the Essentiality of and Recommended Dietary Intakes for Omega-6 and Omega-3 Fatty Acids. *J. Am. Coll. Nutr.* **1999**, *18*, 487–489. [CrossRef]
11. Nesheim, M.; Yaktine, A. (Eds.) Analysis of the balancing of benefits and risks of seafood consumption. In *Seafood Choices: Balancing Benefits and Risks*; National Academies Press: Washington, DC, USA, 2007; pp. 195–216.
12. Carlson, S.E. Docosahexaenoic acid supplementation in pregnancy and lactation. *Am. J. Clin. Nutr.* **2009**, *89*, 678S–684S. [CrossRef] [PubMed]
13. Coletta, J.M.; Bell, S.J.; Roman, A.S. Omega-3 Fatty acids and pregnancy. *Rev. Obstet. Gynecol.* **2010**, *3*, 163–171. [CrossRef] [PubMed]
14. Dimes, M.O. Vitamins and Other Nutrients During Pregnancy. Available online: https://www.marchofdimes.org/pregnancy/vitamins-and-other-nutrients-during-pregnancy.aspx (accessed on 1 March 2019).
15. Pediatrics, A.A.O. Breastfeeding and the use of human milk. *Pediatrics* **2012**, *129*, e827–e841. [CrossRef]
16. US Department of Health and Human Services. 2015–2020 Dietary Guidelines for Americans. Available online: https://health.gov/dietaryguidelines/2015/resources/2015-2020_Dietary_Guidelines.pdf (accessed on 4 March 2019).
17. 2017 EPA-FDA Advice about Eating Fish and Shellfish. Available online: https://www.epa.gov/fish-tech/2017-epa-fda-advice-about-eating-fish-and-shellfish (accessed on 1 March 2019).
18. Papanikolaou, Y.; Brooks, J.; Reider, C.; Fulgoni, V.L. US adults are not meeting recommended levels for fish and omega-3 fatty acid intake: Results of an analysis using observational data from NHANES 2003–2008. *Nutr. J.* **2014**, *13*, 31. [CrossRef] [PubMed]
19. Zhang, Z.; Fulgoni, V.L.; Kris-Etherton, P.M.; Mitmesser, S.H. Dietary Intakes of EPA and DHA Omega-3 Fatty Acids among US Childbearing-Age and Pregnant Women: An Analysis of NHANES 2001-2014. *Nutrients* **2018**, *10*, 416. [CrossRef] [PubMed]
20. Innis, S.M. Perinatal biochemistry and physiology of long-chain polyunsaturated fatty acids. *J. Pediatrics* **2003**, *143*, S1–S8. [CrossRef]
21. Giusto, N.M.; Pasquare, S.J.; Salvador, G.A.; Castagnet, P.I.; Roque, M.E.; Ilincheta de Boschero, M.G. Lipid metabolism in vertebrate retinal rod outer segments. *Prog. Lipid Res.* **2000**, *39*, 315–391. [CrossRef]
22. Bradbury, J. Docosahexaenoic acid (DHA): An ancient nutrient for the modern human brain. *Nutrients* **2011**, *3*, 529–554. [CrossRef]
23. Neuringer, M.; Connor, W.E.; Lin, D.S.; Barstad, L.; Luck, S. Biochemical and functional effects of prenatal and postnatal omega 3 fatty acid deficiency on retina and brain in rhesus monkeys. *Proc. Natl. Acad. Sci. USA* **1986**, *83*, 4021–4025. [CrossRef]
24. Yamamoto, N.; Hashimoto, A.; Takemoto, Y.; Okuyama, H.; Nomura, M.; Kitajima, R.; Togashi, T.; Tamai, Y. Effect of the dietary alpha-linolenate/linoleate balance on lipid compositions and learning ability of rats. II. Discrimination process, extinction process, and glycolipid compositions. *J. Lipid Res.* **1988**, *29*, 1013–1021.
25. Cetin, I.; Alvino, G.; Cardellicchio, M. Long chain fatty acids and dietary fats in fetal nutrition. *J. Physiol.* **2009**, *587*, 3441–3451. [CrossRef]
26. Lauritzen, L.; Brambilla, P.; Mazzocchi, A.; Harsløf, L.B.S.; Ciappolino, V.; Agostoni, C. DHA Effects in Brain Development and Function. *Nutrients* **2016**, *8*, 6. [CrossRef]
27. Schwarzenberg, S.J.; Georgieff, M.K. Advocacy for Improving Nutrition in the First 1000 Days to Support Childhood Development and Adult Health. *Pediatrics* **2018**, *141*, e20173716. [CrossRef]
28. Kitajka, K.; Puskas, L.G.; Zvara, A.; Hackler, L., Jr.; Barcelo-Coblijn, G.; Yeo, Y.K.; Farkas, T. The role of n-3 polyunsaturated fatty acids in brain: Modulation of rat brain gene expression by dietary n-3 fatty acids. *Proc. Natl. Acad. Sci. USA* **2002**, *99*, 2619–2624. [CrossRef] [PubMed]
29. Stillwell, W.; Shaikh, S.R.; Zerouga, M.; Siddiqui, R.; Wassall, S.R. Docosahexaenoic acid affects cell signaling by altering lipid rafts. *Reprod. Nutr. Dev.* **2005**, *45*, 559–579. [CrossRef]
30. Chalon, S. Omega-3 fatty acids and monoamine neurotransmission. *Prostaglandins Leukot. Essent. Fat. Acids* **2006**, *75*, 259–269. [CrossRef]
31. Delion, S.; Chalon, S.; Herault, J.; Guilloteau, D.; Besnard, J.C.; Durand, G. Chronic dietary alpha-linolenic acid deficiency alters dopaminergic and serotoninergic neurotransmission in rats. *J. Nutr.* **1994**, *124*, 2466–2476. [CrossRef]

32. Ahmad, A.; Moriguchi, T.; Salem, N. Decrease in neuron size in docosahexaenoic acid-deficient brain. *Pediatric Neurol.* **2002**, *26*, 210–218. [CrossRef]
33. Coti Bertrand, P.; O'Kusky, J.R.; Innis, S.M. Maternal dietary (n-3) fatty acid deficiency alters neurogenesis in the embryonic rat brain. *J. Nutr.* **2006**, *136*, 1570–1575. [CrossRef]
34. Bergmann, R.L.; Haschke-Becher, E.; Klassen-Wigger, P.; Bergmann, K.E.; Richter, R.; Dudenhausen, J.W.; Grathwohl, D.; Haschke, F. Supplementation with 200 mg/day docosahexaenoic acid from mid-pregnancy through lactation improves the docosahexaenoic acid status of mothers with a habitually low fish intake and of their infants. *Ann. Nutr. Metab.* **2008**, *52*, 157–166. [CrossRef]
35. Judge, M.P.; Harel, O.; Lammi-Keefe, C.J. Maternal consumption of a docosahexaenoic acid-containing functional food during pregnancy: Benefit for infant performance on problem-solving but not on recognition memory tasks at age 9 mo. *Am. J. Clin. Nutr.* **2007**, *85*, 1572–1577. [CrossRef] [PubMed]
36. Dunstan, J.A.; Simmer, K.; Dixon, G.; Prescott, S.L. Cognitive assessment of children at age 2(1/2) years after maternal fish oil supplementation in pregnancy: A randomised controlled trial. *Arch. Dis. Child. Fetal Neonatal Ed.* **2008**, *93*, F45–F50. [CrossRef]
37. Colombo, J.; Gustafson, K.M.; Gajewski, B.J.; Shaddy, D.J.; Kerling, E.H.; Thodosoff, J.M.; Doty, T.; Brez, C.C.; Carlson, S.E. Prenatal DHA supplementation and infant attention. *Pediatric Res.* **2016**, *80*, 656–662. [CrossRef]
38. Innis, S.M. Dietary omega 3 fatty acids and the developing brain. *Brain Res.* **2008**, *1237*, 35–43. [CrossRef]
39. Nordgren, T.M.; Lyden, E.; Anderson-Berry, A.; Hanson, C. Omega-3 Fatty Acid Intake of Pregnant Women and Women of Childbearing Age in the United States: Potential for Deficiency? *Nutrients* **2017**, *9*, 197. [CrossRef]
40. Chin-Lun Hung, G.; Hahn, J.; Alamiri, B.; Buka, S.L.; Goldstein, J.M.; Laird, N.; Nelson, C.A.; Smoller, J.W.; Gilman, S.E. Socioeconomic disadvantage and neural development from infancy through early childhood. *Int. J. Epidemiol.* **2015**, *44*, 1889–1899. [CrossRef]
41. Gil-Sánchez, A.; Demmelmair, H.; Parrilla, J.; Koletzko, B.; Larqué, E. Mechanisms Involved in the Selective Transfer of Long Chain Polyunsaturated Fatty Acids to the Fetus. *Front. Genet.* **2011**, *2*, 57. [CrossRef]
42. Wadhwani, N.; Patil, V.; Joshi, S. Maternal long chain polyunsaturated fatty acid status and pregnancy complications. *Prostaglandins Leukot. Essent. Fat. Acids* **2018**, *136*, 143–152. [CrossRef] [PubMed]
43. Ornoy, A. Prenatal origin of obesity and their complications: Gestational diabetes, maternal overweight and the paradoxical effects of fetal growth restriction and macrosomia. *Reprod. Toxicol.* **2011**, *32*, 205–212. [CrossRef] [PubMed]
44. Gestational Diabetes Mellitus. *Diabetes Care* **2004**, *27*, s88. [CrossRef] [PubMed]
45. American College of Obstetricians and Gynecologists. Hypertension in pregnancy. Report of the American College of Obstetricians and Gynecologists' task force on hypertension in pregnancy. *Obstet. Gynecol.* **2013**, *122*, 1122.
46. Backes, C.H.; Markham, K.; Moorehead, P.; Cordero, L.; Nankervis, C.A.; Giannone, P.J. Maternal preeclampsia and neonatal outcomes. *J. Pregnancy* **2011**, *2011*, 214365. [CrossRef] [PubMed]
47. Di Cianni, G.; Miccoli, R.; Volpe, L.; Lencioni, C.; Del Prato, S. Intermediate metabolism in normal pregnancy and in gestational diabetes. *Diabetes/Metab. Res. Rev.* **2003**, *19*, 259–270. [CrossRef] [PubMed]
48. DeSisto, C.L.; Kim, S.Y.; Sharma, A.J. Prevalence estimates of gestational diabetes mellitus in the United States, Pregnancy Risk Assessment Monitoring System (PRAMS), 2007–2010. *Prev. Chronic Dis.* **2014**, *11*, E104. [CrossRef] [PubMed]
49. Nelson, T.; Shulman, G.; Grainger, D.; Diamond, M.P. Progesterone administration induced impairment of insulin suppression of hepatic glucose production. *Fertil. Steril.* **1994**, *62*, 491–496. [CrossRef]
50. Giorgino, F.; Almahfouz, A.; Goodyear, L.J.; Smith, R.J. Glucocorticoid regulation of insulin receptor and substrate IRS-1 tyrosine phosphorylation in rat skeletal muscle in vivo. *J. Clin. Investig.* **1993**, *91*, 2020–2030. [CrossRef]
51. Buss, C.; Davis, E.P.; Shahbaba, B.; Pruessner, J.C.; Head, K.; Sandman, C.A. Maternal cortisol over the course of pregnancy and subsequent child amygdala and hippocampus volumes and affective problems. *Proc. Natl. Acad. Sci. USA* **2012**, *109*, E1312–E1319. [CrossRef]
52. Xiang, A.H.; Peters, R.K.; Trigo, E.; Kjos, S.L.; Lee, W.P.; Buchanan, T.A. Multiple metabolic defects during late pregnancy in women at high risk for type 2 diabetes. *Diabetes* **1999**, *48*, 848–854. [CrossRef]

53. Kautzky-Willer, A.; Prager, R.; Waldhausl, W.; Pacini, G.; Thomaseth, K.; Wagner, O.F.; Ulm, M.; Streli, C.; Ludvik, B. Pronounced insulin resistance and inadequate beta-cell secretion characterize lean gestational diabetes during and after pregnancy. *Diabetes Care* **1997**, *20*, 1717–1723. [CrossRef]
54. Johns, E.C.; Denison, F.C.; Norman, J.E.; Reynolds, R.M. Gestational Diabetes Mellitus: Mechanisms, Treatment, and Complications. *Trends Endocrinol. Metab. TEM* **2018**, *29*, 743–754. [CrossRef] [PubMed]
55. Solomon, C.G.; Willett, W.C.; Carey, V.J.; Rich-Edwards, J.; Hunter, D.J.; Colditz, G.A.; Stampfer, M.J.; Speizer, F.E.; Spiegelman, D.; Manson, J.E. A prospective study of pregravid determinants of gestational diabetes mellitus. *Jama* **1997**, *278*, 1078–1083. [CrossRef]
56. Kim, C.; Berger, D.K.; Chamany, S. Recurrence of gestational diabetes mellitus: A systematic review. *Diabetes Care* **2007**, *30*, 1314–1319. [CrossRef]
57. Metzger, B.E. Long-term outcomes in mothers diagnosed with gestational diabetes mellitus and their offspring. *Clin. Obstet. Gynecol.* **2007**, *50*, 972–979. [CrossRef]
58. West, N.A.; Crume, T.L.; Maligie, M.A.; Dabelea, D. Cardiovascular risk factors in children exposed to maternal diabetes in utero. *Diabetologia* **2011**, *54*, 504–507. [CrossRef]
59. Zornoza-Moreno, M.; Fuentes-Hernandez, S.; Carrion, V.; Alcantara-Lopez, M.V.; Madrid, J.A.; Lopez-Soler, C.; Sanchez-Solis, M.; Larque, E. Is low docosahexaenoic acid associated with disturbed rhythms and neurodevelopment in offsprings of diabetic mothers? *Eur. J. Clin. Nutr.* **2014**, *68*, 931–937. [CrossRef]
60. Ornoy, A.; Wolf, A.; Ratzon, N.; Greenbaum, C.; Dulitzky, M. Neurodevelopmental outcome at early school age of children born to mothers with gestational diabetes. *Arch. Disease Child. Fetal Neonatal Ed.* **1999**, *81*, F10–F14. [CrossRef]
61. Dionne, G.; Boivin, M.; Seguin, J.R.; Perusse, D.; Tremblay, R.E. Gestational diabetes hinders language development in offspring. *Pediatrics* **2008**, *122*, e1073–e1079. [CrossRef]
62. Dahlquist, G.; Kallen, B. School marks for Swedish children whose mothers had diabetes during pregnancy: A population-based study. *Diabetologia* **2007**, *50*, 1826–1831. [CrossRef]
63. DeBoer, T.; Wewerka, S.; Bauer, P.J.; Georgieff, M.K.; Nelson, C.A. Explicit memory performance in infants of diabetic mothers at 1 year of age. *Dev. Med. Child Neurol.* **2005**, *47*, 525–531. [CrossRef]
64. Fraser, A.; Nelson, S.M.; Macdonald-Wallis, C.; Lawlor, D.A. Associations of existing diabetes, gestational diabetes, and glycosuria with offspring IQ and educational attainment: The Avon Longitudinal Study of Parents and Children. *Exp. Diabetes Res.* **2012**, *2012*, 963735. [CrossRef]
65. Vuong, B.; Odero, G.; Rozbacher, S.; Stevenson, M.; Kereliuk, S.M.; Pereira, T.J.; Dolinsky, V.W.; Kauppinen, T.M. Exposure to gestational diabetes mellitus induces neuroinflammation, derangement of hippocampal neurons, and cognitive changes in rat offspring. *J. Neuroinflamm.* **2017**, *14*, 80. [CrossRef]
66. Wijendran, V.; Bendel, R.B.; Couch, S.C.; Philipson, E.H.; Cheruku, S.; Lammi-Keefe, C.J. Fetal erythrocyte phospholipid polyunsaturated fatty acids are altered in pregnancy complicated with gestational diabetes mellitus. *Lipids* **2000**, *35*, 927–931. [CrossRef]
67. Berghaus, T.M.; Demmelmair, H.; Koletzko, B. Essential fatty acids and their long-chain polyunsaturated metabolites in maternal and cord plasma triglycerides during late gestation. *Biol. Neonate* **2000**, *77*, 96–100. [CrossRef]
68. Thomas, B.A.; Ghebremeskel, K.; Lowy, C.; Offley-Shore, B.; Crawford, M.A. Plasma fatty acids of neonates born to mothers with and without gestational diabetes. *Prostaglandins Leukot. Essent. Fat. Acids* **2005**, *72*, 335–341. [CrossRef]
69. Leveille, P.; Rouxel, C.; Plourde, M. Diabetic pregnancy, maternal and fetal docosahexaenoic acid: A review of existing evidence. *J. Matern. Fetal Neonatal Med.* **2018**, *31*, 1358–1363. [CrossRef]
70. Grygiel-Górniak, B. Peroxisome proliferator-activated receptors and their ligands: Nutritional and clinical implications-a review. *Nutr. J.* **2014**, *13*, 17. [CrossRef]
71. Holdsworth-Carson, S.J.; Lim, R.; Mitton, A.; Whitehead, C.; Rice, G.E.; Permezel, M.; Lappas, M. Peroxisome proliferator-activated receptors are altered in pathologies of the human placenta: Gestational diabetes mellitus, intrauterine growth restriction and preeclampsia. *Placenta* **2010**, *31*, 222–229. [CrossRef] [PubMed]
72. Magnusson, A.L.; Waterman, I.J.; Wennergren, M.; Jansson, T.; Powell, T.L. Triglyceride hydrolase activities and expression of fatty acid binding proteins in the human placenta in pregnancies complicated by intrauterine growth restriction and diabetes. *J. Clin. Endocrinol. Metab.* **2004**, *89*, 4607–4614. [CrossRef]

73. Barrett, H.L.; Kubala, M.H.; Scholz Romero, K.; Denny, K.J.; Woodruff, T.M.; McIntyre, H.D.; Callaway, L.K.; Nitert, M.D. Placental Lipases in Pregnancies Complicated by Gestational Diabetes Mellitus (GDM). *PLoS ONE* **2014**, *9*, e104826. [CrossRef]
74. Gil-Sanchez, A.; Koletzko, B.; Larque, E. Current understanding of placental fatty acid transport. *Curr. Opin. Clin. Nutr. Metab. Care* **2012**, *15*, 265–272. [CrossRef]
75. Segura, M.T.; Demmelmair, H.; Krauss-Etschmann, S.; Nathan, P.; Dehmel, S.; Padilla, M.C.; Rueda, R.; Koletzko, B.; Campoy, C. Maternal BMI and gestational diabetes alter placental lipid transporters and fatty acid composition. *Placenta* **2017**, *57*, 144–151. [CrossRef] [PubMed]
76. Nguyen, L.N.; Ma, D.; Shui, G.; Wong, P.; Cazenave-Gassiot, A.; Zhang, X.; Wenk, M.R.; Goh, E.L.; Silver, D.L. Mfsd2a is a transporter for the essential omega-3 fatty acid docosahexaenoic acid. *Nature* **2014**, *509*, 503–506. [CrossRef] [PubMed]
77. Prieto-Sanchez, M.T.; Ruiz-Palacios, M.; Blanco-Carnero, J.E.; Pagan, A.; Hellmuth, C.; Uhl, O.; Peissner, W.; Ruiz-Alcaraz, A.J.; Parrilla, J.J.; Koletzko, B.; et al. Placental MFSD2a transporter is related to decreased DHA in cord blood of women with treated gestational diabetes. *Clin. Nutr.* **2017**, *36*, 513–521. [CrossRef]
78. Samimi, M.; Jamilian, M.; Asemi, Z.; Esmaillzadeh, A. Effects of omega-3 fatty acid supplementation on insulin metabolism and lipid profiles in gestational diabetes: Randomized, double-blind, placebo-controlled trial. *Clin. Nutr.* **2015**, *34*, 388–393. [CrossRef]
79. Jamilian, M.; Samimi, M.; Kolahdooz, F.; Khalaji, F.; Razavi, M.; Asemi, Z. Omega-3 fatty acid supplementation affects pregnancy outcomes in gestational diabetes: A randomized, double-blind, placebo-controlled trial. *J. Matern. -Fetal Neonatal Med.* **2016**, *29*, 669–675. [CrossRef]
80. Jamilian, M.; Samimi, M.; Mirhosseini, N.; Afshar Ebrahimi, F.; Aghadavod, E.; Taghizadeh, M.; Asemi, Z. A Randomized Double-Blinded, Placebo-Controlled Trial Investigating the Effect of Fish Oil Supplementation on Gene Expression Related to Insulin Action, Blood Lipids, and Inflammation in Gestational Diabetes Mellitus-Fish Oil Supplementation and Gestational Diabetes. *Nutrients* **2018**, *10*, 163. [CrossRef]
81. Zhou, S.J.; Yelland, L.; McPhee, A.J.; Quinlivan, J.; Gibson, R.A.; Makrides, M. Fish-oil supplementation in pregnancy does not reduce the risk of gestational diabetes or preeclampsia. *Am. J. Clin. Nutr.* **2012**, *95*, 1378–1384. [CrossRef] [PubMed]
82. Armaly, Z.; Jadaon, J.E.; Jabbour, A.; Abassi, Z.A. Preeclampsia: Novel Mechanisms and Potential Therapeutic Approaches. *Front. Physiol.* **2018**, *9*, 973. [CrossRef]
83. Jafri, S.; Ormiston, M.L. Immune regulation of systemic hypertension, pulmonary arterial hypertension, and preeclampsia: Shared disease mechanisms and translational opportunities. *Am. J. Physiol. Regul. Integr. Comp. Physiol.* **2017**, *313*, R693–R705. [CrossRef]
84. Cosar, H.; Ozer, E.; Topel, H.; Kahramaner, Z.; Turkoglu, E.; Erdemir, A.; Sutcuoglu, S.; Bagriyanik, A.; Ozer, E.A. Neuronal apoptosis in the neonates born to preeclamptic mothers. *J. Matern. Fetal Neonatal Med.* **2013**, *26*, 1143–1146. [CrossRef]
85. Raghupathy, R. Cytokines as key players in the pathophysiology of preeclampsia. *Med. Princ. Pract.* **2013**, *22* (Suppl. 1), 8–19. [CrossRef]
86. Benyo, D.F.; Miles, T.M.; Conrad, K.P. Hypoxia stimulates cytokine production by villous explants from the human placenta. *J. Clin. Endocrinol. Metab.* **1997**, *82*, 1582–1588. [CrossRef] [PubMed]
87. Loddick, S.A.; Rothwell, N.J. Neuroprotective effects of human recombinant interleukin-1 receptor antagonist in focal cerebral ischaemia in the rat. *J. Cereb. Blood Flow Metab.* **1996**, *16*, 932–940. [CrossRef]
88. Hedtjarn, M.; Leverin, A.L.; Eriksson, K.; Blomgren, K.; Mallard, C.; Hagberg, H. Interleukin-18 involvement in hypoxic-ischemic brain injury. *J. Neurosci.* **2002**, *22*, 5910–5919. [CrossRef]
89. Blomgren, K.; Leist, M.; Groc, L. Pathological apoptosis in the developing brain. *Apoptosis* **2007**, *12*, 993–1010. [CrossRef]
90. Nalivaeva, N.N.; Turner, A.J.; Zhuravin, I.A. Role of Prenatal Hypoxia in Brain Development, Cognitive Functions, and Neurodegeneration. *Front. Neurosci.* **2018**, *12*, 825. [CrossRef]
91. Figueiro-Filho, E.A.; Mak, L.E.; Reynolds, J.N.; Stroman, P.W.; Smith, G.N.; Forkert, N.D.; Paolozza, A.; Ratsep, M.T.; Croy, B.A. Neurological function in children born to preeclamptic and hypertensive mothers—A systematic review. *Pregnancy Hypertens.* **2017**, *10*, 1–6. [CrossRef]
92. Williams, M.; Zingheim, R.W.; King, I.B.; Zebelman, A.M. Omega-3 fatty acids in maternal erythocytes and risk of preeclampsia. *Epidemilogy* **1995**, *6*, 232–237. [CrossRef]

93. Kulkarni, A.V.; Mehendale, S.S.; Yadav, H.R.; Kilari, A.S.; Taralekar, V.S.; Joshi, S.R. Circulating angiogenic factors and their association with birth outcomes in preeclampsia. *Hypertens. Res. Off. J. Jpn. Soc. Hypertens.* **2010**, *33*, 561–567. [CrossRef] [PubMed]
94. Mackay, V.A.; Huda, S.S.; Stewart, F.M.; Tham, K.; McKenna, L.A.; Martin, I.; Jordan, F.; Brown, E.A.; Hodson, L.; Greer, I.A.; et al. Preeclampsia is associated with compromised maternal synthesis of long-chain polyunsaturated fatty acids, leading to offspring deficiency. *Hypertension* **2012**, *60*, 1078–1085. [CrossRef] [PubMed]
95. Wadhwani, N.; Patil, V.; Pisal, H.; Joshi, A.; Mehendale, S.; Gupte, S.; Wagh, G.; Joshi, S. Altered maternal proportions of long chain polyunsaturated fatty acids and their transport leads to disturbed fetal stores in preeclampsia. *Prostaglandins Leukot. Essent. Fat. Acids (PLEFA)* **2014**, *91*, 21–30. [CrossRef]
96. Wang, Y.; Walsh, S.W.; Kay, H.H. Placental tissue levels of nonesterified polyunsaturated fatty acids in normal and preeclamptic pregnancies. *Hypertens. Pregnancy* **2005**, *24*, 235–245. [CrossRef]
97. Rani, A.; Chavan-Gautam, P.; Mehendale, S.; Wagh, G.; Joshi, S. Differential regional fatty acid distribution in normotensive and preeclampsia placenta. *BBA Clin.* **2015**, *4*, 21–26. [CrossRef] [PubMed]
98. Kulkarni, A.V.; Mehendale, S.S.; Yadav, H.R.; Joshi, S.R. Reduced placental docosahexaenoic acid levels associated with increased levels of sFlt-1 in preeclampsia. *Prostaglandins Leukot. Essent. Fat. Acids* **2011**, *84*, 51–55. [CrossRef]
99. Toufaily, C.; Vargas, A.; Lemire, M.; Lafond, J.; Rassart, E.; Barbeau, B. MFSD2a, the Syncytin-2 receptor, is important for trophoblast fusion. *Placenta* **2013**, *34*, 85–88. [CrossRef] [PubMed]
100. Makrides, M.; Duley, L.; Olsen, S.F. Marine oil, and other prostaglandin precursor, supplementation for pregnancy uncomplicated by pre-eclampsia or intrauterine growth restriction. *Cochrane Database Syst. Rev.* **2006**, *3*, CD003402. [CrossRef] [PubMed]
101. Burchakov, D.I.; Kuznetsova, I.V.; Uspenskaya, Y.B. Omega-3 Long-Chain Polyunsaturated Fatty Acids and Preeclampsia: Trials Say "No," but Is It the Final Word? *Nutrients* **2017**, *9*, 1364. [CrossRef] [PubMed]
102. Min, Y.; Djahanbakhch, O.; Hutchinson, J.; Eram, S.; Bhullar, A.S.; Namugere, I.; Ghebremeskel, K. Efficacy of docosahexaenoic acid-enriched formula to enhance maternal and fetal blood docosahexaenoic acid levels: Randomized double-blinded placebo-controlled trial of pregnant women with gestational diabetes mellitus. *Clin. Nutr.* **2016**, *35*, 608–614. [CrossRef]

2

The Impact of Maternal Eating Disorders on Dietary Intake and Eating Patterns during Pregnancy

Annica F. Dörsam [1,*], Hubert Preißl [2], Nadia Micali [3], Sophia B. Lörcher [1], Stephan Zipfel [1] and Katrin E. Giel [1]

1 Department of Psychosomatic Medicine and Psychotherapy, Medical University Hospital Tübingen, 72076 Tübingen, Germany; Sophia.Loercher@med.uni-tuebingen.de (S.B.L.); Stephan.Zipfel@med.uni-tuebingen.de (S.Z.); Katrin.Giel@med.uni-tuebingen.de (K.E.G.)

2 Institute for Diabetes Research and Metabolic Diseases of the Helmholtz Center Munich at the University of Tübingen; fMEG Center; German Center for Diabetes Research (DZD), 72076 Tübingen, Germany; Hubert.Preissl@uni-tuebingen.de

3 Department of Psychiatry, Faculty of Medicine, University of Geneva, 1205 Geneva, Switzerland; nadia.micali@hcuge.ch

* Correspondence: Annica.Doersam@med.uni-tuebingen.de

Abstract: Maternal nutrition in pregnancy has a key influence on optimum fetal health. Eating disorders (EDs) during pregnancy may have detrimental effects on fetal growth and the child's early development. There is limited knowledge concerning the eating behavior, dietary intake and derived nutritional biomarkers as well as the nutrient supplementation in women with EDs during pregnancy. We performed a systematic review according to the PRISMA statement to synthesize current evidence in this field. Of $N = 1203$ hits, 13 full-texts were included in the qualitative synthesis. While women with current Binge Eating Disorder (BED) showed higher energy and fat intakes during pregnancy, women with a lifetime Anorexia Nervosa (AN), Bulimia Nervosa (BN) or both (AN + BN) had similar patterns of nutrient intake and dietary supplement use as healthy women. There is evidence, that women with a history of EDs have a sufficient diet quality and are more likely to be vegetarian. Dieting and bingeing improved substantially with pregnancy. The highlighted differences in the consumption of coffee/caffeine and artificially sweetened beverages as well as the elevated prevalence of iron deficiency anemia in women with a past or active ED during pregnancy might have an important impact on fetal development.

Keywords: anorexia nervosa; bulimia nervosa; binge eating disorder; diet; eating behavior; eating disorders; nutrition; pregnancy; purging

---

1. Introduction

In pregnancy, a lifestyle characterized by regular exercise and a balanced and diverse diet is a significant determinant of the course of pregnancy, the child's development, and the short- and long-term health of the mother and child [1]. In relation to the slight increase in energy intake in the last months of pregnancy, the demand for some vitamins and minerals (including trace elements) increases significantly more [1], usually from the 4th month of pregnancy on [2]. For the nutrients folate and iodine, a markedly increased intake is recommended from the beginning of pregnancy or, ideally, before conception [2]. There is substantial interest in nutrition during pregnancy, due to the extensive research in the area of early nutrition programming [3], arisen from the initial work by Barker ('Fetal Origins of Adult Disease'; FOAD) [4]. Barker's initial concept was later modified to the 'Developmental Origins of Health and Disease' (DOHaD) [5], which postulates that exposure to certain environmental influences during critical periods of development (e.g., intrauterine deficiency or oversupply of nutrients) and growth may have a significant impact on the development of non-communicable diseases (NCDs), such as obesity, diabetes mellitus, cardiovascular and mental disorders, as well as cancer in later life [5–7].

Given that eating disorders (EDs) are characterized by dysfunctional eating behaviors (e.g., caloric restriction, purging behavior), which may result in specific maternal macro- and micronutrient deficiencies, one would predict negative consequences of maternal EDs on the health, growth, and development of the fetus and the newborn infant. Research suggests that up to 7.5% of pregnant women are affected by an ED [8]. EDs include Anorexia Nervosa (AN), Bulimia Nervosa (BN), Binge Eating Disorder (BED) and 'Other Specified Feeding or Eating Disorders' (OSFED) [9]. AN is characterized by an excessive restriction of energy intake, which leads to severe weight loss with a pathological fear of weight gain and a distorted body image [9]. BN is defined by regular episodes of binge eating followed by inappropriate compensatory behaviors such as self-induced vomiting, abuse of laxatives, fasting or excessive exercise to avoid weight gain [9]. BED is associated with recurring episodes of eating significantly more food in a short period of time than most people would eat under comparable conditions, accompanied by feelings of lack of control, guilt, embarrassment or disgust [9].

There is increasing evidence from large cohort studies and register data showing that maternal disordered eating behavior and dysregulated body weight have detrimental effects on the course of pregnancy and birth outcomes. Pregnant women with an active ED are at increased risk of experiencing antepartum hemorrhage [10], hyperemesis gravidarum [11], higher rates of miscarriage [12], caesarean sections, and postpartum depression [13]. The literature on fetal outcomes of women with EDs displays lower [14] and higher birth weights [15,16], intrauterine growth restriction [10], small head circumferences [17], neurobehavioral dysregulations early after birth [18] as well as premature deliveries and perinatal mortality [15]. Disturbances and dysfunctions related to nutrition and eating behaviors which are core symptoms of EDs might contribute to these adverse pregnancy outcomes seen in women with EDs. On the other hand, given that affected women are often unduly preoccupied by eating and weight-control practices, they might have a higher nutritional knowledge, especially in terms of nutrient sources [19]. Therefore, one could also assume that at least subgroups of women with EDs might have a higher diet quality during pregnancy. Although most studies report an improvement in the ED symptomatology during pregnancy [20–23], there is limited knowledge about the actual food intake and overall dietary behavior of pregnant women with EDs.

The present systematic review aims to provide a synthesis of evidence regarding overall nutrition and related issues of pregnant women with a history of EDs. The main research questions are:

1. Do pregnant women with a history of EDs show different dietary intakes and patterns as compared to healthy pregnant women?
2. Do pregnant women with a history of EDs deviate from international dietary recommendations guidelines for pregnancy?
3. Do pregnant women with a history of EDs differ from healthy pregnant women with regard to nutritional biomarkers and dietary supplement intake?
4. Do pregnant women with a history of EDs show dysfunctional eating behaviors, i.e., restrictive eating, dieting, binge eating? Here, we will focus exclusively on behavioral *eating* aspects (which also represent ED symptoms), but not solely on ED symptoms with no direct connection to food intake (e.g., self-induced vomiting).

2. Methods

The review process was conducted according to the 'Preferred Reporting Items for Systematic Reviews and Meta-Analyses' (PRISMA) [24]. Papers were searched on PubMed and PsycInfo and covered a period ranging from 1987 to November 2018. The approach of this systematic review was specified in advance and documented in a protocol.

2.1. *Search Strategy*

Studies were identified by searching electronic databases and scanning reference lists of articles for relevant studies. The search was applied using the scientific databases PubMed and PsycInfo. In addition, we handsearched contents pages of 'The International Journal of Eating Disorders', the 'Journal of Eating Disorders', the 'European Eating Disorders Review', 'Eating Disorders: The Journal of Treatment and Prevention' and 'Nutrients'.

Until November 2018, a search of two databases was performed using the terms 'nutrition', 'food intake', 'eating behavior', 'pregnancy', and 'eating disorders'. As an example, for the PubMed search, the search term was defined as follows:

'(((("nutritional status"[MeSH Terms] OR ("nutritional"[All Fields] AND "status"[All Fields]) OR "nutritional status"[All Fields] OR "nutrition"[All Fields] OR "nutritional sciences"[MeSH Terms] OR ("nutritional"[All Fields] AND "sciences"[All Fields]) OR "nutritional sciences"[All Fields]) OR ("eating"[MeSH Terms] OR "eating"[All Fields] OR ("food"[All Fields] AND "intake"[All Fields]) OR "food intake"[All Fields])) OR ("eating behaviour"[All Fields] OR "feeding behavior"[MeSH Terms] OR ("feeding"[All Fields] AND "behavior"[All Fields]) OR "feeding behavior"[All Fields] OR ("eating"[All Fields] AND "behavior"[All Fields]) OR "eating behavior"[All Fields])) AND ("pregnancy"[MeSH Terms] OR "pregnancy"[All Fields])) AND ("feeding and eating disorders"[MeSH Terms] OR ("feeding"[All Fields] AND "eating"[All Fields] AND "disorders"[All Fields]) OR "feeding and eating disorders"[All Fields] OR ("eating"[All Fields] AND "disorders"[All Fields]) OR "eating disorders"[All Fields]) AND "humans"[MeSH Terms]'.

The first stage of study selection included the removal of duplicate studies, conducted by the paper's first author (A.F.D.). The first and the fourth author (S.B.L.) roughly screened the remaining studies by scanning article titles and abstracts. In the next step, the same two authors performed full text examinations of potentially relevant studies according to the defined eligibility criteria. Disagreements were resolved by discussion between the two investigators; if no agreement could be reached, the last review author (K.E.G.) was consulted.

The first author then extracted information from each included study using a specifically designed data collection sheet. The data collection sheet sought the following variables: (i) study characteristics (including study design, follow-up period, study size, country, funding sources), and the trial's inclusion and exclusion criteria; (ii) characteristics of trial participants (including method of ED diagnosis, gestational week); (iii) type of outcome measures (including dietary quantity and quality, eating patterns, dietary supplement use, nutritional biomarkers, and eating behavior in general), and results (including limitations, strengths, clinical implications and conclusions).

2.2. *Eligibility Criteria*

Eligibility criteria were based on the five PICOS dimensions, i.e., participants (P), interventions (I), comparators (C), outcome (O) and study design (S) [25].

2.2.1. Participants

Participants included pregnant women of any age with a past or current ED. Eating disorders were defined as AN, BN, BED and OSFED, previously known as 'Eating Disorder Not Otherwise Specified' (EDNOS), according to DSM criteria. Pica, an eating disorder that involves the persistent eating of substances that are not food and do not provide nutritional value, was defined as exclusion criterion for this review, as Pica is often described inaccurately as a part of culturally supported or socially normative practices [26]. Pregnant women with additional severe mental disorders (e.g., dementia, schizophrenia) as well as somatic syndromes influencing weight or eating behavior (e.g., diabetes mellitus, epilepsy, Prader-Willi syndrome), or virus infections (e.g., malaria) were excluded from this review.

2.2.2. Interventions

Trials assessing the dietary intake and eating patterns of pregnant women with a history of EDs in comparison to pregnant women without EDs. Dietary intake includes dietary quality, dietary supplement use, and eating behavior in general. Additionally, this review includes studies reporting on nutritional biomarkers of under- or malnutrition.

2.2.3. Comparators

Studies were eligible if a control group was included that consisted of pregnant women without any EDs. If there was no control group assessed, international dietary recommendation guidelines for pregnancy were used as a comparator [1,27,28].

2.2.4. Outcome

Primary outcome measures: Dietary intake in terms of food quantity and food quality, eating patterns regarding different forms of nutrition (e.g., vegetarianism, veganism), dietary supplement use (e.g., vitamin supplements), and nutritional biomarkers (e.g., ferritin). *Secondary outcome measures:* eating behavior in general (e.g., dieting or binge eating).

2.2.5. Study design

Cross-sectional and longitudinal observational studies assessing the dietary intake and eating patterns of pregnant women with a history of EDs. No publication date restrictions were imposed. Unpublished material and abstracts were included; publications in form of book chapters, reviews, case reports/series or dissertations were excluded. This review was limited to studies in English, French or German language.

3. Results

A total of 13 studies were identified for inclusion in this review. Interrater reliability was good, with κ = 0.71. See the flow diagram for an overview of the study selection process (Figure 1).

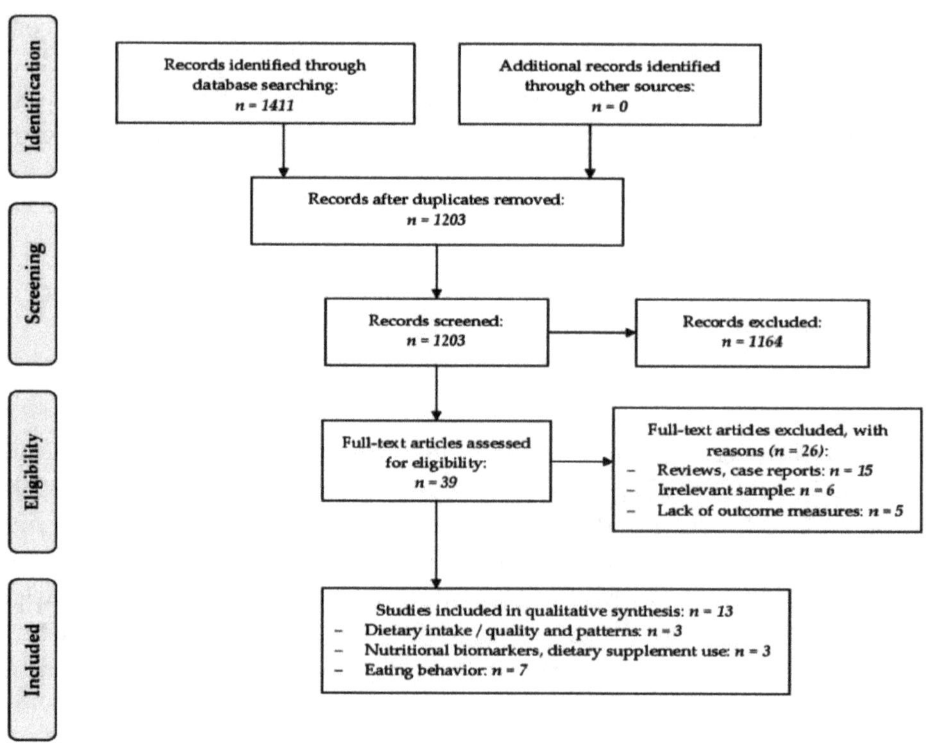

Figure 1. PRISMA flow chart for study inclusion.

We clustered the 13 studies according to the following topics concerning pregnant women with EDs:

1. Dietary intake/quality and patterns ($n = 3$)
2. Nutritional biomarkers and dietary supplement use ($n = 3$)
3. Eating behavior ($n = 7$)

3.1. *Studies Investigating Dietary Intake and Patterns in Pregnant Women with Eating Disorders*

We identified three studies which investigated dietary intakes in pregnancy in women with lifetime EDs [29–31]. All three studies were cross-sectional analyses, using data from large population-based cohort studies (see Table 1). Women with lifetime EDs were compared with control women free of any EDs before or during pregnancy. Maternal history of lifetime EDs was assessed during pregnancy [31] with self-reported questionnaires, either at gestational week (GW) 12 [29], or at six months prior to pregnancy and at GW 18.1 [30]. Dietary information was collected via food frequency questionnaires (FFQs) in the first half of the pregnancy [30,31] and in the third trimester [29]. The FFQ determines the frequency of consumption and the portion size of a wide variety of foods and drinks. Additionally, Micali et al. [29] and Siega-Riz et al. [30] combined related foods into different food groups (e.g., red meat, poultry, sausages/burgers, pies/pasties = 'meat'). Two of the three studies [29,30] examined the exact dietary intake of pregnant women across the ED spectrum in comparison to pregnant women without EDs. Siega-Riz et al. [30] focused on nutrient and food group intakes of pregnant women with BED and BN in the second trimester. Micali et al. [29] examined the dietary intake as well as dietary patterns of pregnant women with AN, BN or both (AN + BN) in the third trimester.

In terms of macronutrient intake, there were no differences to healthy pregnant women in energy, carbohydrate, fat and protein consumption of pregnant women with AN, BN or both in the third trimester [29]. In contrast, women with BED before and during pregnancy showed a higher consumption of total energy and total fat (monounsaturated fatty acids, MUFA; saturated fatty acids, SFA) in the second trimester [30]. Women who developed BED during pregnancy also had a higher total energy and SFA intake [30].

With regard to micronutrient intake through diet, there was very little difference in pregnancy in women with EDs compared with control women [29,30]. In particular, women in the second trimester with BED before and during pregnancy had lower intakes of folate, potassium and vitamin C [30]. This is reflected in the food group consumption, showing lower intakes of fruit and juices in those women [30]. In the third trimester, women with AN and AN + BN had higher folate and potassium intakes; women with AN + BN showed higher intakes of calcium, phosphorus, zinc, and vitamin C and women with BN had a slightly higher vitamin E intake compared to control women [29]. In general, the average mineral and vitamin intakes were satisfying in women with EDs throughout pregnancy [27,28].

In relation to food group consumption, women with BED before and during pregnancy had higher intakes of overall fat (butter, margarines, and oils) and milk desserts in the second trimester [30]. Pregnant women with AN, BN or both in the third trimester were less likely to use butter and drink full-fat milk in favor of skimmed and soya milk [29]. Those women also consumed less meat and fewer potatoes; however, they had a higher intake of soya products and pulses compared to the referent group [29]. Similarly, women with BN before and during pregnancy had a lower intake of high-fat meats in the second trimester [30]. Moreover, a higher consumption of artificially sweetened beverages among women with active and past BN and BED was observed [30]. Women with an active BED showed a slight increase in mean coffee consumption and women with lifetime AN and AN + BN reported a significantly higher coffee consumption (>355 mg caffeine/week) during pregnancy [29,30].

Regarding dietary patterns, women with lifetime EDs scored higher on the vegetarian dietary pattern (high intakes of meat substitutes, pulses, nuts and herbal teas, and high negative intakes of red meat and poultry), which corresponds to their self-report as being vegetarian [29]. Women with a lifetime AN scored higher on the 'traditional' dietary pattern (high loadings for all types of vegetables and red meat and poultry); women with a lifetime AN + BN scored higher on the 'health conscious' (high intake of salad, fruit, rice, pasta, oat and bran-based breakfast cereals, fish, pulses, fruit juices and non-white bread) and the 'traditional' dietary pattern [29].

Nguyen et al. [31] calculated a diet quality score with the data of the FFQs on the basis of the Dutch national dietary guidelines, including 15 components and cut-offs (e.g., vegetables (≥200 g/day), dairy (≥300 g/day), and red meat (≤375 g/week)). After adjustment for socioeconomic and lifestyle factors (maternal age, ethnicity, educational level, BMI, household income, psychiatric symptoms), women with a history of EDs had a significantly higher diet quality score than women unexposed [31].

3.2. *Studies Investigating Maternal Biomarkers of Nutrition and Dietary Supplement Use in Pregnant Women with Eating Disorders*

We identified two studies which assessed maternal biomarkers of nutrition in pregnant women with a history of EDs [15,32], and one study which focused on the dietary supplement use in those women [33] (see Table 2).

Koubaa et al. [32] examined biomarkers of nutrition and stress during early pregnancy in a cohort of women with a previous history of AN or BN in comparison to healthy women. Women with a history of AN showed a significantly higher frequency of anemia (hemoglobin, Hb < 110 g/L), which was related to low levels of maternal serum ferritin in early pregnancy compared to controls ($p < 0.01$). In their large register search study ($n = 4299$), Linna et al. [15] also found an increased occurrence of anemia in women with AN compared to healthy controls.

Regarding dietary supplement use, Dellava et al. [33] performed a cross-sectional analysis of the Norwegian Mother and Child Cohort Study (MoBa). Over 90% of women with an ED diagnosis as well as women without EDs used dietary supplements during pregnancy. Folic acid supplementation was the most common dietary supplement. After adjusting for covariates (maternal age, parity, smoking, household income, and educational level), no significant differences existed across groups for the use of any dietary supplement during pregnancy. However, women with EDNOS-P (purging subtype) were significantly more likely to take iron supplements during pregnancy ($p < 0.04$) [33].

3.3. *Studies Investigating Eating Behavior in Pregnant Women with EDs*

Concerning dysfunctional eating behaviors in pregnant women with a history of EDs, we identified seven relevant studies [20,23,34–38]. These studies provide evidence for a general improvement in dysfunctional eating behaviors during pregnancy in women with a recent or past ED (see Table 3). Women who actively suffered from BN during pregnancy reported an improvement of objective binge episodes with each passing trimester [36,37]. In particular, the frequency of objective binge eating in pregnant women with full or partial AN, BN or BED decreased to 2.9 episodes per 28 days intrapartum compared to 8.7 episodes prepartum [23]. 65% of pregnant women with an active BN, AN or mixed symptoms (AN + BN) who restricted their intake reported that they improved nutritionally or stopped restricting entirely; 56% of those who binged improved during pregnancy [38]. Blais et al. [20] also found a decrease in binge frequency in women with an active BN intrapartum, but no significant differences for binge frequencies and restrictive eating were seen in women with an active AN. For pregnant women with an active AN, BN or both, there was also evidence that bingeing became worse in pregnancy (18%) and that increased impulsivity within food intake resulted in overeating in 12% of those women [38]. Cross-sectional analyses of the Avon Longitudinal Study of Parents and Children (ALSPAC) revealed that 11.3% of women with a recent ED and 4.4% of women with a past ED dieted in late pregnancy, compared to 8% of obese and 2.5% of nonobese control women [34]. Regarding the question of whether they felt a loss of control over eating (LOC) during pregnancy, 72.5% of women with a recent ED and 42.8% of women with a past ED as well as 33.8% of healthy obese women and 36.1% of healthy nonobese women confirmed this question. Especially women with a recent BN were more likely to report LOC in pregnancy compared to all other groups [34].

Table 1. Studies investigating dietary intake/quality/patterns in pregnant women with eating disorders.

Source	Study Design	Country	Sample	ED Diagnosis	*n*	Prevalence of EDs	Outcome	Dietary Information
Nguyen et al., 2017 [31]	Cross-sectional analysis of the Generation R study	Netherlands	Pregnant women with and without a history of any ED	Self-reported questionnaire and clinical diagnoses (subsample; $n = 928$) during pregnancy	6196	9.5% ($n = 591$)	Diet quality score, including 15 components and cut-offs (e.g., vegetables (≥200 g/day), dairy (≥300 g/day), red meat (≤375 g/week))	Semi-quantitative modified 293-item FFQ at 13.6 weeks of gestation (12.4–16.2)
Main findings	Women with a history of EDs had a higher diet quality score than women without EDs							
Micali et al., 2012 [29]	Cross-sectional analysis of the ALSPAC study	United Kingdom	Pregnant women with and without a lifetime AN, BN, and AN + BN (exclusion: non-singleton pregnancies, miscarriage)	Self-reported questionnaire at 12 weeks of gestation	10,137	4.1% ($n = 414$); AN ($n = 151$); BN ($n = 186$); AN + BN ($n = 77$)	Frequency of consumption of various food groups, daily nutrient intakes (macronutrients), and dietary patterns	FFQ at 32 weeks of gestation; 14 food groups, 5 dietary patterns
Main findings (compared to control women)	1. Women with lifetime ED: - 2.8 times more likely to describe themselves as vegetarian - ↑ scoring on 'vegetarian' dietary pattern - ↓ meat, potatoes, SFA (AN, AN + BN) - ↑ soya products, pulses, skimmed and soya milk, fiber - ↓ butter, full-fat milk - ↑ caffeine (>355 mg/day) (esp. AN, AN + BN)					2. Women with a lifetime AN: - ↑ scoring on 'traditional' dietary pattern 3. Women with a lifetime BN: - ↑ bread (1.1 slices/d more), PUFA - ↓ sugar, non-milk extrinsic sugar 4. Women with a lifetime AN + BN: - ↑ scoring on 'health conscious' and 'traditional' dietary pattern		
Siega-Riz et al., 2008 [30]	Cross-sectional analysis of the MoBA study	Norway	Pregnant women with and without lifetime BN and BED	Self-reported questionnaire 6 month before and during pregnancy (18.1 week of gestation)	30,040	6.1% lifetime ED ($n = 1840$); 4.6% active ED ($n = 1393$); BN/BN ($n = 59$); BN/BED ($n = 60$); BED/BED ($n = 650$); none/BED ($n = 624$)	Nutrient and food group intakes	Semi-quantitative FFQ at gestational weeks 15–22; 255 questions, 20 food groups
Main findings (compared to control women)	1. Women with BED before + during pregnancy: - ↑ total energy (2459.0 ± 30.2 kcal vs. 2348.3 ± 4.6 kcal) - ↑ total fat (87.5 ± 1.2 g vs. 80.8 ± 0.2 g) - ↑ MUFA (27.8 ± 0.4 g vs. 26.6 ± 0.1 g) - ↑ SFA (34.2 ± 0.5 g vs. 31.3 ± 0.1 g) - ↓ folate (268.9 ± 3.8 μg vs. 273.4 ± 0.7 μg) - ↓ potassium (4008.1 ± 49 mg vs. 4018.6 ± 7.6 mg) - ↓ vitamin C (155.5 ± 3.7 mg vs. 167.5 ± 0.6 mg) - ↑ butter, margarines, oils, milk desserts, candy, coffee - ↓ fruit, juices, chicken					2. Women with incident BED during pregnancy: - ↑ total energy (2544.1 ± 41.2 kcal vs. 2348.3 ± 4.6 kcal) - ↑ SFA (34.9 ± 0.6 g vs. 31.3 ± 0.1 g) - ↑ cakes, candy, milk desserts, coffee; ↓ juices 3. Women with BN before and during pregnancy: - ↑ yogurt, cheeses - ↓ sweetened beverages, high-fat meats		

Abbreviations: ED: eating disorder; AN: Anorexia Nervosa; BN: Bulimia Nervosa; BED: Binge Eating Disorder; ALSPAC: Avon Longitudinal Study of Parents and Children: MoBa: Norwegian Mother and Child Cohort Study; FFQ: Food Frequency Questionnaire; ↑: higher (consumption); ↓: lower (consumption); SFA: saturated fatty acids; MUFA: monounsaturated fatty acids; PUFA: polyunsaturated fatty acids; BN/BN = BN before and during pregnancy; BN/BED = BN before, BED during pregnancy; BED/BED = BED before and during pregnancy; none/BED = no ED before, BED during pregnancy.

Table 2. Studies investigating nutritional biomarkers and dietary supplement use in pregnant women with eating disorders.

Source	Study Design	Country	Sample	ED Diagnosis	*n*	Prevalence of EDs	Outcome	Main Findings
Koubaa et al., 2015 [32]	Longitudinal cohort study (follow-up period: 1 year)	Sweden	Pregnant, nulliparous non-smoking women with and without a history of AN and BN	Interview according to DSM-IV diagnostic criteria; medical records	96	38.5% ($n = 37$); AN (active AN: $n = 8$; past AN: $n = 12$); BN (active BN: $n = 1$; past BN: $n = 16$)	Maternal serum biomarkers of nutrition and stress at 10 weeks of gestation within a routine blood sample (ferritin, cortisol, TSH, T4, insulin, IGF-I and IGFBP1)	Women with previous AN: - ↑ frequency (70%) of anemia (Hb < 110 g/L) compared to controls (12%) 1. ↓ serum ferritin levels compared to controls
Linna et al., 2014 [15]	Register search study	Finland	Female ED patients and unexposed controls	Attending physicians at the clinic with ICD-10 (AN, BN, atypical AN/BN) and DSM-IV (BED) criteria	4299	15.3% ($n = 657$); AN ($n = 182$); BN ($n = 436$); BED ($n = 39$)	Pregnancy complications (obtained from Medical Birth Register): gestational diabetes mellitus, initiation of insulin treatment, anemia, antenatal corticosteroid treatment, pregnancy-related ICD-10 diagnoses	Anemia was more frequent among women with AN (3.97%) compared with unexposed women (1.54%)
Dellava et al., 2013 [33]	Cross-sectional analysis of the MoBA study	Norway	Pregnant women across eating disorder subtypes compared with a referent group	Self-reported questionnaire at GW 19	37,307	6.3% ($n = 2348$); AN ($n = 34$); BN ($n = 326$); BED ($n = 1944$); EDNOS-P ($n = 44$)	Use of dietary supplements (checklist including 22 specific nutrients, at three time points prior to pregnancy (≥9 weeks, 8–5 weeks and 4–1 week before conception) and eight time periods during pregnancy (GW 1–4, 5–8, 9–12 13–16, 17–20, 21–24, 25–28, and 29+)	Dietary supplement use during pregnancy was as follows (between group differences were not statistically significant): - 91.2% of women with AN - 92.2% of women with BN - 93.2% of women with EDNOS-P (↑ intake of Fe-containing supplements) - 90.6% of women with BED - 93.5% of the women without EDs

Abbreviations: ED: eating disorder; AN: Anorexia Nervosa; BN: Bulimia Nervosa; BED: Binge Eating Disorder; EDNOS-P: Eating Disorder Not Otherwise Specified – Purging subtype; MoBa: Norwegian Mother and Child Cohort Study; TSH: Thyroid-Stimulating Hormone; T4: Free Thyroxine (T4); IGF-I: Insulin-Like Growth Factor I; IGFBP1: IGF Binding Protein 1; Hb: Hemoglobin; Fe: Iron; DSM: Diagnostic and Statistical Manual of Mental Disorders; ICD-10: International Statistical Classification of Diseases and Related Health Problems; GW: gestational week; ↑: higher; ↓: lower.

Table 3. Studies investigating eating behavior in pregnant women with eating disorders.

Source	Study Design	Country	Sample	ED Diagnosis	n	Prevalence of EDs	Outcome	Main Findings
Crow et al., 2008 [23]	Cross-sectional analysis of the McKnight Longitudinal Study of Eating Disorders	United States of America	Pregnant women with full/subthreshold AN, BN or BED	EDE	42	AN (n = 5; 11.9%); BN (n = 15; 35.7%); BED (n = 4; 9.5%); partial AN (n = 5; 11.9%); partial BN (n = 10; 23.8%); partial BED (n = 3; 7.1%)	Eating behaviors and disordered eating cognitions over the course of pregnancy	Frequency of objective binge eating episodes per 28 days intrapartum: 2.9 (vs. 8.7 prepartum)
Micali et al., 2007 [34]	Cross-sectional analysis of the ALSPAC study	United Kingdom	Pregnant women with and without recent/past AN, BN, AN + BN	Self-reported questionnaire at 12 weeks of gestation	12,252	0.5% recent ED (n = 57; 6 AN, 51 BN); 3.2% past ED (n = 395; 167 AN, 158 BN, 70 AN + BN)	18 GW: Self-induced vomiting, laxative use, exercise behavior, shape and weight concern; 32 GW: appraisals about weight gain during pregnancy, dieting, LOC	Dieting in pregnancy: - recent ED: 11.3% - past ED: 4.4% - nonobese controls: 2.5% LOC: - recent ED: 72.5% - past ED: 42.8% - nonobese controls: 36.1% Women with recent BN were more likely to report LOC in pregnancy compared to all other groups
Crow et al., 2004 [35]	Cross-sectional analysis of a longitudinal study (follow-up period: 10 – 15 years)	United States of America	Pregnant women with BN	EDI; SCID; Eating Disorders Questionnaire; self-report of BN symptoms	129	all BN	Bulimic symptoms, alcohol, drug, and tobacco use during pregnancy	Frequency of binge eating during pregnancy was rated as: - decreased by 59.6% - increased by 7.4% - unchanged by 33.0% The prevalence of alcohol use decreased after pregnancy was recognized (35% vs. 14%)
Blais et al., 2000 [20]	Longitudinal Study	United States of America	Pregnant women with AN and BN	LIFE-EAT II every 6 month	82	31,7% AN (AN-R: n = 7; AN-BP: n = 19); 68.3% BN (n = 56)	Pregnancy outcome (live birth, therapeutic/spontaneous abortion), ED symptomatology (restrictive eating, binging, etc.)	BN subjects: ↓ frequency of binging from prepregnancy to post-pregnancy AN subjects: No significant differences were seen for binging frequency and restrictive eating

Table 3. *Cont.*

Source	Study Design	Country	Sample	ED Diagnosis	n	Prevalence of EDs	Outcome	Main Findings
Morgan et al., 1999 [37]	Retrospective analysis	United Kingdom	Pregnant women actively suffering from BN	EDE, SCID	94	all BN	Symptoms of bulimia nervosa and associated psychopathology at conception, each trimester and postnatally	Objective binge episodes improved with each passing trimester of pregnancy
Lemberg et al., 1989 [38]	Longitudinal study	United States of America	Pregnant women with an active AN, BN or mixed symptoms	Retrospective, 55-item questionnaire on ED symptoms and course of pregnancy	43	57% AN-R; 77% BN; 16% combination of both	Eating behaviors both antenatal and postnatal	Women who restricted their intake ($n = 36$): - 65% reported improved nutrition or stopping restricting // complete cessation: 7% Women who binged ($n = 41$): - improvement: 56% // worsening: 18.6% // complete cessation: 14% All women: 12% ↑ impulsivity with food by overeating
Lacey et al., 1987 [36]	Longitudinal study	United Kingdom	Pregnant untreated BN women	St George's Hospital eating disorder unit; DSM-III	20	all BN	Impact of pregnancy on dietary difficulties of the bulimic woman	19 of the 20 subjects reduced frequency of binge eating over the course of pregnancy; only 5 patients were binge eating during the 3rd trimester; 75% having a complete cessation of binging by the 3rd trimester

Abbreviations: ED: eating disorder; AN: Anorexia Nervosa; AN-R: Anorexia Nervosa Restrictive subtype; AN-BP: Anorexia Nervosa Binge-Purge subtype; BN: Bulimia Nervosa; BED: Binge Eating Disorder; LOC: Loss of control over eating; ALSPAC: Avon Longitudinal Study of Parents and Children; EDE: Eating Disorder Examination; Eating Disorder Inventory; Structured Clinical Interview for DSM Axis I Disorders (SCID); LIFE-EAT II: Eating Disorders Longitudinal Interval Follow-up Evaluation; DSM: Diagnostic and Statistical Manual of Mental Disorders; GW: gestational week; ↑: higher; ↓: lower.

4. Discussion

This systematic review analyzed diet quality, nutritional biomarkers and dietary supplement use as well as dysfunctional eating behaviors in women with a current or past ED during pregnancy. Given the fact that, up to now, only three studies have investigated dietary intake and diet quality in women with EDs during pregnancy [29–31], and only one study has investigated nutritional biomarkers [32] and dietary supplement use [33] in pregnant women with EDs, a clear finding of our review is that more research in this area is urgently needed.

4.1. Dietary Intake and Patterns in Pregnant Women with Eating Disorders

Summarizing the current findings of the three relevant studies, there is congruent evidence for an adequate diet in pregnant women with EDs, although there are specific subgroup differences [29–31].

The strengths of these studies are their population-based, longitudinal design, and therefore very large sample sizes. However, all cited studies have a general limitation regarding the examination of food intake with the use of food frequency questionnaires, as they rely on memory and reported intakes, which are subject to measurement errors [39]. Moreover, the items of the FFQ are adapted on the specific diet of a country; thus, carefulness is required regarding participants with different ethnic backgrounds [31]. Another weakness is the use of standard portion sizes to assess nutrient intakes from the FFQs, resulting in imprecise estimates of the actual food quantity [29,30]. It remains unclear whether the FFQ is a valid tool for the dietary assessment in pregnant women with EDs who experience worries and feelings of guilt or embarrassment for not caring for their unborn children, as they may under- or over-report specific food items (e.g., energy-dense foods) [31]. However, several studies conclude that the FFQ is a valid tool for ranking women in accordance with their nutrient intakes during pregnancy [40–42].

Nguyen et al. calculated a higher diet quality score for women with a history of EDs, not differentiating the disorder into active, past or type of ED [31]. Furthermore, the exact dietary data was not presented in the article. Micali et al. examined nutrient and food group intakes of pregnant women with lifetime AN, BN and both [29]; Siega-Riz et al. investigated those of women with active BN and active BED [30]. Consequently, except for the BN group, the other subgroups cannot be compared on the basis of uniform diagnoses between those studies. Nevertheless, the data on dietary intake in pregnant women with a history of AN, BN and AN + BN suggests a relatively good diet quality, supported by a vegetarian dietary pattern with lower intakes of meat and similar protein, fat and carbohydrate intakes compared to controls. However, these results can also be the result of persistent ED symptoms during pregnancy [31]. More precisely, women whose ED cognitions are present in pregnancy might have made more informed choices about a 'healthy' diet that included low caloric foods (e.g., vegetables, skimmed milk) to prevent further weight gain [31] or to avoid 'fattening' foods during an interval when purging episodes may be reduced [30]. If so, those women would have scored higher on the diet quality. An alternative explanation for better nutrition in women with a history of AN, BN or both is an improvement in the ED symptoms during pregnancy, which is suggested by the majority of previous studies in this field [20–23]. This is supported by the notion that, especially during pregnancy, expectant mothers are often highly motivated to optimize their lifestyle [1]. However, women with BED before and during pregnancy showed higher energy and overall fat intakes and lower intakes of some nutrients compared to controls. For women with BED, pregnancy could be a trigger for the continuation or even deterioration of symptoms [22].

The higher consumption of artificially sweetened beverages among women with active and past BN and BED [24] might be a reflection of their ED pattern in reducing added sugars. Summarized data from three very large prospective cohort studies showed several risks which were associated with the consumption of artificially sweetened beverages by pregnant women, including prematurity and the diagnosis of asthma in their children up to the age of seven years [43].

Similarly, the high consumption of caffeine (>355 mg/day), especially in women with AN and AN + BN, is of high concern, since caffeine and coffee consumption during pregnancy might be associated with spontaneous abortion at daily levels of 300 mg caffeine and above in a dose-dependent way (7–19% for every increase in caffeine intake of 100–150 mg/day) [44,45]. Based on limited data, a Cochrane meta-analysis was unable to conclude on the effectiveness of the abstention from caffeine on birth weight or other relevant endpoints [46]. In a clinical sample of ED patients, the main reasons for consuming caffeinated beverages were appetite suppression, feeling of fullness, facilitation with purging, and increasing the metabolic rate to enhance energy expenditure [47]. There is evidence that habitual coffee consumption plays a possible role in weight loss (increased metabolic rate, energy expenditure, lipid oxidation, and lipolytic and thermogenic activities) [48]. However, the American College of Obstetricians (ACOG) and the European Food Safety Authority (EFSA) recommend that pregnant women should drink no more than 200 mg of caffeine per day [49,50].

Lastly, the average intake of all nutrients was sufficient for women with active and past EDs, except for potassium and phosphorus being very high and iron and folate being much lower than recommended in the analyses by Siega-Riz et al. [30]. However, nutrient intakes from supplement use were not included in the analyses.

4.2. Maternal Biomarkers of Nutrition and Dietary Supplement Use in Pregnant Women with Eating Disorders

Both studies that identified nutritional biomarkers during pregnancy showed an increased risk of maternal iron deficiency anemia (IDA) for women with AN during early pregnancy [15,32]. However, data of the nutritional biomarkers throughout pregnancy was not available, since the determination was performed only in one blood sample in early pregnancy [32]. The etiology of anemia is multifactorial and includes insufficient dietary intake of folate, vitamin B_{12} and A, along with iron, which is the most common nutritional cause [51]. According to previous World Health Organization (WHO) reports, on average, about 50% of all cases of anemia in pregnancy were due to iron deficiency [52]. During pregnancy, there is an increased need for iron, because more iron is required for the fetus, placenta and 20% increased erythrocytes in the expectant mother [1]. Iron deficiency in pregnancy increases the risk of premature birth, low birth weight and irreversible or partially reversible neurobehavioral and cognitive impairments [32,51,53–55]. For instance, Koubaa et al. found that maternal serum levels of ferritin in women with a history of AN correlated strongly with impaired memory function in their children at five years of age [32]. Linna et al. did not relate maternal iron status with newborn outcomes, but they reported that maternal AN was associated with several adverse perinatal outcomes (e.g., slow fetal growth, very premature birth, small for gestational age, low birth weight), which could be mediated by low folate or iron intakes during pregnancy [15]. If an IDA is medically diagnosed, iron supplementation in addition to sufficient intake of iron-rich foods is recommended [1]. Therefore, pregnant women with a history of EDs, and particularly of AN, should be closely monitored in terms of nutrient deficiencies.

To our knowledge, the study by Dellava et al. is the only study to date that examined the dietary supplement intake in pregnant women with EDs compared to control women [26]. Unfortunately, it was not possible to determine if women with EDs consumed more or less micronutrients from dietary supplements than women without EDs, since information of the amount of each item contained in the dietary supplements was not collected [26]. It would also be important to know whether women with EDs were instructed by their gynecologist to take dietary supplements [26]. Over 90% of women with EDs used dietary supplements during pregnancy, with folic acid being the most commonly used supplement. Folic acid supplement use was higher during pregnancy than periconceptional for all women [26]. Numerous epidemiological studies and subsequent meta-analyses have shown that a periconceptional folic acid supplementation of 400 μg (alone or in combination with other micronutrients) can reduce the risk of childhood malformations of the nervous system (neural tube defects) [56,57]. However, in the study by Dellava et al., the increase in folic acid supplementation prior to pregnancy in women with and without EDs was likely too late to prevent birth defects associated with folate deficiency according to the Norwegian recommendations [26]. Therefore, involved specialists should motivate women with EDs to supplement critical nutrients (e.g., folate, iron, iodine). Supplements could easily be accepted by these women, as they are not associated with caloric intake [26]. However, in women with purging behavior, it is questionable as to how many supplemented nutrients might be absorbed at the intestinal absorption site.

4.3. Dysfunctional Eating Behavior in Pregnant Women with EDs

In terms of behavioral aspects of eating, pregnancy is associated with an overall improvement in the severity of dysfunctional eating behavior for most women [20,23,34–38]. Reasons for the improvement in eating behavior may include the relief of a sense of responsibility for body weight and shape and the woman's worries about its harming effects on her unborn child [37]. However, pregnancy might also be a trigger for the deterioration of bingeing and overeating [22,38]. After all, every tenth pregnant woman with a recent ED reports restrictive intake, which is worrisome [34]. Reasons for the intensification of dysfunctional eating behaviors may include increased anxiety over weight gain [38]. Furthermore, physiological changes in the course of pregnancy, such as changes in satiety associated with an altered leptin level, may have important influences on eating behavior [58]. The increased rates of LOC, both in women with and without EDs, might be correlated with general ravenous appetite experienced in pregnancy. Interestingly, in the study by Blais et al., pregnancy outcomes (lower live birth rates, higher therapeutic abortion rates) of women with AN and BN were not associated with the maternal age, or the presence of ED symptoms at conception [20].

Additionally, in the postpartum phase, the improvement seems to decline, and dysfunctional eating behaviors tend to return toward prepregnancy levels [29]. Therefore, pregnant women with eating disorders need enhanced intrapartum *and* postnatal support. From a nutritional point of view, the latter is of great importance regarding (breast)feeding practices in women with EDs. For example, in a study with 20 bulimic women, three mothers reported that they restricted the dietary intake of their children within the first year of life [36].

4.4. Strengths and Limitations

This is the first systematic review that has examined pregnancy nutrition and related issues in women with a history of EDs. The strengths of this review are its methodical procedure according to the PRISMA statement and the focus on nutritional aspects of eating disorders during pregnancy. Thus, this review draws attention to important gaps in the eating disorder research.

Given the fact that the studies eligible for this review were very heterogeneous, a quality rating and meta-analysis could not be performed. The articles were ranging over a time span of 30 years; consequently, consistent diagnostic criteria for EDs were not applied. Another major issue is the inadequate diagnostic identification of EDs through self-report in some of the reviewed studies. Therefore, a reporter bias and misclassification of EDs cannot be ruled out. Furthermore, women who reported an ED might have a milder form of ED, since women who suffer from a severe ED might not participate in research studies or might not report their ED accordingly due to potential feelings of sorrow and guilt. Consequently, the prevalence of women with ED and differences in dietary intake might be underestimated. Moreover, it was not possible to ascertain between active and lifetime ED during pregnancy in some studies, resulting in mixed study samples of reduced comparability. There is a limited generalizability in studies that extracted data from the MoBa study, since differences exist between the study sample and the general population in terms of educational level and multivitamin consumption. From the seven studies investigating dysfunctional eating behavior of pregnant women with EDs, three studies had small sample sizes [23,36,38], two studies relied on retrospective recall [35,37] and, unfortunately, only one study included a control group of women without EDs [34].

5. Conclusions and Future Directions

Based on our four research questions investigated in the present systematic review, our main findings are as follows: (1) considering the drawback that dietary intakes were assessed by self-report, pregnant women with a history of EDs show a similar dietary intake to healthy pregnant women; there is evidence that women with EDs have a sufficient diet quality and are more likely to follow a vegetarian dietary pattern. Women with BED seem to be an exception as they show inadequate energy and fat intakes; (2) the startling caffeine and coffee consumption, especially in pregnant women with AN and AN + BN, and the use of artificially sweetened beverages in pregnant women with active and past BN and BED is of high concern and needs further investigation in relation to fetal outcomes; (3) women with AN were at increased risk of experiencing iron deficiency anemia in pregnancy; anyhow, women with EDs did not differ in overall dietary supplement use compared to healthy women; (4) dysfunctional eating behaviors (bingeing, dieting) improved substantially with pregnancy.

We feel that the issue of EDs in pregnancy is still an understudied field. There is still no consistent answer to the underlying biological mechanisms that might explain the increased risk for adverse perinatal outcomes in women with EDs. As outlined above, most of the current evidence in the field is derived from self-report data, which is prone to biases, e.g., due to influences of social desirability or memory gaps. This highlights the need for method combinations, integrating data from self-report, observational data, and in order to elucidate consequences of nutrition practices for fetal development, ideally also from neuropsychological and neurobiological methods [32,59]. For example, fetal magnetoencephalography (fMEG) is a non-invasive method to study fetal brain activity, which has previously revealed evidence that the maternal metabolism might program the fetal brain [60,61]. However, the first step is the adequate assessment and identification of EDs through medical professionals (general practitioner, gynecologist, or fertility specialist), ideally before pregnancy [62]. Paslakis and de Zwaan [62] recently provided clinical recommendations and specific algorithms for the management of pregnant females with EDs and for females with EDs seeking fertility treatment, underlining the importance of an interdisciplinary approach.

Regarding the research gaps concerning pregnant women with EDs, nutrition quality/food intake (including the adherence to a vegan diet), gestational weight gain, gestational diabetes, and dysfunctional behaviors (including substance misuse) are just a few topics which urgently require further investigation. Especially during pregnancy, women with EDs might be highly motivated to change their behavior in favor of their developing child. Therefore, studies on the treatment of EDs during pregnancy are urgently needed to ensure an optimal development of the fetus and to contribute to the prevention of intergenerational transmission of EDs.

Based on the evidence available, the assessment of maternal nutritional status is complex, but especially needed for vulnerable groups like women with EDs during pregnancy. With the exception of women with BED, food intake seems sufficient during pregnancy and dysfunctional eating habits are improved, which is an encouraging finding. Particularly women with active EDs might need nutritional counselling and close monitoring of nutrient deficits. More research is needed to confirm previous studies and to identify treatment interventions that support lasting improvements in eating behaviors and dietary intake in the postpartum phase.

Author Contributions: K.E.G., N.M. and A.F.D. conceived the review topic and research questions. K.E.G. and A.F.D. developed search terms and eligibility criteria. A.F.D. and S.B.L. screened, reviewed and selected the search results, K.E.G. served as a third reviewer for study inclusion. A.F.D. analyzed the included studies and drafted the manuscript. K.E.G., N.M., H.P. and S.Z. critically revised the manuscript.

Acknowledgments: This work was supported by a grant within the fortüne program from the Medical Faculty Tübingen (Project no. F1292064). We acknowledge support by Deutsche Forschungsgemeinschaft and Open Access Publishing Fund of University of Tübingen.

References

1. Koletzko, B.; Cremer, M.; Flothkötter, M.; Graf, C.; Hauner, H.; Hellmers, C.; Kersting, M.; Krawinkel, M.; Przyrembel, H.; Röbl-Mathieu, M.; et al. Diet and lifestyle before and during pregnancy—Practical recommendations of the germany-wide healthy start—Young family network. *Geburtshilfe Frauenheilkd.* **2018**, *78*, 1262–1282. [CrossRef]

2. Berti, C.; Biesalski, H.K.; Gärtner, R.; Lapillonne, A.; Pietrzik, K.; Poston, L.; Redman, C.; Koletzko, B.; Cetin, I. Micronutrients in pregnancy: Current knowledge and unresolved questions. *Clin. Nutr.* **2011**, *30*, 689–701. [CrossRef]
3. Lucas, A. Long-term programming effects of early nutrition—Implications for the preterm infant. *J. Perinatol.* **2005**, *25*, S2. [CrossRef]
4. Barker, D.J. The fetal and infant origins of adult disease. *BMJ (Clin. Res. Ed.)* **1990**, *301*, 1111. [CrossRef]
5. Hoffman, D.J.; Reynolds, R.M.; Hardy, D.B. Developmental origins of health and disease: Current knowledge and potential mechanisms. *Nutr. Rev.* **2017**, *75*, 951–970. [CrossRef]
6. Barker, D.J.P. The origins of the developmental origins theory. *J. Intern. Med.* **2007**, *261*, 412–417. [CrossRef] [PubMed]
7. Gluckman, P.D.; Hanson, M.A.; Cooper, C.; Thornburg, K.L. Effect of in utero and early-life conditions on adult health and disease. *New Engl. J. Med.* **2008**, *359*, 61–73. [CrossRef]
8. Easter, A.; Bye, A.; Taborelli, E.; Corfield, F.; Schmidt, U.; Treasure, J.; Micali, N. Recognising the symptoms: How common are eating disorders in pregnancy? *Eur. Eat. Disord. Rev.* **2013**, *21*, 340–344. [CrossRef] [PubMed]
9. APA. *Diagnostic and Statistical Manual of Mental Disorders*, 5th ed.; APA: Washington, DC, USA, 2013.
10. Eagles, J.M.; Lee, A.J.; Raja, E.A.; Millar, H.R.; Bhattacharya, S. Pregnancy outcomes of women with and without a history of anorexia nervosa. *Psychol. Med.* **2012**, *42*, 2651–2660. [CrossRef]
11. Koubaa, S.; Hallstrom, T.; Lindholm, C.; Hirschberg, A.L. Pregnancy and neonatal outcomes in women with eating disorders. *Obstet. Gynecol.* **2005**, *105*, 255–260. [CrossRef] [PubMed]
12. Micali, N.; Simonoff, E.; Treasure, J. Risk of major adverse perinatal outcomes in women with eating disorders. *Br. J. Psychiatry* **2007**, *190*, 255–259. [CrossRef]
13. Franko, D.L.; Blais, M.A.; Becker, A.E.; Delinsky, S.S.; Greenwood, D.N.; Flores, A.T.; Ekeblad, E.R.; Eddy, K.T.; Herzog, D.B. Pregnancy complications and neonatal outcomes in women with eating disorders. *Am. J. Psychiatry* **2001**, *158*, 1461–1466. [CrossRef]
14. Solmi, F.; Sallis, H.; Stahl, D.; Treasure, J.; Micali, N. Low birth weight in the offspring of women with anorexia nervosa. *Epidemiol. Rev.* **2014**, *36*, 49–56. [CrossRef]
15. Linna, M.S.; Raevuori, A.; Haukka, J.; Suvisaari, J.M.; Suokas, J.T.; Gissler, M. Pregnancy, obstetric, and perinatal health outcomes in eating disorders. *Am. J. Obstet. Gynecol.* **2014**, *211*, e391–e398. [CrossRef]
16. Bulik, C.M.; Von Holle, A.; Siega-Riz, A.M.; Torgersen, L.; Lie, K.K.; Hamer, R.M.; Berg, C.K.; Sullivan, P.; Reichborn-Kjennerud, T. Birth outcomes in women with eating disorders in the norwegian mother and child cohort study (moba). *Int. J. Eat. Disord.* **2009**, *42*, 9–18. [CrossRef]
17. Koubaa, S.; Hallstrom, T.; Hagenas, L.; Hirschberg, A.L. Retarded head growth and neurocognitive development in infants of mothers with a history of eating disorders: Longitudinal cohort study. *BJOG Int. J. Obstet. Gynaecol.* **2013**, *120*, 1413–1422. [CrossRef]
18. Barona, M.; Taborelli, E.; Corfield, F.; Pawlby, S.; Easter, A.; Schmidt, U.; Treasure, J.; Micali, N. Neurobehavioural and cognitive development in infants born to mothers with eating disorders. *J. Child Psychol. Psychiatry* **2017**, *58*, 931–938. [CrossRef]
19. HO, A.S.L.; SOH, N.L.; WALTER, G.; TOUYZ, S. Comparison of nutrition knowledge among health professionals, patients with eating disorders and the general population. *Nutr. Diet.* **2011**, *68*, 267–272. [CrossRef]
20. Blais, M.A.; Becker, A.E.; Burwell, R.A.; Flores, A.T.; Nussbaum, K.M.; Greenwood, D.N.; Ekeblad, E.R.; Herzog, D.B. Pregnancy: Outcome and impact on symptomatology in a cohort of eating-disordered women. *Int. J. Eat. Disord.* **2000**, *27*, 140–149. [CrossRef]
21. Micali, N.; Treasure, J. Biological effects of a maternal ed on pregnancy and foetal development: A review. *Eur. Eat. Disord. Rev.* **2009**, *17*, 448–454. [CrossRef]
22. Bulik, C.M.; Von Holle, A.; Hamer, R.; Knoph Berg, C.; Torgersen, L.; Magnus, P.; Stoltenberg, C.; Siega-Riz, A.M.; Sullivan, P.; Reichborn-Kjennerud, T. Patterns of remission, continuation and incidence of broadly defined eating disorders during early pregnancy in the norwegian mother and child cohort study (moba). *Psychol. Med.* **2007**, *37*, 1109–1118. [CrossRef]
23. Crow, S.J.; Agras, W.S.; Crosby, R.; Halmi, K.; Mitchell, J.E. Eating disorder symptoms in pregnancy: A prospective study. *Int. J. Eat. Disord.* **2008**, *41*, 277–279. [CrossRef]

24. Moher, D.; Liberati, A.; Tetzlaff, J.; Altman, D.G.; The, P.G. Preferred reporting items for systematic reviews and meta-analyses: The prisma statement. *PLoS Med.* **2009**, *6*, e1000097. [CrossRef]
25. Liberati, A.; Altman, D.G.; Tetzlaff, J.; et al. The prisma statement for reporting systematic reviews and meta-analyses of studies that evaluate health care interventions: Explanation and elaboration. *Ann. Intern. Med.* **2009**, *151*, W-65–W-94. [CrossRef]
26. NEDA. PICA. Available online: https://www.nationaleatingdisorders.org/learn/by-eating-disorder/other/pica (accessed on 8 January 2019).
27. Procter, S.B.; Campbell, C.G. Position of the academy of nutrition and dietetics: Nutrition and lifestyle for a healthy pregnancy outcome. *J. Acad. Nutr. Diet.* **2014**, *114*, 1099–1103. [CrossRef]
28. Maternal and Child Nutrition. Public Health Guideline [ph11]. Available online: https://www.nice.org.uk/guidance/qs98/resources/maternal-and-child-nutrition-pdf-2098975759045 (accessed on 8 January 2019).
29. Micali, N.; Northstone, K.; Emmett, P.; Naumann, U.; Treasure, J.L. Nutritional intake and dietary patterns in pregnancy: A longitudinal study of women with lifetime eating disorders. *Br. J. Nutr.* **2012**, *108*, 2093–2099. [CrossRef]
30. Siega-Riz, A.M.; Haugen, M.; Meltzer, H.M.; Von Holle, A.; Hamer, R.; Torgersen, L.; Knopf-Berg, C.; Reichborn-Kjennerud, T.; Bulik, C.M. Nutrient and food group intakes of women with and without bulimia nervosa and binge eating disorder during pregnancy. *Am. J. Clin. Nutr.* **2008**, *87*, 1346–1355. [CrossRef]
31. Nguyen, A.N.; de Barse, L.M.; Tiemeier, H.; Jaddoe, V.W.V.; Franco, O.H.; Jansen, P.W.; Voortman, T. Maternal history of eating disorders: Diet quality during pregnancy and infant feeding. *Appetite* **2017**, *109*, 108–114. [CrossRef]
32. Koubaa, S.; Hallstrom, T.; Brismar, K.; Hellstrom, P.M.; Hirschberg, A.L. Biomarkers of nutrition and stress in pregnant women with a history of eating disorders in relation to head circumference and neurocognitive function of the offspring. *BMC Pregnancy Childbirth* **2015**, *15*, 318. [CrossRef]
33. Dellava, J.E.; Von Holle, A.; Torgersen, L.; Reichborn-Kjennerud, T.; Haugen, M.; Meltzer, H.M.; Bulik, C.M. Dietary supplement use immediately before and during pregnancy in norwegian women with eating disorders. *Int. J. Eat. Disord.* **2011**, *44*, 325–332. [CrossRef]
34. Micali, N.; Treasure, J.; Simonoff, E. Eating disorders symptoms in pregnancy: A longitudinal study of women with recent and past eating disorders and obesity. *J. Psychosom. Res.* **2007**, *63*, 297–303. [CrossRef]
35. Crow, S.J.; Keel, P.K.; Thuras, P.; Mitchell, J.E. Bulimia symptoms and other risk behaviors during pregnancy in women with bulimia nervosa. *Int. J. Eat. Disord.* **2004**, *36*, 220–223. [CrossRef]
36. Lacey, J.H.; Smith, G. Bulimia nervosa: The impact of pregnancy on mother and baby. *Br. J. Psychiatry* **1987**, *150*, 777–781. [CrossRef]
37. Morgan, J.F.; Lacey, J.H.; Sedgwick, P.M. Impact of pregnancy on bulimia nervosa. *Br. J. Psychiatry* **1999**, *174*, 135–140. [CrossRef]
38. Lemberg, R.; Phillips, J. The impact of pregnancy on anorexia nervosa and bulimia. *Int. J. Eat. Disord.* **1989**, *8*, 285–295. [CrossRef]
39. Rodrigo, C.P.; Aranceta, J.; Salvador, G.; Varela-Moreiras, G. Food frequency questionnaires. *Nutr. Hosp.* **2015**, *31*, 49–56.
40. Pinto, E.; Severo, M.; Correia, S.; Dos Santos Silva, I.; Lopes, C.; Barros, H. Validity and reproducibility of a semi-quantitative food frequency questionnaire for use among portuguese pregnant women. *Matern. Child Nutr.* **2010**, *6*, 105–119. [CrossRef]
41. Brantsæter, A.L.; Haugen, M.; Alexander, J.; Meltzer, H.M. Validity of a new food frequency questionnaire for pregnant women in the norwegian mother and child cohort study (moba). *Matern. Child Nutr.* **2008**, *4*, 28–43. [CrossRef]
42. McGowan, C.A.; Curran, S.; McAuliffe, F.M. Relative validity of a food frequency questionnaire to assess nutrient intake in pregnant women. *J. Hum. Nutr. Diet.* **2014**, *27*, 167–174. [CrossRef]
43. Bernardo, W.; Simões, R.; Buzzini, R.; Nunes, V.; Glina, F. Adverse effects of the consumption of artificial sweeteners—Systematic review. *Rev. Da Assoc. Médica Bras.* **2016**, *62*, 120–122. [CrossRef]
44. Li, J.; Zhao, H.; Song, J.-M.; Zhang, J.; Tang, Y.-L.; Xin, C.-M. A meta-analysis of risk of pregnancy loss and caffeine and coffee consumption during pregnancy. *Int. J. Gynecol. Obstet.* **2015**, *130*, 116–122. [CrossRef] [PubMed]

45. Chen, L.-W.; Wu, Y.; Neelakantan, N.; Chong, M.F.-F.; Pan, A.; van Dam, R.M. Maternal caffeine intake during pregnancy and risk of pregnancy loss: A categorical and dose–response meta-analysis of prospective studies. *Public Health Nutr.* **2016**, *19*, 1233–1244. [CrossRef]
46. Jahanfar, S.; Jaafar, S.H. Effects of restricted caffeine intake by mother on fetal, neonatal and pregnancy outcomes. *Cochrane Database Syst. Rev.* **2015**. [CrossRef]
47. Hart, S.; Abraham, S.; Franklin, R.C.; Russell, J. The reasons why eating disorder patients drink. *Eur. Eat. Disord. Rev.* **2011**, *19*, 121–128. [CrossRef]
48. Cano-Marquina, A.; Tarín, J.J.; Cano, A. The impact of coffee on health. *Maturitas* **2013**, *75*, 7–21. [CrossRef] [PubMed]
49. EFSA NDA Panel (EFSA Panel on Dietetic Products, Nutrition and Allergies). Scientific opinion on the safety of caffeine. *EFSA J.* **2015**, *13*, 4102.
50. ACOG. Committee opinion no. 462: Moderate caffeine consumption during pregnancy. *Obstet. Gynecol.* **2010**, *116*, 467–468. [CrossRef] [PubMed]
51. Scholl, T.O. Maternal iron status: Relation to fetal growth, length of gestation, and iron endowment of the neonate. *Nutr. Rev.* **2011**, *69*, S23–S29. [CrossRef]
52. McLean, E.; Cogswell, M.; Egli, I.; Wojdyla, D.; de Benoist, B. Worldwide prevalence of anaemia, who vitamin and mineral nutrition information system, 1993–2005. *Public Health Nutr.* **2009**, *12*, 444–454. [CrossRef]
53. Milman, N. Oral iron prophylaxis in pregnancy: Not too little and not too much! *J. Pregnancy* **2012**, *2012*, 8. [CrossRef]
54. Menon, K.C.; Ferguson, E.L.; Thomson, C.D.; Gray, A.R.; Zodpey, S.; Saraf, A.; Das, P.K.; Skeaff, S.A. Effects of anemia at different stages of gestation on infant outcomes. *Nutrition* **2016**, *32*, 61–65. [CrossRef]
55. Scholl, T.O.; Hediger, M.L.; Fischer, R.L.; Shearer, J.W. Anemia vs iron deficiency: Increased risk of preterm delivery in a prospective study. *Am. J. Clin. Nutr.* **1992**, *55*, 985–988. [CrossRef]
56. De-Regil, L.M.; Peña-Rosas, J.P.; Fernández-Gaxiola, A.C.; Rayco-Solon, P. Effects and safety of periconceptional oral folate supplementation for preventing birth defects. *Cochrane Database Syst. Rev.* **2015**, *12*, 1–254. [CrossRef] [PubMed]
57. U.S. Preventive Services Task Force. Folic acid supplementation for the prevention of neural tube defects: Us preventive services task force recommendation statement. *JAMA* **2017**, *317*, 183–189. [CrossRef] [PubMed]
58. Henson, M.C.; Castracane, V.D. Leptin in pregnancy: An update1. *Biol. Reprod.* **2006**, *74*, 218–229. [CrossRef]
59. Easter, A.; Taborelli, E.; Bye, A.; Zunszain, P.A.; Pariante, C.M.; Treasure, J.; Schmidt, U.; Micali, N. Perinatal hypothalamic-pituitary-adrenal axis regulation among women with eating disorders and their infants. *Psychoneuroendocrinology* **2017**, *76*, 127–134. [CrossRef] [PubMed]
60. Schleger, F.; Linder, K.; Walter, L.; Heni, M.; Brändle, J.; Brucker, S.; Pauluschke-Fröhlich, J.; Weiss, M.; Häring, H.-U.; Preissl, H.; et al. Family history of diabetes is associated with delayed fetal postprandial brain activity. *Front. Endocrinol.* **2018**, *9*, 673. [CrossRef]
61. Fehlert, E.; Willmann, K.; Fritsche, L.; Linder, K.; Mat-Husin, H.; Schleger, F.; Weiss, M.; Kiefer-Schmidt, I.; Brucker, S.; Häring, H.-U.; et al. Gestational diabetes alters the fetal heart rate variability during an oral glucose tolerance test: A fetal magnetocardiography study. *BJOG Int. J. Obstet. Gynaecol.* **2017**, *124*, 1891–1898. [CrossRef]
62. Paslakis, G.; de Zwaan, M. Clinical management of females seeking fertility treatment and of pregnant females with eating disorders. *Eur. Eat. Disord. Rev.* **2019**, 1–9. [CrossRef]

3

The Effects of Vegetarian and Vegan Diet during Pregnancy on the Health of Mothers and Offspring

Giorgia Sebastiani [1,*], Ana Herranz Barbero [1], Cristina Borrás-Novell [1], Miguel Alsina Casanova [1], Victoria Aldecoa-Bilbao [1], Vicente Andreu-Fernández [2], Mireia Pascual Tutusaus [1], Silvia Ferrero Martínez [3], María Dolores Gómez Roig [3] and Oscar García-Algar [1]

1. Neonatology Unit, Hospital Clinic-Maternitat, ICGON, BCNatal, 08028 Barcelona, Spain; HERRANZ@clinic.cat (A.H.B.); CBORRASN@clinic.cat (C.B.-N.); MMALSINA@clinic.cat (M.A.C.); VALDECOA@clinic.cat (V.A.-B.); mireiapascualt@gmail.com (M.P.T.); OGARCIAA@clinic.cat (O.G.-A.)
2. Grup de Recerca Infancia i Entorn (GRIE), Institut d'investigacions Biomèdiques August Pi i Sunyer (IDIBAPS), 08028 Barcelona, Spain; VIANDREU@clinic.cat
3. BCNatal | Barcelona Center for Maternal Fetal and Neonatal Medicine Hospital Sant Joan de Déu, 08028 Barcelona, Spain; sferrero@sjdhospitalbarcelona.org (S.F.M.); lgomezroig@sjdhospitalbarcelona.org (M.D.G.R.)

* Correspondence: GSEBASTI@clinic.cat

Abstract: Vegetarian and vegan diets have increased worldwide in the last decades, according to the knowledge that they might prevent coronary heart disease, cancer, and type 2 diabetes. Althought plant-based diets are at risk of nutritional deficiencies such as proteins, iron, vitamin D, calcium, iodine, omega-3, and vitamin B12, the available evidence shows that well planned vegetarian and vegan diets may be considered safe during pregnancy and lactation, but they require a strong awareness for a balanced intake of key nutrients. A review of the scientific literature in this field was performed, focusing specifically on observational studies in humans, in order to investigate protective effects elicited by maternal diets enriched in plant-derived foods and possible unfavorable outcomes related to micronutrients deficiencies and their impact on fetal development. A design of pregestational nutrition intervention is required in order to avoid maternal undernutrition and consequent impaired fetal growth.

Keywords: vegetarian diets; vegan diets; plant-based diets; nutrition; pregnancy; breastfeeding; human milk; micronutrients; fetal development

---

1. Introduction

Balanced maternal nutrition during pregnancy is imperative for the mother's health status and, consequently, for offspring, and is crucial to maintain an adequate environment for optimal fetal development. According to the theory of "early life programming" environmental factors and lifestyle during pregnancy determine the risk of developing chronic diseases later in life and also influence lifelong health in offspring [1]. Pregnancy requires an increased intake of macro and micronutrients and balanced diet. For that, it offers a critical window of opportunity to acquire dietetic habits that are beneficial for fetal healthy [2].

Pre-pregnancy and pregnancy adherence to food-safety recommendations, according to the updated Dietary Guidelines for American and Mediterranean Diet, should avoid inadequate levels of key nutrients and micronutrients (proteins, iron, folic acid, vitamin D, calcium, iodine, omega-3, and vitamin B12) that may predispose the offspring to chronic condition later in life such as obesity, diabetes, cardiovascular disease, and neurodevelopmental delays [3].

The percentage of vegetarians and vegans in the general population has increased over the last years partly due to evidence that vegetarianism is linked to improved health. Thus, cohort data have shown that low-fat diets enriched with fruit, vegetables, and fiber can lead to a reduction of risk factors for coronary heart diseases, a better lipid profile [4], lower body mass index (BMI) [5], and lower blood pressure [6]. In addition vegetarian diets appear to prevent cancer and type 2 diabetes [7,8]. Nevertheless, some data suggest that vegetarians and vegans may be at greater risk of increased plasma homocysteine levels, an arising risk factor for cardiovascular disease [9,10], and of low bone mineral density, which predisposes to osteoporosis [11]. Plant-based diets are reported to contain less saturated fatty acids, animal protein and cholesterol, and more folate, fibre, antioxidants, phytochemicals, and carotenoids. However, plant-based diets have a low content of essential micronutrients such as iron, zinc, vitamin B 12, vitamin D, omega-3 (n-3) fatty acids, calcium, and iodine. Consequently, the risk of adverse effects due to micronutrient deficiencies that lead to the risk of malnutrition should not be underestimated [12].

The reasons for choosing a vegetarian or vegan lifestyle are variable and range from evidence-based health consciousness to environmental concerns, socioeconomic considerations, ethical grounds, or spiritual/religious beliefs. Medical reasons also exist in some occasions; for instance, women of childbearing age affected by chronic kidney disease (CKD) may be conditioned to the choice of low-protein vegetarian diet [13]. According to the American Dietetic Association, well planned vegetarian diets are safe for all age groups and in all physiological conditions, including childhood, adolescence, pregnancy, and lactation [12,14]. On the contrary, the German Nutrition Society does not recommend vegetarian or vegan diets during pregnancy, lactation, and childhood, due to the inadequate supply of essential nutrients [15].

Vegetarian diets typically comprise of plant foods such as grains, legumes, nuts, seeds, vegetables, and fruit, and exclude all kinds of animal food including meat (pork, beef, mutton, lamb, poultry, game, and fowl), meat products (sausages, salami, and pâté), fish, mollusks, and crustaceans. Vegetarian diets usually include dairy products like eggs and honey. Accordingly, there are two main directions:

(1) Lacto-ovo-vegetarianism (LOV). This excludes meat but includes dairy products, eggs, and honey, together with a wide variety of plant foods. Subcategories are lacto-vegetarianism (LV), which excludes eggs, and ovo-vegetarianism (OV), which excludes dairy products.
(2) Veganism (VEG), which excludes meat, dairy products, eggs, and honey, but includes a wide variety of plant foods [16].

However, some people adhere to other plant-based diets that limit the foods consumed:

- Raw food diet: consisting exclusively of vegetables, including sprouted cereals and pulses, fresh and dried fruits, and seeds, as well as milk and eggs, all of which are mainly eaten raw.
- Fruit diet: consisting exclusively of fresh and dried fruits, seeds, and some vegetables.
- Macrobiotic diet: the strictly vegetarian version of this diet consists of cereals, pulses, vegetables, seaweed, and soy products; while dairy products, eggs, and some vegetables are avoided. Fish is consumed by people who adhere to a macrobiotic diet.

Despite the concrete definition of such categories there is a wide variety of dietary pattern. Vegetarians can be divided into other subgroups: semivegetarians, who are defined as consuming red meat and poultry once per month or more and all meats—including fish—once per month or more, but no more than once per week; pesco-vegetarians, who consume fish once per month or more but all other meats less than once per month; lacto-vegetarians, who consume eggs and dairy once per month or more, but fish and other meats less tan once per month; and lastly, vegans or strict vegetarians are defined as those who do not consume eggs, dairy, or fish [16].

In Europe and North America vegetarians are LOV [17], while Asian Indian vegetarians are mostly lacto-vegetarians [18]. Moreover, it has been described that Chinese vegetarians consume considerably smaller amount of dairy products than Western vegetarians [19].

In 2006, approximately 2.3% of the US adult population (4.9 million people) strictly followed a vegetarian diet, asserting that they never ate meat, fish, or poultry. In 2012 the percentage increased to 5%. Approximately 1.4–2% of the US adult population is vegan [20]. The percentage of young people who are vegetarian is still higher (6–11%), with similar levels of vegetarian teenagers reported in both the United Kingdom and Australia [21]. On the basis of dietary recall data from the 1999–2004 National Health and Nutrition Examination Survey (NHANES), 7.5% of American women were reported adhering to a vegetarian diet [22]. The distribution of women of childbearing age who follow a vegetarian diet is different between developed and developing countries. In developing countries, the prevalence of vegetarian diet may increase due to poverty and economic reasons. In India, 20–30% of the total population is considered to be vegetarian for religious reasons, but normally they do not eat meat because of economic causes. In developed countries, vegetarians comprehend more women than men, and tend to be of higher educational or socioeconomic status, with low probabilities to plan children, and generally they are under 40 years of age. There are also variations between ethnic groups. In the United Kingdom, people of non-White ethnic origin are more likely to indicate themselves as vegetarian than white (15% vs. 6% of white respondents) [23].

Despite the assessment of the importance of a healthy diet in pregnancy, data have demonstrated that women don't change diet during pregnancy, so optimal preconception dietary pattern is determinant for a healthy pregnancy [24]. In addition, the period of lactation is extremely important for growing patterns of infants and the effectiveness of breastfeeding depends on maternal nutritional status. The lack of macro- and micronutrient intake during lactation may lead to the reduction of micronutrients and energy content in breast milk that could lead to severe illness in breastfed infant [25].

The aim of this narrative review was to analyze the existing studies in humans focused on the effects of vegetarian (LOV) and vegan (VEG) diets during pregnancy on maternal outcomes and nutritional status and on fetal healthiness and complications, valuing the risks and benefits of such nutritional choice. Moreover our aim was to study the period of lactation and breast milk composition of vegetarian and vegan mothers and if the breastfeeding is safe for optimal child growth, because there are no specific clinical guidelines about lactation for vegetarian mothers. The publications reviewed in this paper mainly concern plant-based diets as LOV and VEG. Consequently, the results mainly pertain to these diets, which are generally defined as "vegetarian". We did not assess studies about raw food, fruit, and macrobiotic diets. A research for English written articles was performed using MEDLINE/PubMed/Cochrane databases (since 2000 up to 31 December 2018). The research was based on the combination of the following keywords: vegetarian diet, vegan diet, plant-based nutrition, pregnancy outcomes, fetal development, vegetarian/vegan, and breastfeeding/human milk, combined with words related to nutritional status and to the nutrients of interest (protein, vitamin B12, folate, calcium, iron, zinc, iodine, and n-3 fatty acids). Studies were identified and examined for methodology and key results. Researches about preconception period were also analyzed. Review team members screened titles and abstracts and selected articles that seemed pertinent to the topics, excluding those not in English or not concerned with humans. The full papers were read to select potentially eligible articles and to assess the scientific merit and relevance of each paper valued. The manuscripts were also analyzed according with the type of study (case–control, review, longitudinal cohort, and cross-sectional), type of diets, number of cases, and possible bias. We performed a narrative review because we expected high heterogeneity of results and lack of randomised trials in pregnant vegetarians in the literature. We included American Dietetic Association Guidelines in pregnancy and International Guidelines for vegetarian and vegan diets; moreover, we also included scientific papers about the nutritional status of mothers, reflecting fetal nutrition and possible detrimental effects on fetal development. We included few data before 2000, only those with crucial results.

Especially, our main goal was to highlight if vegetarian or vegan diets could be considered safe for the mother's health and for offspring during pregnancy and lactation. We also focused on the effect of these dietary patterns on the lack of micronutrients in order to find a target therapy that could avoid fetal complication.

2. Review

2.1. International Guidelines for a Healthy Nutrition in Pregnancy: Omnivores and Vegetarians (see Table S1)

Pregnancy is a critical period during which the mother requires different amount of nutrients for healthy gestation, in order to promote optimal fetal development and to avoid the "reprogramming" of fetal tissue, predisposing the infant to lifelong chronic conditions [26]. Preconception body mass index (BMI) is determinant to avoid adverse outcomes during pregnancy. Overweight and caloric excess are related to maternal and fetal health risk including diabetes, preeclampsia and cardiovascular disease, so gestational weight gain during pregnancy must be kept into the normal range recommended [27]. On the contrary, low BMI and malnourished mothers could impair fetal development and nutrients supply, leading to adverse birth outcomes, physical and cognitive delays in childhood, and metabolic disorders in adulthood [28].

In the course of normal gestation plasma volume expands, producing a decrease of vitamins and minerals concentrations; however, plasma lipids and cholesterol arise. During early gestation the fat stores of mothers increase, whereas the last gestation is characterized by increased insulin resistance: these are metabolic changes essential to support fetal growth [29].

According to the 2015–2020 Dietary Guidelines for Americans (DGA), pregnant women have to consume a variety of foods to maintain energy and nutrient requirements and to gain recommended amounts of weight. According to the Dietary Reference Intakes (DRIs) and Institute of Medicine (IOM), caloric necessities are no higher than the estimated energy requirement for nonpregnant women until the second trimester. The extra energy requirement per day is 340 kcal in the second trimester and 452 kcal in the third trimester (IOM), or 260 kcal and 500 kcal, respectively (according to European Food Safety Authority—EFSA) [30,31]. The Guidelines recommend practicing moderate intensity physical activity during pregnancy for benefits to both the mother and fetus [32].

All pregnant women need appropriate nutritional supplementation. Iron supplementation is essential for iron deficiency anemia during gestation [33]. Folic acid consumption of 600 mcg/day from fortified foods and dietary supplements is needed to avoid neural tube defects (NTD) [34]. In addition adequate levels of vitamin D (600 UI/day), choline (450 mg/day), and iodine (220 mcg/day) are needed for normal fetal growth and brain development [35–37]. During a normal pregnancy the efficiency of calcium absorption increases, so the intake of calcium is equal to a nonpregnant woman of the same age. During pregnancy and lactation, adequate calcium intake is considered to be 1000 mg/day. Women with calcium intakes less than 500 mg/day need additional amounts to achieve maternal and fetal bone requirements [38]. Supplementary Materials Table S1 shows the daily nutrients requirements of the principal macro- and micronutrients during pregnancy and lactation, as well as a comparison between the American Guidelines, IOM, EFSA, and International Federation of Gynecology and Obstetrics (FIGO) [39,40].

The Physicians Committee for Responsible Medicine suggests that vegetarian pregnant women have to follow the recommendations for protein intake and should increase up to 25 g of protein each day to reach 1.1 g/kg/day as in pregnancy the demand of protein increases [40,41]. The recommendations are to consume daily portions of dark green vegetables (1–2 servings), other vegetables and fruits (4–5 servings), bean and soy products (3–4 servings), whole grains (six or more servings), and nuts, seeds, and wheat germ (1–2 servings). Vegetarians should include sources of protein, iron, and vitamin B-12 intake, as well as calcium and vitamin D if avoiding milk products. Charts listed in these guidelines are useful for substituting beans, tofu, nuts, eggs, and seeds for meats, and include alternative food sources for calcium if milk and dairy products are rejected [3,41].

2.2. *International Guidelines for Vegetarian and Vegan Diets*

According to the Academy of Nutrition and Dietetics a well planned plant-based eating pattern could be appropriate for all stages of life if adequate and healthy recommendations are followed. For example, in the vegetarian population, if the diet includes a variety of plant products, it would provide the same protein quality as a diet that included meat. Venti et al. provided a modified food guide pyramid for vegetarian and vegan diets [42]. According to these recommendations, the normal intake of protein is 0.8 g/kg/day for an adult woman who follows diets containing high quality protein such as egg, meat, milk, or fish. If dairy products, whole grains, beans, nuts, and seeds are the primary protein sources in the diet, the protein digestibility falls, so the recommendation for dietary protein should increase 20% for vegetarian adult woman until 1 g/kg/day. The protein quality of foods is assessed by their Protein Digestibility Corrected Amino Acid Score (PDCAAS), which measures the score for amino acid digestibility. Values close to 1 correspond to animal products supplying all nine essential amino acids, while values below 0.7 are typical of plant foodstuffs. Even if the score is lower, the combination of more vegetable foods with different amino acid composition could enhance the overall quality of their protein component [31].

According to Messina's guide for North American vegetarians, this population have to consume more legumes, nuts, tofu, beans, seeds, fortified breakfast cereals, milk, cheese or yogurt, and fortified soymilk, which are good sources of vitamin B12, vitamin D, iron, and calcium (the recommendation is the intake of 1200 to 1500 mg/day of calcium, 20% more than omnivores). People who adhere to vegan diets would have to intake daily supplements of vitamin D, vitamin B12, and calcium because the average of these nutrients is insufficient [43].

Although the vegetarian and vegan population tries to compensate the adequate intake of micronutrients, these types of diets limit their amounts. Alfa-linolenic acid (omega-3 or ALA) derives from foods such as flax seeds, chia seeds, mungo beans, walnuts, and canola and soybean oils, so vegetarians consume an abundance of ALA. One teaspoonful of walnuts, soybeans, and mungo beans or one teaspoonful of flaxseed oil or ground flaxseed will supply the daily requirement of ALA. High temperature damages this oil, so it should not be fried. Linoleic acid (n-6 or LA) is derived from nuts, seeds, leafy vegetables, grains, and vegetable oils (corn, safflower, sesame, and sunflower). Unsaturated fatty acids are crucial for cell membrane function and the production of eicosanoids (thromboxanes, leukotrienes, prostaglandins, and prostacyclins). LA (n-6) is converted to arachidonic acid (AA) and ALA (n-3) is converted to eicosapentaenoic acid (EPA) and docosahexaenoic acid (DHA). High intake of LA (n-6) inhibits the synthesis of DHA from ALA (n-3). Consequently, a balanced ratio intake of n-6 and n-3 as 1:2 or 1:3 would be most advantageous for vegetarians. To improve the conversion of ALA to more physiologically active fatty acids like EPA and DHA is essential for the development of brain and nervous system. Vegetarians should guarantee that their diet contains sufficient proteins, pyridoxine, biotin, calcium, copper, magnesium, and zinc. In addition, they should reduce intake of n-6 fatty acids and trans fatty acids that inhibit such conversion, by limiting consumption of processed and deep-fried foods, and alcohol [44]. However, people who adhere to vegetarian or vegan diets steadily show low plasma EPA or DHA, especially vegans compared to nonvegetarians [45].

Moreover vegetarian diets have been associated with iron deficiency but not to iron deficiency anemia so the recommendation for vegetarians is to enrich the diet with iron-fortified breads and cereals, beans and lentils, raisins, and blackstrap molasses, as well as sources of vitamin C, like tomatoes and citrus fruits for optimal iron absorption, cooked in cast iron pans [46]. The iron from vegetarian diets is less available for absorption because these diets contain nonheme iron from plants that is worst absorbed than heme iron contained in animal food like meat. In contrast the absorption of nonheme iron in vegetarian people is high to compensate low body iron stores compared to nonvegetarians. The mean iron absorption from a vegetarian diet is estimated 10% compared to 18% of a diet containing meat. Moreover, nonheme iron absorption is inhibited by whole grains, legumes, and nuts because they contain phytic acid so a balanced diet is needed [47]. Zinc deficiency is also common in people who adhere to vegetarian diets due to the inhibition of zinc absorption from plant food with phytic acid, an inhibitor of zinc bioavailability, so the recommendation is a 50% greater intake of zinc [48]. Calcium intake is high in LOV but vegans show low intake of calcium than recommended. Calcium can be found in low-oxalate (high bioavailability) foods such as bokchoi, broccoli, Chinese cabbage, collards, kale, okra, turnip greens, and soy products. Other foods with slightly less calcium bioavailability are fortified soymilk, sesame seeds, almonds, and red and white beans. Calcium bioavailability from plant foods can be affected by oxalates and phytates, which are inhibitors of calcium absorption; for example spinach and rhubarb have a low calcium bioavailability, whereas kale, broccoli, and bokchoi have high calcium bioavailability. Another important calcium source is water, in particular, hard water that has high calcium and magnesium levels derived from groundwater, particularly from limestone and dolomite [31]. If dietary intake of calcium is low, calcium supplemention should be recommended in divided doses [49–51].

Low vitamin D is the most common deficiency among LOV and vegan people so they may need sun exposure, food fortified with vitamin D, and daily supplements to maintain adequate serum levels. Good sources of vitamin D are found in fish liver oils, fatty fish, and egg yolks, but vitamin content in these foods varies. However, reaching adequate levels of vitamin D from fortified foods is a challenge for vegans because few plant foods are fortified with this vitamin. In such cases, especially in vegan population, vitamin D supplements seem to be the most adequate way to ensure correct vitamin D status [52].

Vegetarian diets are at serious risk of vitamin B12 depletion and/or deficiency, an essential micronutrient that plays a specific role in the synthesis of DNA and red blood cell division and in one carbon metabolism. Vitamin B12 is an essential nutrient that transfers the methyl group in a methionine synthase-requiring reaction, converting homocysteine to methionine. It is essential for the synthesis of energy in mitochondria and for erythropoiesis in the bone marrow. In addition, it is also necessary for the synthesis of myelin and the maintenance of neural axons. Vitamin B12, also called cobalamin, is found in adequate ranges only in animal and dairy foods. If the consumption of animal foods is absent as seen in vegetarian diets it results in low intake and cobalamin deficiency due to its scarce presence in plant foods, although vegetarians consume some fortified foods as cereals and soy products. This deficiency generates hematological alterations, impairment of erythropoiesis, and neurologically-poor outcomes as it plays a key role in neuronal myelinization [53]. The DRI for Vitamin B12 is 2.4 μg/day for adults [54]. The European Food Safety Authority (EFSA) Panel on Dietetic Products, Nutrition and Allergies established an Adequate Intake (AI) of cobalamin nearly 4 μg/day for adults [55]. A high intake of plant-based foods may result in high folate levels, which may cause vitamin B-12 depletion by rectifying the hematologic alterations that are present with vitamin B12 insufficiency. A high prevalence of deficiency, assessed by methylmalonic acid and/or holotranscobalamin II levels, is frequent among vegetarians, and a high prevalence of increased concentration of homocysteine. Vegan subjects reported the most compromised status of vitamin B12 because they do not consume eggs, yoghurt, cheese, and milk, which are natural sources of cobalamin. Chronic low intake of vitamin B12 can lead to a depletion status, and this progressive deficiency may become clinically evident after years, resulting in permanent neurologic damage [56–58].

2.3. *The Effects of Vegetarian and Vegan Diets during Pregnancy on Maternal Nutritional Profile (see Table S2)*

Vegetarian and vegan diets have been considered a nutritional challenge during pregnancy, and they require strong awareness to achieve complete intake of essential nutrients, as such, these diets are at risk of nutritional deficiencies. As described, several studies have demonstrated the insufficient supply of essential nutrients such as vitamin B12, vitamin D, calcium, zinc, iron, proteins, essential fatty acids, and iodine in vegetarian and vegan diets [46]. Here we discuss the published evidence of the effect of plant food diets on maternal nutritional profile. The choice of vegetarian or vegan diet is always in preconception, period so well adjusted preconception nutrition is essential for healthy pregnancy. The nutritional pattern depends on the socioeconomic status of the mother, ethnicity, and the reason for choosing vegetarian diets. If the choice is not cultural but is due to ethical beliefs and good socioeconomic status, the probability of a balanced diet increases [59]. In a case–control poblational study called the KOALA Birth Cohort Study (a prospective cohort of 2834 mother–infant pairs in the Netherlands), vegetarian pregnant women who chose organic foods, had higher education and calculated good intake of macro- and micronutrients for a balanced diet [60]. In the same cohort, vegetarian pregnant women had lower BMI if compared to women following a conventional dietary pattern, and lower prevalence of overweight and obesity 4–5 years after delivery [61]. Generally it is difficult to verify the effect of such diets and to separate them from other determinant factors such as ethnicity, lifestyles, or smoking.

2.3.1. Vitamin B12

A recent review shows that there is a high prevalence of vitamin B12 depletion or deficiency among vegetarians [62]. During pregnancy the intestinal absorption of vitamin B12 increases; absorption is better in small amounts and frequent intervals as fetal needs are not high. Vitamin B12 derived from maternal tissue stores does not cross the placenta, but the absorbed vitamin B12 is transferred across the placenta. Low maternal serum concentration of vitamin B12 during the first trimester is a risk factor for NTD and poor maternal outcomes such as preeclampsia, macrocytic anemia, and neurological impairment [63]. The estimated average requirement (EAR) of vitamin B12 is 2.2 μg/day for pregnancy and 2.4 μg/day for lactation [39]. Many people with vitamin B12 deficiency present signs of clinical anemia or mild anemia. The macrocytosis may be masked by a concomitant disorder, such as iron deficiency, thalassemias, or typical high folate levels in vegetarian women [63]. Dietary deficiency of vitamin B12 is frequent in some developing countries or population with marginal status like India, the Middle East, Africa, China, and Central America [64].

In the prospective PREFORM study in Toronto ($n = 368$), the prevalence of suboptimal B12 status (serum total B12 <210 pmol/L) was 35% at 12–16 gestational weeks and 43% at delivery; the prevalence of B12 deficiency (serum total B12 <148 pmol/L) was 17% and 38%, respectively. Maternal dietary vitamin B12 intake during pregnancy was weakly associated with maternal vitamin B12 levels [65]. Another prospective longitudinal study conducted during pregnancy showed that the prevalence of B12 deficiency increased between the second and third trimester from 8% to 35% in healthy pregnant women with B12 intake >RDA (2.6 μg/day). This decrement of plasma total B12 during pregnancy could be the consequence of increased metabolic rate, active B12 transport across the placenta, and hemodilution [66], so it is important to distinguish if very low serum vitamin B12 in pregnancy represents a true deficiency or an exaggerated physiological fall.

Koebnick et al., in a longitudinal cohort study, compared serum vitamin B12 and homocysteine concentrations in pregnant women consuming a LOV diet, low meat diet (LMD = <300 g/wk), or a diet with larger amounts of meat (>300 g/wk). Dietary vitamin B12 intake, serum levels of vitamin B12, and plasma total homocysteine concentrations were measured once in each trimester. This data included 27 pregnant LOV, 43 pregnant low meat consumers and 39 pregnant controls who consumed more meat as a 'Western diet' (WD). The following criteria were used to consider "low serum concentration of vitamin B12"; <130 pmol/L in the first trimester, <120 pmol/L in the second trimester, and <100 pmol/L in the third trimester. The prevalence of B12 deficiency, based on these cutoffs in at least one trimester, was found to be 39% of LOV, 9% of low-meat eaters, and 3% of the control group. Also, the odds ratio of having a low serum B12 during at least one trimester was 3.9 (95% confidence interval, 1.9–6.1) times higher among LOV and 1.8 (1.0–3.9) times higher among low meat consumers compared with the odds among women of control group. The deficiency rate for women was 33% in the first trimester, 17% in the second, and 39% in the third trimesters. The limitations of this study are that the sample did not include vegan participants, the inclusion of a small population, and that some comparisons were more cross-sectional than longitudinal due to the study design. Moreover high folate intake and folate supplementation during pregnancy may cover the real effects of low vitamin B12 intake on plasma. The higher deficiency in vegetarian pregnant women in the third trimester pointed out a depletion of vitamin B12 stores instead of expanded blood volume.

The authors recommend a higher intake of vitamin B-12 of more than 3.0 mcg/daily for pregnant women consuming a LOV diet [67].

Gibson et al. conducted a cross-sectional study in 99 pregnant women from Ethiopia and included participants whose diet was based on either maize (*Zea mays* L.) and fermented enset (*Enset ventricosum*) products that are the major staple foods consumed. As in the Sidama Zone of Southern Ethiopia, animal products often provide <1% of total energy, this low intake of animal products is coincident with infections and bacterial overgrowth, meaning that pregnant women in Sidama are at high risk of vitamin B-12 deficiency and possibly of folate deficiency. They described that 23% of pregnant women had low plasma vitamin B12 (<150 pmol/L), but 62% had elevated plasma methylmalonic acid (MMA) (>271 nmol/L). None had elevated plasma cystathionine or total homocysteine. Even though they were diagnosed with vitamin B-12 deficiency, there were no signs of macrocytic anemia. This data was limited by the small sample and it was conducted in a specific population [68]. In a cross-sectional study conducted in 284 Canadian pregnant women in Vancouver, the authors found that pregnant South Asian women had suboptimal B12 status (11.5%) or B12 deficiency (61.5%) and showed more MMA plasma concentrations. Plasma total B12 concentration was positively associated with age, education, and B12 supplements. Pre-pregnancy BMI was the strongest independent predictor of plasma total B12 concentration. One limitation of this data was the absence of a dietary assessment to quantify B12 intake, as this specific population promoted vegetarianism [69]. A study conducted in small sample of pregnant Indian women showed that hyperhomocystinemia leads to global DNA hypermethylation in vegetarian population due to low dietary intake of vitamin B-12 during pregnancy and that this could predispose to cardiovascular risk and obesity [70]. All these studies provide evidence that vegetarian and vegan pregnant women are at high risk of vitamin B12 depletion.

On the contrary, a longitudinal case–control study recruited 109 participants and showed that high folate intake in LOV pregnant women and low risk of folate deficiency [71].

2.3.2. Vitamin D and Calcium

Plasma levels of vitamin D during pregnancy depend on sunlight exposure and intake of foods high in vitamin D, fortified foods, or supplements. During pregnancy there is not an increment of vitamin D requirements. Vitamin D deficiencies exist among the general population, especially those with dark skin and vegetarians. Data from the third NHANES indicate that ~42% of African American women and 4% of white women show vitamin D insufficiency [72]. Vegan diets have shown lower average intakes of vitamin D than lacto-vegetarians and omnivores [73]. Sachan et al. performed a cross-sectional data describing the levels of serum vitamin D, calcium, and parathormone (PTH) in 207 urban and rural pregnant women (84.3% of urban and 83.6% of rural women). They found vitamin D values below the cutoff (<22.5 ng/mL) and low calcium intake in the population who does not consume meat. In this study, 14% of the mothers had biochemical osteomalacia [74]. Another data found similar results in Iranian pregnant women at the delivery [75]. Dasgupta et al. recruited a total of 50 pregnant female aged 20–40 years of the Northern Eastern Part of India and assessed vitamin D during the first trimester. Nearly 42% of the cases had vitamin D deficiency and 14% had vitamin D insufficiency in the first trimester; 63.63% who had 25(OH)D levels <20 ng/mL were vegetarians. They did not find any association between vitamin D levels and multivitamin supplements or dietary calcium intake [76]. These studies were limited by the recruitment of a specific population.

During pregnancy and lactation, adequate calcium intake is considered to be 1000 mg/day. Vegetarians and vegans should consume 1200 to 1500 mg/day of calcium, 20% more than omnivores. Pregnant and lactating women should consume a minimum of eight servings of calcium-rich foods [12].

Despite recommendations about a good intake during pregnancy, vegetarian pregnant women are at high risk of vitamin D deficiency and may suffer bone impairment, osteoporosis, and hypocalcemia [77]. In a population-based cross-sectional survey conducted in Shaanxi Province in Northwest China, pregnant women who followed a vegetarian pattern had low calcium intake [78].

2.3.3. Iron

During pregnancy, mild anemia is physiologic as a consequence of the normal hemodilution status. During the second and third trimesters of pregnancy there is a rise in maternal blood volume and iron transportation to the placenta and fetus, showing an increased necessity for iron. Iron absorption from plant (nonheme) and animal (heme) supply is improved during pregnancy and increases with each trimester. Inhibitors of iron absorption include calcium, coffee, and fiber. Vitamin C can help to enhance absorption by reducing the inhibitory effects of phytate. [79,80]. The average of dietary iron needed in pregnancy is dependent on maternal preconception stores and estimated requirements are shown in Table S1.

A systematic review and meta-analysis showed that vegetarian population exhibits lower stores of iron compared to nonvegetarian [81]. In pregnant vegetarian women the results are controversial. A British study, conducted in a cohort of 1274 pregnant women aged 18–45 years, showed that vegetarians had adequate iron intakes from diet and they followed the recommended iron supplementation during the first and second trimesters of pregnancy more than nonvegetarians [82]. Sharma et al. described a high prevalence of anemia in Indian pregnant women because of very low frequency of meat eating. However, this study was cross-sectional and limited to a specific population [83].

2.3.4. Essential Fatty Acids

LA (n-6) and ALA (n-3) are polyunsaturated fatty acids which are obtained from food sources. LA (n-6) is converted to arachidonic acid (AA), and ALA is converted to EPA and DHA. DHA is an important component of neural and retinal membranes. It accumulates in the brain and retina during the end of gestation and early postnatal life. Polyunsaturated fatty acids are transferred via the placenta to the developing fetus from the mother's plasma. Adequate provision of DHA is thought to be essential for optimal visual and neurologic development during early life [84]. A significant percentage of women of childbearing age in Europe are vegetarian and the majority of the population in countries such as India. This group is particularly at risk as the exclusion of meat or fish from the diet may determine very low intakes of DHA. According to a more comprehensive database and improved questionnaire, vegetarian women can achieve higher intakes of DHA (30 mg/day) [85]. For example, women consuming diets with marine products or eating marine oil supplements can reach very high intakes of DHA (>1000 mg/day). The adequate ingestion of DHA is especially important in the last stage of pregnancy as placenta is able to channel the uptake of DHA to the fetus [86].

The literature regarding DHA levels in pregnancy is limited. Pregnant and lactating women increase the necessity of a source of preformed DHA. Lower proportions of DHA have been found in the fetal plasma of vegetarian mothers if compared with mothers who are omnivores [87].

2.3.5. Zinc

Zinc is less bioavailable and it is likely to be present in lower ranges when obtained from plant-derived compared to animal food sources [47]. Vegetarians usually have lower zinc consumption compared with omnivores and their serum zinc levels are lower but in the normal range [88].

During pregnancy the need of Zinc increases so women are encouraged to enhance the intake of zinc and adopting food preparation methods which improve its absorption (soaking, germination fermentation, and sourdough leavening of bread) and reduce phytate levels in zinc rich foods [89].

Although high zinc intake is essential during pregnancy, the consequences of zinc deficiency are not described, so it has been postulated that the body adapts the absorption according to the average intake [90]. The current recommendation of dietary intake for zinc in pregnant women aged 19–50 years is 11 mg/day [48]. A meta-analysis compared the dietary zinc intake of pregnant vegetarian and nonvegetarian (NV) groups: the zinc intake of vegetarians was found to be lower than that of NV (-1.38 ± 0.35 mg/day; $p < 0.001$); the exclusion of low meat eaters from the analysis revealed a greater difference (-1.53 ± 0.44 mg/day; $p = 0.001$). Neither vegetarian nor NV groups met the recommended dietary allowance (RDA) for zinc. In contrast, the evidence evaluated in this systematic review suggests that there is no difference between groups in biomarkers of zinc status (concentrations of zinc in serum/plasma, urine, and hair) or in functional outcomes associated with pregnancy (period of gestation and birth weight) [91].

2.3.6. Iodine, Magnesium

Vegetarian or vegan diets may result in low iodine intake because the main dietary sources of iodine are meat, fish, and dairy products, but iodine in the salt could avoid the risk of deficiency [92].

An adequate magnesium status during pregnancy is essential for fetal development. Serum magnesium levels physiologically decrease during pregnancy due to high demand, higher renal excretion, and haemodilution. In a longitudinal study conducted in 108 healthy pregnant women, significant higher dietary magnesium intakes were observed in pregnant women consuming a plant-based diet (508,714 mg/day for LOV and 504,711 mg/day for low-meat eaters) than in pregnant women consuming a control diet (41,279 mg/day). Urinary magnesium excretion was higher in LOV, followed by low-meat eaters, when compared to the control group [93]. So vegetarian or vegan diets result in high magnesium levels.

2.3.7. Proteins

Proteins demand during pregnancy and lactation increases up to 71 g/day (1.1–1.2 g/kg/day) compared to 46 g/day (0.8 g/kg/day) for nonpregnant women. Protein deposition in maternal and fetal tissues increases throughout pregnancy, much more during the third trimester. Enhanced protein synthesis occurs, combined with decreased amino acid catabolism and urea synthesis. The increment of circulating plasma amino acids is a conservation mechanism for retention of protein during a period of increased demand. Additional protein is needed in pregnancy to reach the estimated 21 g/day deposited in fetal, placental, and maternal tissues during the second and third trimesters. Proteins derived from plants are sufficient to reach these needs. Legumes, nuts, tofu, and eggs are good sources of proteins. Soy protein can reach adequate protein needs as animal protein. Cereals content is low in lysine, so this essential amino acid can be acquired by the intake of more beans and soy products. An increase in all sources of protein can compensate a low lysine average [63]. Pregnant women who adhere to vegan diet are at higher risk of protein deficiency so additional protein is indicated for the vegan diet in the second and third trimesters: 25 g of protein may be added by including 1.5 cups of lentils or 2.5 cups of soy milk per day [94].

2.4. The Effects of Vegetarian and Vegan Diets during Pregnancy on Mother's Health (see Table S3)

2.4.1. Preeclampsia (PE)

Studies about the effects of vegetarian and vegan diet on maternal outcome have yielded incongruent results. The most ancient retrospective data conducted by Carter et al. [95], in 775 vegan mothers in "the Farm"—a vegan community in Summertown, Tennessee—reported only one case of preeclampsia (0.13%).

PE may be caused by a relative prostacyclin deficiency secondary to an excessive production of thromboxane A2. A vegan diet (low in AA) might provide protection against this condition, especially if the conversion of LA to AA is inhibited by decreased activity of the enzyme delta-6-desaturase. Another observational prospective study enrolled 1.538 pregnant Washington state residents and used food frequency questionnaire (FFQ) to assess maternal dietary intake three months before and during pregnancy [96]. They reported that dietary fiber might reduce dyslipidaemia, a condition related to PE. In the group of fiber intake the relative risk (RR) of PE for women in the highest ($\geq$21.2 g/day) vs. the lowest quartile (<11.9 g/day) was 0.28 (95% CI = 0.11–0.75). The same was for water-soluble fiber and insoluble fiber.

Vegetarian diet combined with physical activity seems to reduce the risk of PE. A longitudinal study conducted in 238 black pregnant women from Congo showed that the incidence of arterial hypertension was 4.6% overall (2.9% of whom had PE and 1.7% of whom showed transient hypertension). Women who did not usually consume daily servings of vegetables during pregnancy (33.3%) showed higher frequency of PE compared to women who consumed more than three servings of vegetables per day (3.7%) [97]. In a case–control study, conducted in 172 preeclamptic pregnant women and 339 normotensive controls, the authors described that foods that were beneficial in decreasing the risk of preeclampsia were fruits, vegetables, cereals, dark bread, and low-fat dairy products for their high content of fiber, calcium, and potassium [98]. Despite the evidence support the protective effect of plant based diets on PE, these results might be read with caution because PE is a multifactorial condition.

2.4.2. Gestational Diabetes

Vegetarian diets and high intake of fiber could avoid the development of Gestational Diabetes (GD). In a prospective cohort study of 13,110 pregravid women of Nurses' Health Study II (USA) the authors conducted a self-reported FFQ. They described 758 cases of GD in an 8-year period. Dietary total fiber and cereal and fruit fiber were negatively associated with GD risk after adjustment. Each 10 g/day increment in total fiber intake was associated with 26% (95% CI 9–49) reduction in GD risk. Each 5 g/day increment in cereals was linked to a 23% (9–36) risk reduction and fruit fiber with a 26% (5–42) risk reduction. The combination of high-glycemic load and low-cereal fiber diet was linked to a 2.15-fold (1.04–4.29) increased risk of GD [99]. Another randomized controlled clinical trial included 52 women with GD who were randomly assigned to receive control (n = 26) vs. DASH (Dietary Approaches to Stop Hypertension) diet (n = 26) only for four weeks. The control diet was composed of 45–55% carbohydrates, 15–20% protein, and 25–30% fat. The DASH diet was rich in fruits, vegetables, whole grains, low-fat dairy products, lower saturated fats, cholesterol, and refined grains with a total of 2400 mg/day of sodium. In addition, the DASH diet is low energy-dense and contains high amounts of dietary fiber, phytoestrogens, potassium, calcium, magnesium, and folic acid. Women who consumed the control diet had more incidence of cesarean section—46.2% vs. 80.8% of control group—as well as less need for insulin after intervention: 23% vs. 73% for control group [100]. Assaf et al. [101] conducted a case–control study of 697 normoglycemic women who were randomized (at 8–12 weeks of gestation) in control group (337), of which fat consumption was limited to 30% of total caloric intake, or the intervention group (360), where a MedDiet was offered, enhanced with Extra Virgin Olive Oil (EVOO) and pistachios (40–42% fats of total caloric intake). The composite outcome was defined as having one event of emergency C-section, perineal trauma, pregnancy-induced hypertension and preeclampsia, prematurity, large for gestational age (LGA), and small for gestational age (SGA). The authors found a significant reduction in the risk of composite outcome in the group who received the MedDiet enhanced with EVOO and nuts. The data involved an Indian population and found that Indian vegetarians display a high prevalence of GD; however this concern is of a specific population with high susceptibility to diabetes [102]. Moreover a cross-sectional study in India enrolled 995 white British pregnant women, described that low circulating levels of vitamin B12 were correlated to high maternal BMI and high insulin resistance (assessed by HOMA method) [103].

Nevertheless, a recent Cochrane review showed that dietary interventions in pregnancy for preventing gestational diabetes mellitus need more high-quality evidence to determine their potential effects in pregnancy [104]. In addition, according to a systematic review of observational studies on gestational weight gain (GWG), the intake of carbohydrates and vegetarian diets was associated with lower GWG, contrary to diets with higher intakes of proteins, animal fats, and energy-dense foods, suggesting that plant-based dietary patterns could be beneficial in preventing GWG and consequently GD [105].

2.4.3. Preterm Delivery

Data correlating preterm delivery and vegetarian diets are controversial. A retrospective study conducted in Australia analyzed maternal dietary patterns in the 12 months before conception on fetal growth and preterm delivery [106]. They studied three patterns: (1) high-protein/fruit (characterized by fish, meat, chicken, fruit, and some whole grains); (2) high-fat/sugar/takeaway (takeaway foods, potato chips, and refined grains); and (3) vegetarian-type (vegetables, legumes, and whole grains). A 1-SD (standard deviation) increase in the scores on the high-protein/fruit pattern was associated with decreased likelihood of preterm birth, whereas the reverse direction was apparent for the high-fat/sugar/takeaway pattern. A 1-SD increase in the scores on the high fat/sugar/takeaway pattern was also associated with shorter gestation and low birth length. A longitudinal prospective study conducted on Danish National Birth Cohort enrolled 35,530 nonsmoking women, investigated the association of maternal intake of a Mediterranean-type diet (MD) assessed by FFQ and preterm birth [107]. MD was defined as fish twice a week or more, use of olive or rape seed oil, consumption of five fruits and vegetables a day, ate meat (other than poultry and fish) at most twice a week, and drank at most two cups of coffee a day. For early preterm birth Odds ratio was 0.61 (95% CI: 0.35–1.05) in women fulfilling all criteria for MD and 0.28 (0.11–0.76) in women with none, adjusted for possible confounders (parity, BMI, maternal height, socioeconomic status and cohabitant status). So MD during pregnancy may reduce the risk of early delivery in Danish women. Data including the Norwegian Mother and Child Cohort Study (MoBa) enrolled 26,115 pregnant women using FFQ and divided them in three groups: 569 of full criteria of MD, 25,397 1–4 criteria of MD, and 159 none criteria. No differences were found in preterm birth (OR: 0.73; 95% CI: 0.32, 1.68). A significantly lower rate of preterm birth was found in women with fish intake twice or more a week (OR: 0.84; 95% CI: 0.74, 0.95) [108]. A randomized clinical trial conducted in Norway on 290 pregnant White women (BMI 19–32), analyzed the effect of a cholesterol-lowering diet on maternal, cord, and neonatal plasma lipids and pregnancy outcomes [109]. Maternal total and low-density lipoprotein (LDL) cholesterol levels were lowered in the intervention compared with the control group, but lipid levels in cord blood and in neonates born to mothers in the intervention versus the control groups did not differ. Preterm birth (< 37 weeks) was lower in the intervention group (RR 0.10; 95% CI 0.01–0.77). In addition a prospective data performed in Denmark found the relationship of low consumption of seafood with a strong risk of preterm delivery and low birth weight, OR = 3.6 (95% confidence interval 1.2 to 11.2) showing that low plasma concentration of EPA and DHA during pregnancy is a strong risk factor for subsequent early preterm birth in Danish women [110,111].

2.4.4. Consequences of Unbalanced Nutrition on Mother's Mental Health

Recently, maternal depression has been linked to inadequate nutrition during pregnancy. Pregnant women are particularly vulnerable to the adverse effects of poor nutrition on mood because pregnancy and lactation increase nutrient requirements. Plausible links between nutrition and mood have been reported for folate, vitamin B12, calcium, vitamin D, iron, selenium, zinc, and PUFAs, which are required for the biosynthesis of several neurotransmitters such as serotonin, dopamine, and norepinephrine [112]. Numerous studies have found a positive association between low n-3 levels and a higher incidence of maternal depression. The two n-3 fatty acids most correlated to brain development and function are EPA and DHA, of which, the latter is the most prominent in the brain. Nevertheless the current evidence from randomised controlled trials is inconclusive [113]. A recent study assessed that self-reported postpartum depression was more prevalent among vegetarians than omnivorous subjects, probably due to inadequate micronutrients intake [114].

2.5. The Effects of Vegetarian and Vegan Diets during Pregnancy on Fetal Outcomes (see Table S4)

Fetal outcomes depend on a balanced interchange between maternal nutrients, placental transport and fetal growth factors. Maternal undernutrition may lead impairment of fetal development due to nutrient limitations and decreased nutrient source for fetal growth, changes in placental functions, and epigenetic modifications in the fetal genome. Macro- and micronutrients may directly regulate DNA stability and phenotypic adaptation by influencing the availability of methyl donors thereby modulating epigenetics mechanisms. In animal models, the metabolism of amino acids (glycine, histidine, methionine, and serine) and vitamins (B6, B12, and folate) provide methyl donors for DNA and protein methylation, emphasizing the critical role of balanced nutrient supply through placenta [115].

Dietary patterns may involve very different foods that contain a multitude of nutrients with interactive functions. Many of them are also correlated, so it is difficult to separate their effects. Thus, the cumulative effects of nutrients may be easier to identify than those of a single nutrient.

The increase of women adopting vegetarian or vegan diets has raised concerns about these risks during pregnancy. Nevertheless, the effect of vegetarian or vegan diets on fetal anthropometrics differs considerably between studies. Many studies have found positive correlation between birth weight (BW) and maternal intake of certain food items such as milk, fruits, and green leafy vegetables [116,117]. A recent review included papers that assessed diet by FFQ and studied the association among different dietary patterns and BW. Authors found that the patterns positively associated with BW were labeled "nutrient dense", "protein-rich", "health conscious", and "Mediterranean". Those negatively associated with BW were labeled "Western", "processed", "vegetarian", "transitional", and "wheat products". The dietary patterns "Western" and "wheat products" were also associated with higher risk of SGA babies, whereas a "traditional" pattern in New Zealand was inversely associated with having a SGA baby [118]. Wen et al. [119] found an association between vegetarian diet and lower fetal growth during the second trimester. In a prospective data reported by Reddy et al. [120], birth weight and head circumference and length were lower in the infants born from South Asian vegetarians, even after adjusting for maternal height, duration of gestation, parity, gender of infants, and smoking habits. A systematic review of the literature performed by Murphy et al. [121], studied the associations of consumption of fruits and vegetables during pregnancy with infant birth weight or SGA births. This data identified limited evidence of a positive association between fruit and vegetable consumption during pregnancy and birth weight.

On the contrary, there are data demonstrating a protective effect of plant-based dietey patterns on anthropometric fetal development explained by the high content of vitamins in such diets. A case–control study enrolled 787 pregant women and assessed fruit and vegetable consumption during pregnancy using FFQ (in-person interview). The authors reported that women with lower intake of vegetables during the first trimester had higher incidence of SGA and no association was found between fruit consumption and birth outcomes [122]. Four multiethnic birth cohorts in Canada (the NutriGen Alliance) involving 3997 pairs of full-term neonates and mothers assessed dietary patterns by FFQ. Among White Europeans, a plant-based dietary pattern was inversely associated with birth weight and increased risk of SGA. Not adjusted for cooking methods (among South Asians) maternal consumption of a plant-based diet was associated with a higher birth weight [123]. The heterogeneus results may be due to the different dietary context between developed or developing Countries and most of the included studies concerning low BW provided no maternal information on body mass index or gestational weight gain for vegetarians or controls. Other prospective studies showed that average birthweights of infants born from vegetarian mothers do not differ significantly from omnivorous mothers. Clinical relevance of these data is at least doubtful and the heterogeneity of the results suggests the presence of confounding factors. As fetal growth is directly affected by maternal protein intake, pregnant women need to consume an optimal variety of food plants in vegetarian or vegan diets to achieve the same biodisponibility of proteins of omnivorous population as several studies have demonstrated [124–126].

Micronutrients such as vitamin B12 and zinc are deficient in vegetarian and vegan diets, as the main source are animal products [127]. It has been suggested that the supposed lower BW observed among infants born from mothers who adhere to vegetarian diets may be related to poor nutritional status with regard to iron or vitamin B12. As is highlighted in Fikawati et al.'s longitudinal study, infants may be born as well with low vitamin B12 stores if the maternal intake during pregnancy is inadequate [124]. Maternal B12 status is a key determinant of infant B12 status and is an independent factor for NTD [128]. A recent review demonstrated an association between vitamin B12 status, low BW and preterm delivery [129]. The effects of vegetarian diet on the development of NTD are contradictory [130,131]. Although the direct effect on fetal development has not been well described, vegetarian women may include extra sources of vitamin B12 in their diet to avoid fetal depletion.

Iron deficiency during pregnancy has been associated with low BW and neonatal anemia [132]. Iron derived from meat has better bioavailability than iron provided by plants, therefore vegetarian and vegan women should take a higher content of iron to avoid depletion of internal stores [94]. In fact, a British study found that iron deficiency during pregnancy was not higher in vegetarians and that iron intake was higher in vegetarian women during the first trimester [82], probably due to an awareness of risks and a consequent well planned diet. A recent review showed that vitamin D deficiency is also linked to fetal poor growth and vegetarians are at risk of vitamin D deficiency [133].

An increased risk of hypospadias has been associated to vegetarian or vegan diet during pregnancy, based in the increased intake of phytoestrogens. It was first reported in one prospective study, which obtained an adjusted OR of 4.99 (2.10–11.88) in vegetarian women compared to their omnivorous counterparts. However, this work failed to demonstrate a relationship between the incidence of hypospadias and the intake of soya products, which were supposed to be the first source of phytoestrogens in this lifestyle [134]. Another Scandinavian prospective case–control study reported an increased risk of hypospadias in women with diets excluding meat and fish diet. The study was based in the hypothesis that the lack of some essential amino acids may produce a deficiency during organogenesis [135]. However, these large and well-designed studies had the limitation that their conclusions were based on indirect correlations derived from retrospectively self-administered questionnaires. On the contrary, more recent works, which have focused on the relationship of nutrients to estrogen metabolism and the quantity of phytoestrogens in the diet to hypospadias, have not found positive correlation [136,137]. Furthermore, one Italian study found a positive correlation between hypospadias and a frequent consumption of fish during pregnancy [138]. This contradictory data, together with other studies, suggest that the imbalance of some nutrients or the intake of food contaminants may play roles in the genesis of hypospadias; however, at this point in time, there is not enough information to conclude that vegetarian or vegan diets increase the risk of disruption during the genital organogenesis [139,140].

Plant-based and vegetarian diets, characterized by a high consumption of fruits and vegetables and low or no intakes of cured meat and smoked fish, which represent the principal exogenous dietary sources of nitrate, nitrite, and N-nitroso compounds, associated with a higher risk of developing NTD, would be protective to the risk of congenital malformations [92]. However, it has been described that pickled vegetables are also a source of nitrite and NOCs. A study showed the association between maternal periconceptional consumption of pickled vegetables and NTD in four Chinese countries [141]. They found that >6 pickled vegetable meals/wk increased the risk of NTD, compared with less frequent (i.e., <1 meal/week) consumption. In addition, the authors showed that maternal intake (>1 meal/week) of meat, eggs, or milk had protective effect against the risk of NTD, so the literature is controversial.

2.6. The Effects of Vegetarian and Vegan Diet on the Composition of Human Milk

Vegetarian diets differ between individuals: without good information and well planned diets, vegetarians may be at risk for some deficiencies during pregnancy and consequently during breastfeeding period. In the Table S1 we recollected the daily nutrient requirements during pregnancy and lactation. Although vegetarian diets are usually rich in carbohydrates, the need to develop energy reserves during lactation increases demand for more calories. Both vegetarian and nonvegetarian mothers need caloric reserves to reach sufficient energy average for breastfeeding during the postpartum period [142]. The composition of human milk changes dynamically and can vary according to many maternal factors, such as diet and nutritional status. A recent study analyzed the association of maternal nutrition and body composition with human milk composition. They did not find a significant statistical relationship between human milk composition and nutrients in women's diet during the first six months of lactation. For women in the third month postpartum, they observed moderate to strong correlations between total protein content in milk and the body composition measures such as percentage of fat mass, fat-free mass, and muscle mass. The variance in milk fat content was related to body mass index (BMI), with a significant positive correlation in the first month postpartum. These findings suggest that maternal body composition may be associated with the nutritional value of human milk, with independence of type of diet [143]. Nutritional supplements do not change milk composition in observational studies maybe due to compensatory physiological mechanisms that conserve stable milk macronutrient composition related to the nutritional modifications of maternal diet [144]. Also protein concentration in human milk does not vary in relation to maternal intake of vegetal or animal proteins [145]. Nevertheless, Agostoni et al. [146] reported that animal proteins, compared to plant proteins, are associated with positive psychomotor development indices for infants and young children.

Vegetarian mothers might have low pre-pregnancy nutritional status that can lead to low maternal fat stores for lactation. Fikawati et al. [147] conducted a longitudinal data on mother–infant breastfeeding pairs in Indonesia. They followed 42 pairs of vegetarian and 43 pairs of nonvegetarian. Sociodemographic characteristics did not differ between the two dietary groups except in maternal parity. Vegetarian mothers had lower pre-pregnancy BMI but higher pregnancy weight gain compared to nonvegetarian. This study showed that vegetarian mothers had significantly lower BMI during lactation than nonvegetarian and the breastfeeding had no effect on infant weight and length but had significant effect on mothers' BMI and weight loss. The mothers in the nonvegetarian group in this study had a significantly greater energy intake compared with the vegetarians. Without adequate intake of energy during lactation the postpartum nutritional profile of vegetarian mothers decreased, so the maternal nutritional stores are sacrificed to support infant normal growth.

Low maternal vitamin B-12 intake during lactation can lead to low vitamin B12 content in breast milk which can cause permanent neurological disabilities in infants with low vitamin B12 levels. Maternal vitamin B12 status is the major factor affecting the severity of cobalamin deficiency in breast-fed infants and vegetarian and vegan population are at increasing risk [148]. In regions where animal source food consumption is low and prenatal supplementation is not common, infants are at risk of vitamin B12 deficiency, as shown in prospective data which found that maternal and infant serum/plasma and breast milk total vitamin B12 concentrations were significantly higher among Canadian mothers compared to Cambodian mothers [149]. Breastfed infants of mother who adhere to vegan diets are at increased risk of vitamin B12 deficiency [150]. Pawlak et al. [151], conducted a cross-sectional study in which 74 vegan, vegetarian, and nonvegetarian women were recruited. The prevalences of low vitamin B-12 (<310 pmol/L) were 19.2% for vegans, 18.2% for vegetarians, and 15.4% for nonvegetarians, which was independent of diet. Approximately 85% of participants categorized as having low vitamin B-12 were taking vitamin B12 supplements at doses in excess of the Recommended Dietary Allowance but this study had limitation of small sample.

Specific fatty acids that form the total lipid fraction are influenced by maternal nutrition. Fatty acids intake derives from the maternal plasma, or they synthesized endogenously by the mammary glands. Both of these sources are influenced by maternal diet composition [143].

The breast milk of vegetarians and particularly vegans in the United Kingdom showed lower DHA levels if compared to omnivores, but in the United States, vegetarians do not have lower levels of DHA in breast milk lipids, probably due to higher ingestion of ALA from soybean oil or preformed DHA [63]. Compared to nonvegetarians, the breast milk of vegetarians was found to have more than twice the amount of LA and ALA, but less than half the amount of DHA [84]. The levels of DHA in human milk augment with DHA supplementation. Supplementation with DHA during lactation is more useful to raise DHA content in breast milk than supplementing only during pregnancy [152]. A recent review analyzed 13 low- and middle-income countries and showed that the content of DHA in breast milk was very low in populations living mainly on plant-based diets but higher in fish-eating countries [153].

A cross-sectional observational study of 74 lactating women following a vegan (n = 26), vegetarian (n = 22), or omnivore (n = 26) diet pattern was conducted in the United States [154]. They found that breast milk from vegans had significantly higher unsaturated fat and total omega-3 fats, and lower saturated fats, trans fats, and omega-6 to omega-3 ratios than vegetarian and omnivore. DHA concentrations in breast milk were low regardless of maternal diet pattern, and were reflective of low seafood intake and supplement use. Supplement use was relatated to high DHA levels. The study was limited to small sample. The vegan diet contains essentially no ARA and DHA, as plants thought to have fatty acids (such as hempseed, rapeseed, flaxseeds, soy beans, and walnuts) are poorly converted into DHA by the body [155].

In addition, in the developed world, vitamin D deficiency is most frequently diagnosed exclusively in breastfed infants of vegetarian or vegan mothers [156].

More data are needed to evaluate the milk composition of mother following vegetarian or vegan diets.

2.7. *Vegetarian and Vegan Diet during Pregnancy and Lactation: Target Therapy and Health Intervention*

Specific dietary interventions before, during, and after gestation that are aimed in improving diet quality and setting appropriate intakes of macro- and micronutrients are important to avoid maternal health impairment with consequent physical and neurological fetal abnormalities.

The Mediterranean diet pattern, characterized by low total fat (<30% of energy), low saturated fat (<10% of energy), high complex carbohydrates (but relatively low total carbohydrate), and high dietary fiber intake, is generally considered healthy for all people, and has been recommended as a good preconception and pregnancy diet. The intake of pulses, green leafy vegetables, cereals, and fruit that is associated with best adherence to the Mediterranean diet provides a relatively high intake of folate, which is particularly important in the preconception period. Following a Mediterranean diet also increases the likelihood of achieving adequate intakes of zinc, B vitamins, vitamin A, vitamin E, magnesium, and vitamin C [40].

A strict plant-based diet is suitable during pregnancy but it must be well planned in order to provide all the energy requirements and meet critical nutrients, such as protein, fiber, omega-3, fatty acids, zinc, iodine, calcium, vitamin D, and vitamin B12. The vegetarian-type pattern is not associated to any outcome as preterm birth, BW or SGA if requirements are met [106,127]. Educational resources and food recommendations help vegetarians to consume adequate and complete diets. Some tools could be used for educating vegetarian patients as recording dietary intake by food diaries, providing charts that list of different sources of nutrients or sample menus [63]. Providers should regularly assess a woman's diet and her energy intake [121]. Guidelines on what to eat during pregnancy and lactation are essentially the same for vegetarians as for meateaters, but women who choose restricted diets may need to consume supplements or fortified food in order to reach the recommended requirements [9].

2.7.1. Proteins

Protein needs are particularly high during pregnancy and lactation. Although protein requirements are easily met in a vegan diet, it is recommended an increase by 10% of protein intake during pregnancy [157]. Adding 1.5 cups of lentils or 2.5 cups of soy milk per day could cover additional protein need [94]. Essential amino acids can be full obtained from both grains and legumes. An increase in all sources of protein can compensate for low lysine intake [63]. Lysine is an amino acid that can be more readily obtained from beans and soy and less readily obtained from cereals.

Some plant foods, such as soy, lupines, spinach, pseudocereals (buckwheat, quinoa, and amaranth), and hemp seeds, have all the essential amino acids in similar proportions to animal foods. But some other foods, such as antinutritional factors or fiber, interfere in the absorption of plant proteins. Plant proteins have low digestibility (on average 85%) [157]. If protein consumption in a vegan diet is well planned, no differences in infant birth weight in vegan mothers in comparison with omnivorous mothers have been observed [16]. Balanced energy and protein supplementation reduce the risk of stillbirth and SGA, but high-protein supplementation is not recommended [158]. Plasma quantization of amino acids could be performed in a laboratory to detect deficiencies [159].

2.7.2. Fibers

Fiber intake is recommended in pregnancy because it improves the richness of microbiota and avoids constipation but an excessive consume can difficult the meeting of appropriate nutrient and energy absorption. Therefore, during second and third trimester, alternative foods are preferred (fruits and vegetables, refined grains, peeled beans, and high-protein, high-energy, fiber-free foods such as soy milk, tofu, and soy yoghurt) [157].

2.7.3. Fatty acids/Omega-3

Due to the limited vegetable sources of DHA, pregnant vegetarian women are encouraged to consume an algae-based supplement. ALA is the only *n*-3 fatty acid present in plant foods (flaxseeds, hempseeds, chia seeds, walnuts, and their oils), but ALA elongation to EPA and DHA is limited, and influenced by diet. High dietary LA intake, excessive intakes of trans fatty acids, inadequate intakes of energy, protein, pyridoxine, biotin, calcium, copper, magnesium, or zinc can impair EPA and DHA synthesis [16]. A balanced intake of *n*-3 and *n*-6 fatty acids is important in order to produce sufficient amounts of DHA and EPA. Vegans and vegetarians can be at a disadvantage in balancing this ratio, because they may limit sources of ALA (n-3) or DHA in their diet, and they typically consume an abundance of LA [63]. Good plant sources of omega-3 fatty acids include ground flaxseeds and flaxseed oil, ground chia seeds, and walnuts. Seed oils rich in omega-6, trans fats (margarine), and tropical oils (coconut, palm, and palm kernel oils), which are rich in saturated fats, should be avoided in order to maintain an optimal omega-6/omega-3 ratio and favor the conversion of ALA into polyunsaturated fatty acids (PUFAs). Olive oil has a low influence in this ratio and, in addition to flaxseed oil, and should be the only additional oil to use as omga-3 source. In a recent Cochrane review, the authors studied supplement of omega-3 fatty acids in pregnant women. They found increased prolonged gestation > 42 weeks from 1.6% to 2.6% in women who received omega-3 LCPUFA compared with no omega-3 (moderate-quality evidence); reduced risk of perinatal death (moderate-quality evidence); fewer neonatal care admissions (moderate-quality evidence); reduced risk of low BW babies (15.6% versus 14% (high-quality evidence)); and a small increase in LGA babies (moderate-quality evidence). PE might possibly be reduced with omega-3 LCPUFA but with low-quality evidence. No differences were found for SGA or intrauterine growth restriction. It seems reasonable to recommend a daily supplementation of DHA for all pregnant women [160]. Even at the pregestational level, an intake of adequate amounts of n–3 PUFAs and DHA plays a major role; indeed, small variations in the habitual maternal dietary composition before pregnancy are likely to be more effective in improving the delivery of long-chain PUFAs to the fetus than large dietary changes in the late stages of pregnancy [92]. In these stages, a daily intake of 100 to 200 mg microalgae-derived DHA supplement is suggested [157].

2.7.4. Zinc

Vegetarians should be encouraged to consume more dietary zinc than the Population Reference Intake (PRI) suggested for omnivores, especially when the dietary phytate/zinc ratio is high [16]. Legumes, soy, nuts, seeds, and grains are all rich in zinc [157]. Zinc absorption can be improved by adopting food preparation methods (soaking, germination fermentation, sourdough leavening of bread) that reduce phytate levels in zinc rich foods. Zinc-fortified foods (e.g., breakfast cereals) can also be used. Zinc-rich foods should be eaten together with foods that contain organic acids such as fruit, and vegetables of Brassicaceae family [16] in order to improve zinc absorption.

2.7.5. Iodine

Vegan diets could provide low intake of iodine, although iodine deficiencies are quite uncommon in Western countries. Iodized salt is the safest way to reach iodine requirements in vegan pregnant and lactating women. Iodized salt varies among countries. The estimated average requirement for iodine in pregnant women is 200 μg/day [157]. Higher salt intake during pregnancy in vegans is considered harmless because of the low incidence of hypertension in this population, and can facilitate to meet the iodine requirements. Another option can be an algae-derived supplement.

2.7.6. Iron

Iron supplementation is only recommended if iron status has been shown to be low by appropriate blood tests [16]. A well planned vegan diet can meet iron needs. Iron content in vegan diets is in nonheme form, with lower bioavailability than heme-forms from animal sources (1–34% and 15–35%, respectively). During pregnancy it is recommended a daily consumption of iron rich foods as soy, beans, seeds, nuts, and green leafy vegetables as well as vitamin-C in combination. Some cooking considerations and food preparations should also improve iron absorption [157].

2.7.7. Calcium

A vegan diet can protect calcium stocks by increasing absorption [94]. Therefore, supplementation is rarely needed. Vegetarians and vegans should consume 1200 to 1500 mg/day of calcium, which is ~20% more calcium than that recommended for omnivores [63]. Ideally, low-oxalate foods (high bioavailability), such as broccoli or bokchoi, must be preferred. Other foods with slightly less calcium bioavailability are fortified soymilk, sesame seeds, almonds, and red and white beans. Another important source of calcium is hard water. Most of the varied diets above 2400 kcal should completely cover calcium needs [157]. Villar et al. [161] conducted a randomized clinical trial in 8325 pregnant women with dietary calcium intake <600 mg/day. In the intervention group the intake was 1.5 g/day calcium. They did not find differences in PE. They found a reduction of severe preeclamptic complications index. Preterm delivery was reduced only in women <20 years. Neonatal mortality rate was lower in the calcium group. Another data from Cochrane database evaluated calcium supplementation (≥1 g/day) during pregnancy in 13 studies. This supplement was associated with a significant reduction in the risk of preeclampsia, particularly for women with low calcium diets but the significant reduction in the risk of PE associated with calcium supplementation might be overestimated (small effect, high heterogeneity and publication bias) [162]. The World Health Organization recommends 1.5 g to 2 g of calcium daily for pregnant women with low dietary calcium intake [40].

2.7.8. Vitamin D

Vegans must rely strongly on ultraviolet B rays—the band of ultraviolet that causes synthesis of vitamin D-3—from direct sunlight, to obtain sufficient vitamin D. Extending sunlight exposure and consuming vitamin D fortified foods may be appropriate strategies to avoid possible vitamin D deficiencies [92]. Adequate levels of this molecule and the maintenance of proper metabolism during pregnancy need to be emphasized because some beneficial effects have been reported. For example vitamin D enhances insulin responsiveness for glucose transport, through the modulation of insulin receptor expression. Vitamin D induces insulin secretion and decreases insulin resistance preventing gestational diabetes. In addition, it plays a critical role in the regulation of blood pressure and electrolyte and plasma volume homeostasis; therefore, normal serum vitamin D levels help to prevent hypertension and PE through suppression of the renin–angiotensin system [163]. Nevertheless, excess vitamin D may also have detrimental effects because it might decrease progesterone concentrations causing a preterm labor or impair fertility outcomes, so supplementation should be selective [164].

Vitamin D supplements are the usual remedy for meeting the recommended requirements (15 μg/day). Good sources of vitamin D are found in fish, liver oils, fatty fish, and egg yolks, but vitamin content in these foods varies by the time of year [63]. Plant sources of vitamin D are beans, broccoli, and leafy greens, but its content of this molecule without fortification is low, except for some wild mushrooms that contain a relevant concentration of this vitamin; therefore, vegetarian and vegan women are at risk of vitamin D deficiency. These source of vitamin D can be further fortified with calcium supplements, including cow's milk, some soymilk products, and some breakfast cereals. Serum levels of vitamin D are easily measured if there is concern regarding intake of this essential nutrient [94]. Optimal serum 25-OH vitamin levels for pregnant women are above 75 nmol/L (30 ng/mL). Most of prenatal vitamins contain insufficient vitamin D in order to prevent infant vitamin D deficiency, so to get the recommended doses of 1000 to 2000 IU per day, are considered safe in pregnancy [157]. A recent Cochrane review underlines that supplementing pregnant women with vitamin D in a single or continued dose increases serum 25-hydroxyvitamin-D, and may reduce the risk of preeclampsia, low BW, and preterm delivery. However, when vitamin D and calcium are combined, the risk of preterm birth is increased. Further studies are needed to evaluate vitamin D supplementation and the correct dose during pregnancy [165].

2.7.9. Vitamin B12

Vitamin B12 is not found in plant sources, and therefore must be obtained through animal consumption or via supplements [94]. Since vitamin B12 deficiency may appear in pregnant vegetarian women, in particular vegans, an adequate B12 status should be improved, so the use of B12 supplements is necessary. Pregnant and lactating vegans should be advised to supplement their diets with 4 μg/d of vitamin B12 [150]. Foods fortified with vitamin B12 include meat substitute products, breakfast cereals, soymilks, tofu, cereals, and nutritional yeast. Seaweed and tempeh are generally not reliable sources of vitamin B12. Four servings daily of vitamin B12-fortified foods are recommended in pregnancy and lactation [63]. Even if common pre- and postnatal multivitamins contain 100% of the RDA for vitamin B12, they are not positively associated with B12 concentration in breastmilk of vegetarian women because only a fraction of the B12 they provide is absorbed. Pregnant and lactating vegetarian and vegan mothers should be encouraged to take an individual B12, supplement and dissolve it under the tongue or chew it slowly in order to increase absorption [157]. In the case of vitamin B12 deficiency, the majority of clinical studies suggest starting with high parenteral doses of B12, after which oral treatment is continued. Considering the importance of adequate intake of vitamin B12 during pregnancy and considering that supplementation is not toxic, an ingestion of higher dose of B12 supplement (50 μg/day) would ensure correct vitamin status [92]. Vitamin B12 status (serum B12, along with homocysteine and folic acid) should be regularly checked throughout pregnancy also in women with optimal B12 levels in the first trimester, and it is necessary to adjust supplementation schemes according to the laboratory results [157].

3. Limitations

The present study corresponds to a descriptive review in which the majority of papers evaluated maternal dietary intake through a food frequency questionnaire. The main limitations of these questionnaires are the different food list and the possible mistakes of reporting.

Most studies analyzed in this review concluded that vegetarian and/or vegan diets exert diverse effects on pregnant outcome and nutritional profile. However, some of them describe specific populations in India or Africa with lower economic status and particular idiosyncrasy. For that, ethnicity and poverty have to be taken into account as a cause of an unbalanced diet, micronutrient deficiency, and poor pregnancy outcome. Furthermore, epidemiological and biochemical studies need to be done in Western countries to corroborate the conclusions obtained in African and/or Asian regions.

Mother undernutrition could be multifactorial, so it is important to mention the difficulties to determine the molecular mechanisms promoted by each micronutrient which may affect specifically the maternal nutritional profile.

4. Conclusions

Diet is one of the most significant lifestyle-related factors in determining health state and predisposing the offspring to develop several diseases. Vegetarian and vegan diets are emerging worldwide due to the evidence that plant-based dietary patterns reduce the risk of coronary heart disease, high blood pressure, type 2 diabetes, and cancer. Pregnancy is a critical window of opportunity to provide dietetic habits that are beneficial for fetal healthy. It is also an exclusive condition in which the requirements of energy and micronutrients intake increase to maintain the supply of essential nutrients for fetal development. Each stage of fetal growth is dependent on appropriate maternal nutrient transfer, so a balanced diet is essential to avoid fetal complications. The choice of vegetarian or vegan diet is always in the preconception period due to ethical reasons or poor social condition, so a well-adjusted preconception nutrition is essential for healthy pregnancy. Available data demonstrated that micronutrients insufficiency and caloric restriction are more common in developing countries, where vegetarian diets are chosen because of socioeconomic reasons. On the contrary in developed countries, the consciousness and the concern of a balanced diet is taken more into account. Generally it is difficult to verify the effects of such diets on pregnancy outcomes and to separate them from other confounding factors such as ethnicity, lifestyles or smoking.

Although more high quality evidence is needed, balanced plant-based diets rich in fibers and low in fat are considered to be protective against poor pregnancy outcomes such as PE, DG, and preterm delivery. However, these protective effects disappear if micronutrients deficiencies emerge. Moreover unbalanced dietary patterns with lack of macro- and micronutrients such as proteins, vitamin B12, vitamin D, calcium, DHA, and iron are at more risk of fetal impairment (low BW, neurological disabilities, and fetal malformations). Maternal undernutrition may potentially alter fetal growth trajectory by modifying placental weight and nutrient transfer capacity; depending on the severity of the nutritional deprivation and on the timing of depletion. Thus, plant-based diets during pregnancy and lactation require a strong awareness for a complete intake of essential key nutrients and vitamin supplements, according to international guidelines.

In addition, during breastfeeding both vegetarian and nonvegetarian mothers need caloric reserves to reach sufficient energy average. The composition of human milk changes dynamically and may vary according to many maternal factors, such as nutritional status. Nutritional supplements do not change milk composition in observational studies, also proteins concentration in human milk does not vary in relation to maternal intake of vegetal or animal proteins, but maternal body composition may be associated with the nutritional value of human milk. So maternal undernutrition, producing lack of vitamin B12, vitamin D, calcium, and DHA during lactation may lead to low vitamin content in breast milk, which can cause permanent neurological disabilities in infants or low bone mineralization.

Finally, the current manuscript supports the evidence that maternal nutritional status is the key condition for health benefits of plant-based diets. Vegetarians and vegans are at risk of nutritional deficiencies, but if the adequate intake of nutrients is upheld, pregnancy outcomes are similar to those reported in the omnivorous population. So updated evidence highlights that well-balanced vegetarian and vegan diets should be considered safe for the mother's health and for offspring during pregnancy and lactation. In this regard, specific dietary interventions before, during, and after gestation that are aimed at improving diet quality and adjusting appropriate intakes of macro- and micronutrients might avoid maternal health impairment, mental diseases during pregnancy, and consequent physical and neurological fetal disabilities. The vegetarian-type pattern should be considered safe and it is not associated with preterm birth, BW, or SGA if the requirements are met. Therefore, healthcare professionals might have knowledge about plant-based diets characteristics in order to implement balanced dietary patterns, enhancing supplement intake, and paying attention to critical nutrients to avoid dangerous health outcomes. Further large-scale observational studies would help to define correlations between plant-based diets, gestation, and health, and might be suitable to design pregestational nutrition intervention strategies.

Author Contributions: All authors contributed to the work reported. G.S. carried out the reference search of bibliographic source, selecting papers, and Writing—Original Draft Preparation; she made the tables and the review of manuscript. A.H.B., C.B.-N., M.A.C., V.A.-B., M.P.T., and S.F.M. contributed to the bibliographic source and elaboration of the initial manuscript and tables. V.A.-F. supervised the methodology and reviewed the manuscript. M.D.G.R. and O.G.-A. performed the final check of the manuscript from a gynaecologist's and neonatologist's point of view, respectively.

Acknowledgments: This work was supported by grant from Red de Salud Materno-Infantil y del Desarrollo (SAMID) (RD16/0022/0002) from Instituto de Salud Carlos III, Madrid (Spain).

References

1. Fall, C.H. Fetal programming and the risk of noncommunicable disease. *Indian. J. Pediatr.* **2013**, *80* (Suppl. 1), S13–S20. [CrossRef] [PubMed]
2. Barker, D.J.P.; Bergmnann, R.L.; Ogra, P.L. (Eds.) *The Window of Opportunity: Pre-Pregnancy to 24 Months of Age*; Karger, Nestle Nutrition Institute: Basel, Switzerland, 2008; pp. 1–266.
3. Procter, S.B.; Campbell, C.G. Position of the Academy of Nutrition and Dietetics: Nutrition and Lifestyle for a Healthy Pregnancy Outcome. *J. Acad. Nutr. Diet.* **2014**, *114*, 1099–1103. [CrossRef] [PubMed]
4. Wang, F.; Zheng, J.; Yang, B.; Jiang, J.; Fu, Y.; Li, D. Effects of Vegetarian Diets on Blood Lipids: A Systematic Review and Meta-Analysis of Randomized Controlled Trials. *J. Am. Heart. Assoc.* **2015**, *27*, e002408. [CrossRef] [PubMed]
5. Rosell, M.; Appleby, P.; Spencer, E.; Key, T. Weight gain over 5 years in 21,966 meat-eating, fish-eating, vegetarian, and vegan men and women in EPIC-Oxford. *Int. J. Obes.* **2006**, *30*, 1389–1396. [CrossRef] [PubMed]
6. Berkow, S.E.; Barnard, N.D. Blood pressure regulation and vegetarian diets. *Nutr. Rev.* **2005**, *63*, 1–8. [CrossRef] [PubMed]
7. Khan, N.; Afaq, F.; Mukhtar, H. Cancer chemoprevention through dietary antioxidants: Progress and promise. *Antioxid. Redox. Signal.* **2008**, *10*, 475–510. [CrossRef] [PubMed]
8. Jenkins, D.J.; Kendall, C.W.; Marchie, A.; Jenkins, A.L.; Augustin, L.S.; Ludwig, D.S.; Barnard, N.D.; Anderson, J.W. Type 2 diabetes and the vegetarian diet. *Am. J. Clin. Nutr.* **2003**, *78*, 610S–616S. [CrossRef] [PubMed]
9. Phillips, F. Vegetarian nutrition. *British Nutrition Foundation. Nutr. Bull.* **2005**, *30*, 132–167. [CrossRef]
10. Chang-Claude, J.; Hermann, S.; Eilber, U.; Steindorf, K. Lifestyle determinants and mortality in German vegetarians and health-conscious persons: Results of a 21-year follow-up. *Cancer Epidemiol. Biomark. Prev.* **2005**, *14*, 963–968. [CrossRef] [PubMed]
11. Ho-Pham, L.T.; Nguyen, N.D.; Nguyen, T.V. Effect of vegetarian diets on bone mineral density: A Bayesian meta-analysis. *Am. J. Clin. Nutr.* **2009**, *90*, 943–950. [CrossRef] [PubMed]
12. Position of the American Dietetic Association: Vegetarian diets. *J. Amer. Diet. Assoc.* **2009**, *109*, 1266–1282. [CrossRef]
13. Piccoli, G.B.; Attini, R.; Vasario, E.; Gaglioti, P.; Piccoli, E.; Consiglio, V.; De Agostini, C.; Oberto, M.; Trodos, T. Vegetarian supplemented low-protein diets. A safe option for pregnant CKD patients: Report of 12 pregnancies in 11 patients. *Nephrol. Dial. Transplant.* **2011**, *26*, 196–205. [CrossRef] [PubMed]
14. U.S. Department of Agriculture; U.S. Department of Health and Human Services. *Dietary Guidelines for Americans 2010*, 7th ed.; U.S. Government Printing Office: Washington, DC, USA, 2010.
15. Richter, M.; Boeing, H.; Grünewald-Funk, D.; Heseker, H.; Kroke, A.; Leschik-Bonnet, E.; Oberritter, H.; Strohm, D.; Watzl, B.; The German Nutrition Society (DGE). Vegan Diet Position of the German Nutrition Society (DGE). *Ernaehrungs. Umschau. Int.* **2016**, *4*, 92–102.

16. Agnoli, C.; Baroni, L.; Bertini, I.; Ciappellano, S.; Fabbri, A.; Papa, M.; Pellegrini, N.; Sbarbati, R.; Scarino, M.L.; Siani, V.; et al. Nutrition, Metabolism & Cardiovascular Diseases Position paper on vegetarian diets from the working group of the Italian Society of Human Nutrition. *Nutr. Metab. Cardiovasc. Dis.* **2017**, *27*, 1037–1052. [PubMed]
17. Davey, G.K.; Spencer, E.A.; Appleby, P.N.; Allen, N.E.; Knox, K.H.; Key, T.J. Epic-oxford: Lifestyle characteristics and nutrient intakes in a cohort of 33 883 meat-eaters and 31 546 non meat-eaters in the UK. *Public Health Nutr.* **2003**, *6*, 259–269. [CrossRef] [PubMed]
18. Jayanthi, V. Vegetarianism in India. *Perit. Dial. Int.* **2001**, *21*, S322–S325. [PubMed]
19. Lee, H.Y.; Woo, J.; Chen, Z.Y.; Leung, S.F.; Peng, X.H. Serum fatty acid, lipid profile and dietary intake of Hong Kong Chinese omnivores and vegetarians. *Eur. J. Clin. Nutr.* **2000**, *54*, 768–773. [CrossRef] [PubMed]
20. Stahler, C. How Often Do Americans Eat Vegetarian Meals? And How Many Adults in the U.S. Are Vegetarian? Available online: http://www.vrg.org/journal/vj2011issue4/vj2011issue4poll.php (accessed on 10 October 2017).
21. Vegetarian Resource Group. How Many Youth Are Vegetarians? How Many Kids Don't Eat Meat? *Veg. J.* **2005**, *4*, 26–27.
22. Farmer, B.; Larson, B.T.; Fulgoni, V.L., III; Rainville, A.J.; Liepa, G.U. A vegetarian dietary pattern as a nutrient-dense approach to weight management: An analysis of the national health and nutrition examination survey 1999–2004. *J. Am. Diet. Assoc.* **2011**, *111*, 819–827. [CrossRef] [PubMed]
23. Sabate, J.; Ratzin-Turner, R.A.; Brown, J.E. Vegetarian Diets: Descriptions and Trends. In *Vegetarian. Nutrition*; CRC Series in Modern Nutrition; CRC: Boca Raton, FL, USA, 2001; pp. 3–18.
24. Crozier, S.R.; Robinson, S.M.; Godfrey, K.M.; Cooper, C.; Inskip, H.M. Women's dietary patterns change little from before to during pregnancy. *J. Nutr.* **2009**, *139*, 1956–1963. [CrossRef] [PubMed]
25. Allen, L.H. Multiple micronutrients in pregnancy and lactation: An overview. *Am. J. Clin. Nutr.* **2005**, *81*, 1206S–1212S. [CrossRef] [PubMed]
26. Shapira, N. Prenatal nutrition: A critical window of opportunity for mother and child. *Womens Health* **2008**, *4*, 639–656. [CrossRef] [PubMed]
27. Rasmussen, K.M.; Yaktine, A.L. (Eds.) *Weight Gain During Pregnancy: Reexamining the Guidelines*; National. Academies. Press: Washington, DC, USA, 2009.
28. Black, R.E.; Victora, C.G.; Walker, S.P.; Bhutta, Z.A.; Christian, P.; de Onis, M.; Ezzati, M.; Grantham-McGregor, S.; Katz, J.; Martorell, R.; et al. Maternal and child undernutrition and overweight in low-income and middle-income countries. *Lancet* **2013**, *382*, 427–451. [CrossRef]
29. Academy of Nutrition and Dietetics. Practice Paper of the Academy of Nutrition and Dietetics: Nutrition and Lifestyle for a Healthy Pregnancy Outcome. Available online: http://www.eatright.org/members/practicepapers/ (accessed on 22 May 2014).
30. US Department of Agriculture. Dietary Guidelines for Americans, 2015–2020. Available online: http://www.cnpp.usda.gov/dgas2010-policydocument.htm (accessed on 3 March 2019).
31. EFSA (European Food Safety Authority). *Dietary Reference Values for Nutrients: Summary Report*; EFSA Supporting Publication: London, UK, 2017.
32. US Department of Health and Human Services. Physical activity for women during pregnancy and the postpartum period. In *2008 Physical Activity Guidelines for Americans*; Office of Disease Prevention & Health Promotion: Washington, DC, USA, 2008; pp. 41–42.
33. Gautam, C.S.; Saha, L.; Sekhri, K.; Saha, P.K. Iron deficiency in pregnancy and the rationality of iron supplements prescribed during pregnancy. *Medsc. J. Med.* **2008**, *10*, 283–288.
34. Centers for Disease Control and Prevention. Folic Acid: Recommendations. Available online: http://www.cdc.gov/ncbddd/folicacid/recommendations.html (accessed on 24 September 2012).
35. Thorne-Lyman, A.; Fawzi, W.W. Vitamin D during pregnancy and maternal, neonatal and infant health outcomes: A systematic review and meta-analysis. *Paediatr. Perinat. Epidemiol.* **2012**, *26* (Suppl. 1), 75–90. [CrossRef] [PubMed]
36. Caudill, M.A. Pre- and postnatal health: Evidence of increased choline needs. *J. Am. Diet. Assoc.* **2010**, *110*, 1198–1206. [CrossRef] [PubMed]
37. Obican, S.G.; Jahnke, G.D.; Soldin, O.P.; Scialli, A.R. Teratology public affairs committee position paper: Iodine deficiency in pregnancy. *Birth Defects Res.* **2012**, *94 Pt A*, 677–682. [CrossRef]

38. Hacker, A.N.; Fung, E.B.; King, J.C. Role of calcium during pregnancy: Maternal and fetal needs. *Nutr. Rev.* **2012**, *70*, 397–409. [CrossRef] [PubMed]
39. Kominiarek, M.A.; Rajan, P. Nutrition Recommendations in Pregnancy and Lactation. *Med. Clin. North. Am.* **2016**, *100*, 1199–1215. [CrossRef] [PubMed]
40. Hanson, M.A.; Bardsley, A.; De-Regil, L.M.; Moore, S.E.; Oken, E.; Poston, L.; Ma, R.C.; McAuliffe, F.M.; Maleta, K.; Purandare, C.N.; et al. The International Federation of Gynecology and Obstetrics (FIGO) recommendations on adolescent, preconception, and maternal nutrition: "Think Nutrition First". *Int. J. Gynaecol. Obstet.* **2015**, *131*, S213–S253. [CrossRef]
41. Physicians Committee for Responsible Medicine Website. Vegetarian Diets for Pregnancy. Available online: www.pcrm.org/health/veginfo/pregnancy.html (accessed on 28 March 2007).
42. Venti, C.A.; Johnston, C.S. Modified Food Guide Pyramid for Lactovegetarians and Vegans. *J. Nutr.* **2002**, *132*, 1050–1054. [CrossRef] [PubMed]
43. Messina, V.; Melina, V.; Mangels, A.R. A new guide for North American Vegetarians. *J. Am. Diet. Assoc.* **2003**, *103*, 771–775. [CrossRef] [PubMed]
44. Davis, B.C.; Kris-Etherton, P.M. Achieving optimal essential fatty acid status in vegetarians: Current knowledge and practical implications. *Am. J. Clin. Nutr.* **2003**, *78*, 640S–646S. [CrossRef] [PubMed]
45. Welch, A.; Shakya-Shrestha, S.; Lentjes, M.; Wareham, N.; Khaw, K. Dietary intake and status of n-3 polyunsaturated fatty acids in a population of fish-eating and non fish-eating meat-eaters, vegetarians, and vegans and the precursor-product ratio of a-linolenic acid to long-chain n-3 polyunsaturated fatty acids: Results from the EPIC-Norfolk cohort. *Am. J. Clin. Nutr.* **2010**, *92*, 1040–1051. [PubMed]
46. Position of the Academic of Nutrition and Dietetics: Vegetarian diets. *J. Acad. Nutr. Diet.* **2015**, *115*, 801–810. [CrossRef] [PubMed]
47. Hunt, J.R. Bioavailability of iron, zinc, and other trace minerals from vegetarian diets 1-4. *Am. J. Clin. Nutr.* **2003**, *78*, 633–642. [CrossRef] [PubMed]
48. Foster, M.; Chu, A.; Petocz.; Samman, S. Effect of vegetarian diets on zinc status: A systematic review and meta-analysis of studies in humans. *J. Sci. Food. Agric.* **2013**, *93*, 2362–2371. [CrossRef] [PubMed]
49. Institute of Medicine. Dietary Reference Intakes for Calcium and Vitamin D. Available online: http://www.iom.edu/Reports/2010/Dietary-Reference-Intakes-for-calcium-and-vitamin-D.aspx (accessed on 17 October 2013).
50. Larsson, C.L.; Johansson, G.K. Dietary intake and nutritional status of young vegans and omnivores in Sweden. *Am. J. Clin. Nutr.* **2002**, *76*, 100–106. [CrossRef] [PubMed]
51. Weaver, C.M.; Proulx, W.R.; Heaney, R. Choices for achieving adequate dietary calcium with a vegetarian diet. *Am. J. Clin. Nutr.* **1999**, *70*, 543S–548S. [CrossRef] [PubMed]
52. Crowe, F.L.; Steur, M.; Allen, N.E.; Appleby, P.N.; Travis, R.C.; Key, T.J. Plasma concentrations of 25-hydroxyvitamin D in meat eaters, fish eaters, vegetarians and vegans: Results from the EPIC-Oxford study. *Public Health Nutr.* **2011**, *14*, 340–346. [CrossRef] [PubMed]
53. Rizzo, G.; Laganà, A.S.; Rapisarda, A.M.C.; La Ferrera, G.M.G.; Buscema, M.; Rossetti, P.; Nigro, A.; Muscia, V.; Valenti, G.; Sapia, F.; et al. Vitamin B12 among vegetarians: Status, assessment and supplementation. *Nutrients* **2016**, *8*, 767. [CrossRef] [PubMed]
54. Otten, J.J.; Hellwig, J.P.; Meyers, L.D. *Dietary Reference Intakes: The Essential Guide to Nutrient Requirements*; Institute of Medicine of the National Academies: Washington, DC, USA, 2006.
55. Panel on Dietetic Products, Nutrition, and Allergies. Scientific opinion on dietary reference values for cobalamin (Vitamin B12). *EFSA J.* **2015**, *13*, 4150.
56. Pawlak, R.; Lester, S.E.; Babatunde, T. The prevalence of cobalamin deficiency among vegetarians assessed by serum vitamin B12: A review of literature. *Eur. J. Clin. Nutr.* **2014**, *68*, 541–548. [CrossRef] [PubMed]
57. Obersby, D.; Chappell, D.C.; Dunnett, A.; Tsiami, A.A. Plasma total homocysteine status of vegetarians compared with omnivores: A systematic review and metaanalysis. *Br. J. Nutr.* **2013**, *109*, 785–794. [CrossRef] [PubMed]
58. Herrmann, W.; Schorr, H.; Obeid, R.; Geisel, J. Vitamin B-12 status, particularly holotranscobalamin II and methylmalonic acid concentrations, and hyperhomocysteinemia in vegetarians. *Am. J. Clin. Nutr.* **2003**, *78*, 131–136. [CrossRef] [PubMed]

59. Northstone, K.; Emmett, P.; Rogers, I. Dietary patterns in pregnancy and associations with socio-demographic and lifestyle factors. *Eur. J. Clin. Nutr.* **2008**, *62*, 471–479. [CrossRef] [PubMed]
60. Simões-Wüst, A.P.; Moltó-Puigmartí, C.; Van, Dongen; Martien, C.J.M.; Dagnelie, P.C.; Thijs, C. Organic food consumption during pregnancy is associated with different consumer profiles, food patterns and intake: The KOALA Birth Cohort Study. *Public Health Nutr.* **2017**, *20*, 2134–2144.
61. Simões-Wüst, A.P.; Kummeling, I.; Mommers, M.; Huber, M.A.; Rist, L.; van de Vijver, L.P.; Dagnelie, P.C.; Thijs, C. Influence of alternative lifestyles on self-reported body weight and health characteristics in women. *Eur. J. Public Health* **2013**, *24*, 321–327. [CrossRef] [PubMed]
62. Pawlak, R.; James, P.S.; Raj, S.; Cullum-Dugan, D.; Lucus, D. How prevalent is vitamin B12 deficiency among vegetarians? *Nutr. Rev.* **2013**, *71*, 110–117. [CrossRef] [PubMed]
63. Penney, D.S.; Miller, K.G. Nutritional Counseling for Vegetarians During Pregnancy and Lactation. *J. Midwifery Women's Health* **2008**, *53*, 37–44. [CrossRef] [PubMed]
64. Stabler, S.P.; Allen, R.H. Vitamin B12 deficiency as a worldwide problem. *Annu. Rev. Nutr.* **2004**, *24*, 299–326. [CrossRef] [PubMed]
65. Visentin, C.E.; Masih, S.P.; Plumptre, L.; Schroder, T.H.; Sohn, K.J.; Ly, A.; Lausman, A.Y.; Berger, H.; Croxford, R.; Lamers, Y.; et al. Low serum vitamin B-12 concentrations are prevalent in a cohort of pregnant Canadian women. *J. Nutr.* **2016**, *146*, 1035–1042. [CrossRef] [PubMed]
66. Koebnick, C.; Heins, U.A.; Dagnelie, P.C.; Wickramasinghe, S.N.; Ratnayaka, I.D.; Hothorn, T.; Pfahlberg, A.B.; Hoffmann, I.; Lindemans, J.; Leitzmann, C. Longitudinal concentrations of vitamin B(12) and vitamin B(12)-binding proteins during uncomplicated pregnancy. *Clin. Chem.* **2002**, *48*, 928–933. [PubMed]
67. Koebnick, C.; Hoffmann, I.; Dagnelie, P.C.; Heins, U.A.; Wickramasinghe, S.N.; Ratnayaka, I.D.; Gruendel, S.; Lindemans, J.; Leitzmann, C. Long-Term Ovo-Lacto Vegetarian Diet Impairs Vitamin B-12 Status in Pregnant Women. *J. Nutr.* **2004**, *134*, 3319–3326. [CrossRef] [PubMed]
68. Gibson, R.S.; Abebe, Y.; Stabler, S.; Allen, R.H.; Westcott, J.E.; Stoecker, B.J.; Krebs, N.F.; Hambidge, K.M. Zinc, gravida, infection, and iron, but not vitamin B-12 or folate status, predict hemoglobin during pregnancy in Southern Ethiopia. *J. Nutr.* **2008**, *138*, 581–586. [CrossRef] [PubMed]
69. Jeruszka-Bielak, M.; Isman, C.; Schroder, T.H.; Li, W.; Green, T.J.; Lamers, Y. South Asian Ethnicity is related to the highest risk of vitamin B12 deficiency in pregnant canadian women. *Nutrients* **2017**, *23*, 317. [CrossRef] [PubMed]
70. Gadgil, M.S.; Joshi, K.S.; Naik, S.S.; Pandit, A.N.; Otiv, S.R.; Bhushan, K.; Patwardhan, B.K. Association of homocysteine with global DNA methylation in vegetarian Indian pregnant women and neonatal birth anthropometrics. *J. Matern. Fetal Neonatal Med.* **2014**, *27*, 1749–1753. [CrossRef] [PubMed]
71. Koebnick, C.; Heins, U.A.; Hoffmann, I.; Dagnelie, P.C.; Leitzmann, C. Folate status during pregnancy in women is improved by long-term high vegetable intake compared with the average western diet. *J. Nutr.* **2001**, *131*, 733–739. [CrossRef] [PubMed]
72. Nesby-O'Dell, S.; Scanlon, K.S.; Cogswell, M.E.; Gillespie, C.; Hollis, B.W.; Looker, A.C.; Allen, C.; Doughertly, C.; Gunter, E.W.; Bowman, B.A. Hypovitaminosis D prevalence and determinants among African American and white women of reproductive age: Third Health and Nutrition Examination Survey, 1988–1944. *Am. J. Clin. Nutr.* **2002**, *76*, 187–192. [CrossRef] [PubMed]
73. Smith, A.M. Veganism and osteoporosis: A review of the current literature. *Int. J. Nurs. Pract.* **2006**, *12*, 302–306. [CrossRef] [PubMed]
74. Sachan, A.; Gupta, R.; Das, V.; Agarwal, A.; Awasthi, P.K.; Bhatia, V. High prevalence of vitamin D deficiency among pregnant women and their newborns in northern India. *Am. J. Clin. Nutr.* **2005**, *81*, 1060–1064. [CrossRef] [PubMed]
75. Kazemi, A.; Sharifi, F.; Jafari, N.; Mousavinasab, N. High prevalence of vitamin D deficiency among pregnant women and their newborns in an Iranian population. *J. Womens Health* **2009**, *18*, 835–839. [CrossRef] [PubMed]
76. Dasgupta, A.; Saikia, U.; Sarma, D. Status of 25(OH)D levels in pregnancy: A study from the North Eastern part of India. *Indian J. Endocrinol. Metab.* **2012**, *16* (Suppl. 2), S405–S407. [PubMed]
77. Elsori, D.H.; Hammoud, M.S. Vitamin D deficiency in mothers, neonates and children. *J. Steroid. Biochem. Mol. Biol.* **2018**, *175*, 195–199. [CrossRef] [PubMed]
78. Yang, J.; Dang, S.; Cheng, Y.; Qui, H.; Mi, B.; Jiang, Y.; Yan, H. Dietary intakes and dietary patterns among pregnant women in Northwest China. *Public Health Nutr.* **2017**, *20*, 282–293. [CrossRef] [PubMed]

79. Graves, B.S.; Barger, M.K. A "conservative" approach to iron supplementation during pregnancy. *J. Midwifery Women's Health* **2001**, *46*, 159–166. [CrossRef]
80. Williamson, C. Nutrition in pregnancy. *Nutr. Bull.* **2006**, *31*, 28–59. [CrossRef]
81. Haider, L.M.; Schwingshackl, L.; Hoffmann, G.; Ekmekcioglu, C. The effect of vegetarian diets on iron status in adults: A systematic review and meta-analysis. *Crit. Rev. Food. Sci. Nutr.* **2018**, *58*, 1359–1374. [CrossRef] [PubMed]
82. Alwan, N.A.; Greenwood, D.C.; Simpson, N.A.; McArdle, H.J.; Godfrey, K.M.; Cade, J.E. Dietary iron intake during early pregnancy and birth outcomes in a cohort of British women. *Hum. Reprod.* **2011**, *26*, 911–919. [CrossRef] [PubMed]
83. Sharma, J.B.; Soni, D.; Murthy, N.S.; Malhotra, M. Effect of dietary habits on prevalence of anemia in pregnant women of Delhi. *J. Obs. Gynaecol. Res.* **2003**, *29*, 73–78. [CrossRef]
84. Jensen, C.L. Effects of n-3 fatty acids during pregnancy and lactation. *Am. J. Clin. Nutr.* **2006**, *83*, S1452–S1457. [CrossRef] [PubMed]
85. Masson, L.F.; McNeill, G.; Tomany, J.O.; Simpson, J.A.; Peace, H.S.; Wei, L.; Grubb, D.A.; Bolton-Smith, C. Statistical approaches for assessing the relative validity of a food-frequency questionnaire: Use of correlation coefficients and the kappa statistic. *Public Health Nutr.* **2003**, *6*, 313–321. [CrossRef] [PubMed]
86. Haggarty, P. Effect of placental function on fatty acid requirements during pregnancy. *Eur. J. Clin. Nutr.* **2004**, *58*, 1559–1570. [CrossRef] [PubMed]
87. Sanders, T.A.B. Essential fatty acid requirements of vegetarians in pregnancy, lactation and infancy. *Am. J. Clin. Nutr.* **1999**, *70*, 555S–559S. [CrossRef] [PubMed]
88. Foster, M.; Samman, S. Vegetarian diets across the lifecycle: Impact on zinc intake and status. *Adv. Food. Nutr. Res.* **2015**, *74*, 93–131. [PubMed]
89. Baroni, L.; Goggi, S.; Battino, M. VegPlate: A Mediterranean-Based Food Guide for Italian Adult, Pregnant, and Lactating Vegetarians. *J. Acad. Nutr. Diet.* **2018**, *118*, 2235–2243. [CrossRef] [PubMed]
90. King, J.C. Determinants of maternal zinc status during pregnancy. *Am. J. Clin. Nutr.* **2000**, *71*, 1334S–1343S. [CrossRef] [PubMed]
91. Foster, M.; Herulah, U.; Prasad, A.; Petocz, P.; Samman, S. Zinc Status of Vegetarians during Pregnancy: A Systematic Review of Observational Studies and Meta-Analysis of Zinc Intake. *Nutrients* **2015**, *7*, 4512–4525. [CrossRef] [PubMed]
92. Pistollato, F.; Sumalla Cano, S.; Elio, I.; Masias Vergara, M.; Giampieri, F.; Battino, M. Plant-Based and Plant-Rich Diet Patterns during Gestation: Beneficial Effects and Possible Shortcomings. *Adv. Nutr. An. Int. Rev. J.* **2015**, *6*, 581–591. [CrossRef] [PubMed]
93. Koebnick, C.; Leitzmann, R.; García, A.L.; Heins, U.A.; Heuer, T.; Golf, S.; Katz, N.; Hoffmann, I.; Leitzmann, C. Long-term effect of a plant-based diet on magnesium status during pregnancy. *Eur. J. Clin. Nutr.* **2005**, *59*, 219–225. [CrossRef] [PubMed]
94. Tyree, S.; Baker, B.R.; Weatherspoon, D. On veganism and pregnancy. *Int. J Child. Educ.* **2012**, *27*, 43–49.
95. Carter, J.P.; Furman, T.; Robert Hutcheson, H. Preeclampsia and reproductive performance in a community of vegans. *South. Med. J.* **1987**, *80*, 692–697. [CrossRef] [PubMed]
96. Qiu, C.; Coughlin, K.B.; Frederick, I.O.; Sorensen, T.K.; Williams, M.A. Dietary fiber intake in early pregnancy and risk of subsequent preeclampsia. *Am. J. Hypertens.* **2008**, *21*, 903–909. [CrossRef] [PubMed]
97. Longo-Mbenza, B.; Kadima-Tshimanga, B.; Buassa-bu-Tsumbu, B.; M'Buyamba, K., Jr. Diets rich in vegetables and physical activity are associated with a decreased risk of pregnancy induced hypertension among rural women from Kimpese, DR Congo. *Niger. J. Med.* **2008**, *17*, 45–49. [PubMed]
98. Frederick, I.O.; Williams, M.A.; Dashow, E.; Kestin, M.; Zhang, C.; Leisenring, W.M. Dietary fiber, potassium, magnesium and calcium in relation to the risk of preeclampsia. *J. Reprod. Med.* **2005**, *50*, 332–344. [PubMed]
99. Zhang, C.; Liu, S.; Solomon, C.G.; Hu, F.B. Dietary fiber intake, dietary glycemic load, and the risk for gestational diabetes mellitus. *Diabetes Care* **2006**, *29*, 2223–2230. [CrossRef] [PubMed]
100. Asemi, Z.; Samimi, M.; Tabassi, Z.; Esmaillzadeh, A. The effect of DASH diet on pregnancy outcomes in gestational diabetes: A randomized controlled clinical trial. *Eur. J. Clin. Nutr.* **2014**, *68*, 490–495. [CrossRef] [PubMed]
101. Assaf-Balut, C.; García de la Torre, N.; Duran, A.; Fuentes, M.; Bordiú, E.; del Valle, L.; Familiar, C.; Valerio, J.; Jiménez, I.; Herraiz, M.A.; et al. A Mediterranean Diet with an Enhanced Consumption of Extra Virgin Olive Oil and Pistachios Improves Pregnancy Outcomes in Women Without Gestational Diabetes Mellitus:

A Sub-Analysis of the St. Carlos Gestational Diabetes Mellitus Prevention Study. *Ann. Nutr. Metab.* **2019**, *74*, 69–79. [CrossRef] [PubMed]

102. Arora, G.P.; Thaman, R.G.; Prasad, R.B.; Almgren, P.; Brons, C.; Groop, L.C.; Vaag, A.A. Prevalence and risk factors of gestational diabetes in Punjab, North India: Results from a population screening program. *Eur. J. Endocrinol.* **2015**, *173*, 257–267. [CrossRef] [PubMed]
103. Knight, B.A.; Shields, B.M.; Brook, A.; Hill, A.; Bhat, D.S.; Hattersley, A.T.; Tajnik, C.S. Lower Circulating B12 Is Associated with Higher Obesity and Insulin Resistance during Pregnancy in a Non-Diabetic White British Population. *PLoS ONE.* **2015**, *10*, 8. [CrossRef] [PubMed]
104. Muktabhant, B.; Lawrie, T.A.; Lumbiganon, P.; Laopaiboon, M.; Ta, L.; Lumbiganon, P.; Laopaiboon, M.; Tieu, J.; Shepherd, E.; Middleton, P. Dietary advice interventions in pregnancy for preventing gestational diabetes mellitus (Review). *Cochrane Database Syst. Rev.* **2017**, *1*, CD007145.
105. Streuling, I.; Beyerlein, A.; Rosenfeld, E.; Schukat, B.; von Kries, R. Weight gain and dietary intake during pregnancy in industrialized countries—A systematic review of observational studies. *J. Perinat. Med.* **2011**, *39*, 123–129. [CrossRef] [PubMed]
106. Grieger, J.A.; Grzeskowiak, L.E.; Clifton, V.L. Preconception Dietary Patterns in Human Pregnancies Are Associated with Preterm Delivery. *J. Nutr.* **2014**, *144*, 1075–1080. [CrossRef] [PubMed]
107. Mikkelsen TB Association between a Mediterranean diet and risk of preterm birth among Danish women: A prospective cohort study. *Acta Obs. Gynecol. Scand.* **2008**, *87*, 325–330. [CrossRef] [PubMed]
108. Haugen, M.; Meltzer, H.M.; Brantsaeter, A.L.; Mikkelsen, T.; Østerdal, M.L.; Alexander, J.; Olsen, S.F.; Bakketeig, L. Mediterranean-type diet and risk of preterm birth among women in the Norwegian Mother and Child Cohort Study (MoBa): A prospective cohort study. *Acta Obs. Gynecol. Scand.* **2008**, *87*, 319–324. [CrossRef] [PubMed]
109. Khoury, J.; Henriksen, T.; Christophersen, B.; Tonstad, S. Effect of a cholesterol-lowering diet on maternal, cord, and neonatal lipids, and pregnancy outcome: A randomized clinical trial. *Am. J. Obs. Gynecol.* **2005**, *193*, 1292–1301. [CrossRef] [PubMed]
110. Olsen, S.F.; Secher, N. Low consumption of seafood in early pregnancy as a risk factor for preterm delivery: Prospective cohort study. *BMJ* **2002**, *324*, 447. [CrossRef] [PubMed]
111. Olsen, S.F.; Halldorsson, T.I.; Thorne-Lyman, A.L.; Strøm, M.; Gørtz, S.; Granstrøm, C.; Nielsen, P.H.; Wohlfahrt, J.; Lykke, J.A.; Langhoff-Roos, J.; et al. Plasma Concentrations of Long Chain N-3 Fatty Acids in Early and Mid-Pregnancy and Risk of Early Preterm Birth. *Ebiomedicine* **2018**, *35*, 325–333. [CrossRef] [PubMed]
112. Leung, B.M.; Kaplan, B.J. Perinatal depression: Prevalence, risks, and the nutrition link—A review of the literature. *J. Am. Diet. Assoc.* **2009**, *109*, 1566–1575. [CrossRef] [PubMed]
113. Gould, J.F.; Best, K.; Makrides, M. Perinatal nutrition interventions and post-partum depressive symptoms. *J. Affect. Disord.* **2017**, *15*, 2–9. [CrossRef] [PubMed]
114. Hogg-Kollars, S.; Mortimore, D.; Snow, S. Nutrition health issues in self-reported postpartum depression. *Gastroenterol. Hepatol. Bed Bench* **2011**, *4*, 120–136. [PubMed]
115. Cetin, I.; Mando, C.; Calabrese, S. Maternal predictors of intrauterine growth restriction. *Curr. Opin. Clin. Nutr. Metab. Care* **2013**, *16*, 310–319. [CrossRef] [PubMed]
116. Olsen, S.F.; Halldorsson, T.I.; Willett, W.C.; Knudsen, V.K.; Gillman, M.W.; Mikkelsen, T.B.; Olsen, J.; NUTRIX Consortium. Milk consumption during pregnancy is associated with increased infant size at birth: Prospective cohort study. *Am. J. Clin. Nutr.* **2007**, *86*, 1104–1110. [CrossRef] [PubMed]
117. Rao, S.; Yajnik, C.S.; Kanade, A.; Fall, C.H.; Margetts, B.M.; Jackson, A.A.; Shier, R.; Joshi, S.; Rege, S.; Lubree, H.; et al. Intake of micronutrient-rich foods in rural Indian mothers is associated with the size of their babies at birth: Pune maternal nutrition study. *J. Nutr.* **2001**, *131*, 1217–1224. [CrossRef] [PubMed]
118. Kjøllesdal, M.K.R.; Holmboe-Ottesen, G. Dietary Patterns and Birth Weight—A Review. *AIMS Public Health* **2014**, *1*, 211–225. [CrossRef] [PubMed]
119. Wen, X.; Justicia-Linde, F.; Kong, K.; Zhang, C.; Chen, W.; Epstein, L. Associations of diet and physical activity with the three components of gestational weight gain. *Am. J. Epidemiol.* **2013**, *11*, S11–S81.
120. Reddy, S.; Sanders, T.A.B.; Obeid, O. The influence of maternal vegetarian diet on essential fatty acid status of the newborn. *Eur. J. Clin. Nutr.* **1994**, *48*, 358–368. [PubMed]

121. Murphy, M.M.; Stettler, N.; Smith, K.M.; Reiss, R. Associations of consumption of fruits and vegetables during pregnancy with infant birth weight or small for gestational age births: A systematic review of the literature. *Int. J. Womens. Health* **2014**, *6*, 899–912. [CrossRef] [PubMed]
122. Ramón, R.; Ballester, F.; Iñiguez, C.; Rebagliato, M.; Murcia, M.; Esplugues, A.; Marco, A.; García de la Hera, M.; Vioque, J. Vegetable but not fruit intake during pregnancy is associated with newborn anthropometric measures. *J. Nutr.* **2009**, *139*, 561–567. [CrossRef] [PubMed]
123. Zulyniak, M.A.; De Souza, R.J.; Shaikh, M.; Desai, D.; Lefebvre, D.L.; Gupta, M.; Wilson, J.; Wahi, G.; Subbarao, P.; Becker, A.B.; et al. Does the impact of a plant-based diet during pregnancy on birth weight differ by ethnicity? A dietary pattern analysis from a prospective Canadian birth cohort alliance. *BMJ* **2017**, *7*, e017753. [CrossRef] [PubMed]
124. Fikawati, S.; Syafiq, A.; Wahyuni, D. Nutrient intake and pregnancy outcomes among vegetarian mothers in Jakarta, Indonesia. *Veg. Nutr. J.* **2013**, *20*, 15–25.
125. Robic, T.; Benedik, E.; Bratanic, B.; Fidler Mis, N.; Rogelj, I.; Golja, P. Body composition in (NON) vegetarian pregnant women and their neonates. *Clin. Nutr. Suppl.* **2012**, *7*, 108. [CrossRef]
126. Gomez Roig, M.D.; Mazarico, E.; Ferrero, S.; Montejo, R.; Ibanez, L.; Grima, F.; Vela, A. Differences in dietary and lifestyle habits between pregnant women with small fetuses and appropriate-for- gestational-age fetuses. *J. Obs. Gynaec. Res.* **2017**, *43*, 1145–1151. [CrossRef] [PubMed]
127. Piccoli, G.; Clari, R.; Vigotti, F.; Leone, F.; Attini, R.; Cabiddu, G.; Mauro, G.; Castelluccia, N.; Colombi, N.; Capizzi, I.; et al. Vegan-vegetarian diets in pregnancy: Danger or panacea? A systematic narrative review. *BJOG* **2015**, *122*, 623–633. [CrossRef] [PubMed]
128. Molloy, A.M. Should vitamin B_{12} status be considered in assessing risk of neural tube defects? *Ann. N. Y. Acad. Sci.* **2018**, *1414*, 109–125. [CrossRef] [PubMed]
129. Molloy, A.M.; Kirke, P.N.; Brody, L.C.; Scott, J.M.; Mills, J.L. Effects of folate and vitamin B12 deficiencies during pregnancy on fetal, infant, and child development. *Food. Nutr. Bull.* **2008**, *29* (Suppl. 2), S101–S111. [CrossRef] [PubMed]
130. Larsen, P.S.; Nybo Andersen, A.M.; Uldall, P.; Bech, B.H.; Olsen, J.; Hansen, A.V.; Strandberg-Larsen, K. Maternal vegetarianism and neurodevelopment of children enrolled in The Danish National Birth Cohort. *Acta Paediatr.* **2014**, *103*, e507–e509. [CrossRef] [PubMed]
131. Deb, R.; Arora, J.; Meitei, S.Y.; Gupta, S.; Verma, V.; Saraswathy, K.N.; Saran, S.; Kalla, A.K. Folate supplementation, MTHFR gene polymorphism and neural tube defects: A community based case control study in North India. *Metab. Brain Dis.* **2011**, *26*, 241–246. [CrossRef] [PubMed]
132. Haider, B.A.; Olofin, I.; Wang, M.; Spiegelman, D.; Ezzati, M.; Fawzi, W.W. Anaemia, prenatal iron use, and risk of adverse pregnancy outcomes: Systematic review and meta-analysis. *BMJ* **2013**, *346*, 3443. [CrossRef] [PubMed]
133. Hu, Z.; Tang, L.; Xu, H.L. Maternal Vitamin D Deficiency and the Risk of Small for Gestational Age: A Meta-analysis. *Iran. J. Public. Health* **2018**, *47*, 1785–1795. [PubMed]
134. North, K.; Golding, J. A maternal vegetarian diet in pregnancy is associated with hypospadias. The ALSPAC Study Team. Avon Longitudinal Study of Pregnancy and Childhood. *BJU* **2000**, *85*, 107–113. [CrossRef]
135. Akre, O.; Boyd, H.A.; Ahlgren, M.; Wilbrand, K.; Westergaard, T.; Hjalgrim, H.; Nordenskjöld, A.; Ekbom, A.; Melbye, M. Maternal and gestational risk factors for hypospadias. *Environ. Health Perspect.* **2008**, *116*, 1071–1076. [CrossRef] [PubMed]
136. Carmichael, S.L.; Cogswell, M.E.; Ma, C.; Gonzalez-Feliciano, A.; Olney, R.S.; Correa, A.; Shaw, G.M.; National Birth Defects Prevention Study. Hypospadias and maternal intake of phytoestrogens. *Am. J. Epidemiol.* **2013**, *178*, 434–440. [CrossRef] [PubMed]
137. Carmichael, S.L.; Ma, C.; Feldkamp, M.L.; Munger, R.G.; Olney, R.S.; Botto, L.D.; Shaw, G.M.; Correa, A. Nutritional factors and hypospadias risks. *Paediatr. Perinat. Epidemiol.* **2012**, *26*, 353–360. [CrossRef] [PubMed]
138. Giordano, F.; Carbone, P.; Nori, F.; Mantovani, A.; Taruscio, D.; Figa Talamanca, I. Maternal diet and the risk of hypospadias and cryptorchidism in the offspring. *Paediatr. Perinat. Epidemiol.* **2008**, *22*, 249–260. [CrossRef] [PubMed]
139. Christensen, J.S.; Asklund, C.; Skakkebæk, N.E.; Jørgensen, N.E.; Andersen, H.R.; Jørgensen, T.M.; Olsen, L.H.; Høyer, A.P.; Moesgaard, J.; Thorup, J.; et al. Association between organic dietary choice during

pregnancy and hypospadias in offspring: A study of mothers of 306 boys operated on for hypospadias. *J. Urol.* **2013**, *189*, 1077–1082. [CrossRef] [PubMed]

140. De Kort, C.A.; Nieuwenhuijsen, M.J.; Mendez, M.A. Relationship between maternal dietary patterns and hypospadias. *Paediatr. Perinat. Epidemiol.* **2011**, *25*, 255–264. [CrossRef] [PubMed]
141. Li, Z.W.; Zhang, L.; Ye, R.W.; Liu, J.M.; Pei, L.J.; Zheng, X.Y.; Ren, A.G. Maternal periconceptional consumption of pickled vegetables and risk of neural tube defects in offspring. *Chin. Med. J.* **2011**, *124*, 1629–1633. [PubMed]
142. Wilson, P.R.; Pugh, L.C. Promoting nutrition in breastfeeding women. *J. Obs. Gynecol. Neonatal Nurs.* **2005**, *34*, 120–124. [CrossRef] [PubMed]
143. Bzikowska-Jura, A.; Czerwonogrodzka-Senczyna, A.; Olędzka, G.; Szostak-Węgierek, D.; Weker, H.; Wesołowska, A. Maternal Nutrition and Body Composition During Breastfeeding: Association with Human Milk Composition. *Nutrients* **2018**, *27*, 10. [CrossRef] [PubMed]
144. Keikha, M.; Bahreynian, M.; Saleki, M.; Kelishadi, R. Macro- and micronutrients of human milk composition: Are they related to maternal diet? A comprehensive systematic review. *Breastfeed. Med.* **2017**, *12*, 517–527. [CrossRef] [PubMed]
145. Boniglia, C.; Carratu, B.; Chiarotti, F.; Giammarioli, S.; Sanzini, E. Influence of maternal protein intake on nitrogen fractions of human milk. *Int. J. Vitam. Nutr. Res.* **2003**, *73*, 447–452. [CrossRef] [PubMed]
146. Agostoni, C.; Decsi, T.; Fewtrell, M.; Goulet, O.; Kolacek, S.; Koletzko, B.; Michaelsen, K.F.; van Goudoever, J. Complementary feeding: A commentary by the ESPGHAN committee on nutrition. *J. Pediatr. Gastroenterol. Nutr.* **2008**, *46*, 99–110. [CrossRef] [PubMed]
147. Fikawati, S.; Syafiq, A.; Irawati, A.; Karima, K. Comparison of Lactational Performance of Vegetarian and Non-Vegetarian Mothers in Indonesia. *Malays. J. Nutr.* **2014**, *20*, 15–25.
148. Honzik, T.; Adamovicova, M.; Smolka, V.; Magner, M.; Hruba, E.; Zeman, J. Clinical presentation and metabolic consequences in 40 breastfed infants with nutritional vitamin B12 deficiency—What have we learned? *Eur. J. Paediatr. Neurol.* **2010**, *14*, 488–495. [CrossRef] [PubMed]
149. Chebaya, P.; Karakochuk, C.D.; March, K.M.; Chen, N.N.; Stamm, R.A.; Kroeun, H.; Sophonneary, P.; Borath, M.; Shahab-Ferdows, S.; Hampel, D.; Barr, S.I.; et al. Correlations between Maternal, Breast Milk, and Infant VitaminB12 Concentrations among Mother-Infant Dyads in Vancouver, Canada and Prey Veng, Cambodia: An Exploratory Analysis. *Nutrients* **2017**, *9*, 270. [CrossRef] [PubMed]
150. Pawlak, R. To vegan or not to vegan when pregnant, lactating or feeding young children. *Eur. J. Clin. Nutr.* **2017**, *71*, 1259–1262. [CrossRef] [PubMed]
151. Pawlak, R.; Vos, P.; Shahab-Ferdows, S.; Hampel, D.; Allen, L.H.; Perrin, M.T. Vitamin B-12 content in breast milk of vegan, vegetarian, and nonvegetarian lactating women in the United States. *Am. J. Clin. Nutr.* **2018**, *108*, 525–531. [CrossRef] [PubMed]
152. Boris, J.; Jensen, B.; Salvig, J.D.; Secher, N.J.; Olsen, S.F. A randomized controlled trial of the effect of fish oil supplementation in late pregnancy and early lactation on the n-3 fatty acid content in human breast milk. *Lipids* **2004**, *39*, 1191–1196. [CrossRef] [PubMed]
153. Michaelsen, K.F.; Dewey, K.G.; Perez-Exposito, A.B.; Nurhasan, M.; Lauritzen, L.; Roos, N. Food sources and intake of n-6 and n-3 fatty acids in lowincome countries with emphasis on infants, young children (6–24 months), and pregnant and lactating women. *Matern. Child. Nutr.* **2011**, *7* (Suppl. 2), 124–140. [CrossRef] [PubMed]
154. Perrin, M.T.; Pawlak, R.; Dean, L.L.; Christis, A.; Friend, L. A cross-sectional study of fatty acids and brain-derived neurotrophic factor (BDNF) in human milk from lactating women following vegan, vegetarian, and omnivore diets. *Eur. J. Nutr.* **2018**. [CrossRef] [PubMed]
155. Blanchard, D.S. Omega 3: Fatty acid supplementation in perinatal settings. *Am. J. Matern. Child Nurs.* **2006**, *31*, 250–256. [CrossRef]
156. Baatenburg de Jong, R.; Bekhof, J.; Roorda, R.; Zwart, P. Severe nutritional vitamin deficiency in a breast-fed infant of a vegan mother. *Eur. J. Pediatr.* **2005**, *164*, 259–260. [CrossRef] [PubMed]
157. Baroni, L.; Goggi, S.; Battaglino, R.; Berveglieri, M.; Fasan, I.; Filippin, D.; Griffith, P.; Rizzo, G.; Tomasini, C.; Tosatti, M.A.; et al. Vegan Nutrition for Mothers and Children: Practical Tools for Healthcare Providers. *Nutrients* **2018**, *20*, 5. [CrossRef] [PubMed]
158. Ota, E.; Hori, H.; Mori, R.; Farrar, D. Antenatal dietary education and supplementation to increase energy and protein intake. *Cochrane Database Syst. Rev.* **2015**. [CrossRef] [PubMed]

159. Manta-vogli, P.D.; Schulpis, K.H.; Dotsikas, Y.; Yannis, L. The significant role of amino acids during pregnancy: Nutritional support. *J. Matern. Fetal Neonatal Med.* **2018**, *30*, 1–7. [CrossRef] [PubMed]
160. Middleton, P.; Shepherd, E.; Makrides, M. Omega-3 fatty acid addition during pregnancy. *Cochrane Database Syst. Rev.* **2018**, *15*, CD003402. [CrossRef] [PubMed]
161. Villar, J.; Abdel-Aleem, H.; Merialdi, M.; Mathai, M.; Ali, M.M.; Zavaleta, N.; Purwar, M.; Hofmeyr, J.; Thi Nhu Ngoc, N.; Campódonico, L.; et al. World Health Organization randomized trial of calcium supplementation among low calcium intake pregnant women. *Am. J. Obs. Gynecol.* **2006**, *194*, 639–649. [CrossRef] [PubMed]
162. Hofmeyr, G.J.; Lawrie, T.A.; Atallah, A.N.; Duley, L.; Torloni, M.R. Calcium supplementation during pregnancy for preventing hypertensive disorders and related problems. [Review][Update of Cochrane Database Syst. Rev. 2010;(8):CD001059; PMID: 20687064]. *Cochrane Database Syst. Rev.* **2014**, *6*, CD001059.
163. Colonese, F.; Laganà, A.S.; Colonese, E.; Sofo, V.; Salmeri, F.M.; Granese, R.; Triolo, O. The pleiotropic effects of vitamin D in gynaecological and obstetric diseases: An overview on a hot topic. *Biomed. Res. Int.* **2015**, *2015*, 986281. [CrossRef] [PubMed]
164. Laganà, A.S.; Vitale, S.G.; Ban Frangež, H.; Vrtačnik-Bokal, E.; D'Anna, R. Vitamin D in human reproduction: The more, the better? An evidence-based critical appraisal. *Eur. Rev. Med. Pharm. Sci.* **2017**, *21*, 4243–4251.
165. De-Regil, L.M.; Palacios, C.; Lombardo, L.K.; Peña-Rosas, J.P. Vitamin D supplementation for women during pregnancy. *Cochrane Database Syst. Rev.* **2016**. [CrossRef] [PubMed]

4

Supplementation of Plants with Immunomodulatory Properties during Pregnancy and Lactation—Maternal and Offspring Health Effects

Aneta Lewicka [1], Łukasz Szymański [2], Kamila Rusiecka [3], Anna Kucza [3], Anna Jakubczyk [4], Robert Zdanowski [3] and Sławomir Lewicki [3,*]

1 Laboratory of Epidemiology, Military Institute of Hygiene and Epidemiology, Kozielska 4, 01-163 Warsaw, Poland
2 Department of Microwave Safety, Military Institute of Hygiene and Epidemiology, Kozielska 4, 01-163 Warsaw, Poland
3 Department of Regenerative Medicine and Cell Biology, Military Institute of Hygiene and Epidemiology, Kozielska 4, 01-163 Warsaw, Poland
4 Department of Biochemistry and Food Chemistry, University of Life Sciences, Skromna 8, 20-704 Lublin, Poland
* Correspondence: slawomir.lewicki@wihe.pl

Abstract: A pregnant woman's diet consists of many products, such as fruits, vegetables, cocoa, tea, chocolate, coffee, herbal and fruit teas, and various commercially available dietary supplements, which contain a high number of biological active plant-derived compounds. Generally, these compounds play beneficial roles in women's health and the development of fetus health. There are, however, some authors who report that consuming excessive amounts of plants that contain high concentrations of polyphenols may negatively affect the development of the fetus and the offspring's health. Important and problematic issues during pregnancy and lactation are bacterial infections treatment. In the treatment are proposals to use plant immunomodulators, which are generally considered safe for women and their offspring. Additional consumption of biologically active compounds from plants, however, may increase the risk of occurrences to irreversible changes in the offspring's health. Therefore, it is necessary to carry out safety tests for immunomodulators before introducing them into a maternal diet. Here, we present data from animal experiments for the four most-studied plants immunomodulators genus: *Rhodiola*, *Echinacea*, *Panax*, and *Camellia*, which were used in maternal nutrition.

Keywords: immunomodulators; maternal nutrition; pregnancy; *Rhodiola*; *Echinacea*; *Panax*; *Camellia*

1. Introduction

The antibiotic treatments of bacterial infections during pregnancy and lactation are very problematic because of their negative effects on embryo and newborn development. The food and drug administration agency divided all known antibiotics into five groups (A, B, C, D, X) depending on the potential risk of harmful effects on the offspring. In general, only group A antibiotics are considered to be safe when used during pregnancy and lactation [1]. Prenatal exposure to the antibiotics from the remaining groups may modify the immunological system of the offspring. The offspring of mothers treated during pregnancy with the group B antibiotics, such as penicillin and cephalosporin, showed, after pathogen stimulation, a decrease of the specific immune response and increase of the nonspecific immune response [2]. Also, prenatal treatment with antibiotics increased the risk of childhood asthma and obesity [3].

The alternative therapy, which could potentially support or even replace antibiotic treatment, would be the use of plant-derived immunomodulators. Nowadays, there are more than 300 plants which exhibit beneficial properties for humans. Plant-derived compounds which affect the immune system belong to chemical groups of compounds such as: alkaloids (i.e., leonurine [4], piperine [5], and sophocarpine [6]), terpenoids (i.e., ginsan [7] or oleanolic acid [8]), polysaccharides (from licorice *Glycyrrhiza uralensis Fisch* [9], or from *Lentinus edodes* [10]), lactones (from *Datura quercifolia* [11] or sesquiterpene lactones from *Loranthus parasiticus*), and essential oils (Z-ligustilide [12] or Tetramethylpyra-zine [13]). However, the most well-known and numerous group of immune-affecting compounds belongs to flavonoids, which are divided into flavones, flavanones, flavanols, flavonols, catechins, isoflavones, and anthocyanins [14].

Some of the flavonoids, such as genistein or quercetin, are commonly-used supplements in human nutrition [15,16]. Plant-derived immunomodulators affect the immune system in various ways: [1] directly by affecting the immune cell functions in both adaptive and innate immunity [17] and by direct anti-microbial, anti-viral, or anti-fungal properties [18] o r [2] indirectly by modulation of non-immune cell function [19], reduction of inflammation [20], the influence of cytokines secretion [21], or modulation of angiogenesis [22].

Most importantly, plant-derived immunomodulators are generally considered as safe for humans and therefore are a good alternative for the use of most synthetic immunomodulators, which cause various side effects. This statement is mostly true for people in a normal state of life, however, for pregnant women and their offspring, this can become dangerous. Several researchers had shown that theobromine and cocoa catechins administered to pregnant mice affected embryonic angiogenesis and morphology and function of some of their progeny organs, among them the lymphoid system and kidneys [23–27]. Therefore, before the recommendation of supplementation of plant-derived immunomodulators in the maternal diet, experiments on animals should be performed. Here, we presented data from animal experiments for the four most-studied plants' immunomodulators genus, *Rhodiola*, *Echinacea*, *Panax*, and *Camellia*, which were used in maternal nutrition. The summarized effects of Rhodiola, *Echinacea*, Ginseng, and Camellia, or its extracts supplemented in pregnancy and/or lactation on mothers and offspring health, are presented in Table 1.

Table 1. Summarized effects of *Rhodiola*, *Echinacea*, Ginseng, and Camellia, or its extracts, supplemented in pregnancy and/or lactation on mothers and offspring health.

Herb or Extract	Key Substances	Pharmacological Action	
		Mother	Offspring
Rhodiola	phenylethanoid salidroside and tyrosol, phenolic acids (i.e., chlorogenic, ferulic, ellagic and p-coumaric), and flavonoids (i.e., fisetin, naringenin, kaempferol, epicatechin, luteolin, quercetin, epigallocatechin and (+)-catechin)	reduces the percentage of cells with a respiratory burst in granulocytes (supplementation with RKW) [28] increases in the percentage of granulocytes and monocytes in the blood with the respiratory burst (supplementation with RKW-A) [28] contributes to changes in spleen morphology and structure [29] increases the concentration of VEGF and bFGF [30] reduces the number of CD4 + and CD19 + cells and the total number of NK cells [31]	increases hemoglobin concentration (about 0.6 mg/dL) [32] decreases in the mean percentage of lymphocytes in peripheral blood, and an increase in the mean percentage of granulocytes [32] decreases in the percentage of CD3+ cells and CD4+ [32] increases the concentration of IL-10 in the serum [33] stimulate the phagocytosis process [32] significant difference in tissue localization and the number of CD8+ cells [34] contributes to a higher number of CD8+ cells in the central part of the spleen [34] influence cell proliferation in response to mitogen supplementation (LPS, PHA and ConA) [29] decreases the number of apoptotic cells [35] decreases the concentration of VEGF in the sera [30]
Echinacea	alkamides, ketoalkenes, caffeic acid derivatives, polysaccharides, glycoproteins, and caftaric acid	does not affect hematological and reproductive parameters [36] no influences on the enzyme results [37] decreases the level of crude protein in colostrum [37] decreases the level of antibodies in the plasma [37] decreases the number of spleen lymphocytes and nucleated erythroid cells [38] contributes to more frequent miscarriages in the early stages of pregnancy [38]	decreases the number of embryos in litter and significantly diminished VEGF and bFGF content of embryos tissue [39] increases phagocytic activity in blood [40] increases bacterial diversity [40] non-teratogenic, does not increase the risk of malformations [41–43]
Ginseng	polysaccharides, flavonoids, fatty acids, peptides, and saponins (mainly ginsenosides)	increases the total IgG concentration in milk and serum of sows, which was associated with elevated levels of cytokines: IL-2, IL-6, TNF- α, and IFN-γ [44] stimulates the effect of isolated lymphocytes after pokeweed mitogen stimulation [45] stimulates the innate immunity in cows with *Staphylococcus aureus* infection [46] increases phagocytosis, oxidative burst activity of blood neutrophils and number of monocytes [46]	increases IL-2 and TNF-α concentration in the piglets' serum [44] reduces the incidence of schizophrenia in the offspring [47] alleviates the toxic effects of phthalates and bisphenol A [48] reverses the negative effect of dexamethasone on the synthesis of testosterone in Leydig cells [49] teratogenic effect [50]

Table 1. *Cont.*

Herb or Extract	Key Substances	Pharmacological Action	
		Mother	Offspring
Camellia	epigallocatechin, epicatechin, epicatechin gallate	increases the ratio of IL-10/TNF-α and IL-1β in mesenteric adipose tissue and causes a decrease in catalase in the liver [51] inhibits the penetration of macrophages and increases the expression of AMPK (during lactation) [52] contributes to alterations in urinary calcium, creatinine, and urea during the prenatal period, nephrotoxicity [53] increases levels of proinflammatory cytokines and decreases anti-inflammatory cytokines levels in serum [53] decreases of hemoglobin concentration and loss of the biconcave structure of erythrocytes [54] increases of WBC level in the mother's blood and induced significant changes in the histology of liver and serum enzymes [54] decreases the level of folic acid [55] increases the efficacy of oral nifedipine treatment in severe pregnancy-induced preeclampsia [56] may be associated with an increased risk of pre-eclampsia [57]	increases the risk of premature birth [58] risk factor for low birth weight of offspring [59] protect against dyslipidemia, glucose intolerance, and fat accumulation [60] pro-inflammatory effect on the adipose tissue (not on a high-fat diet) [60] decreases the retroperitoneal adipose tissue relative weight and SOD activity but increases adiponectin, LPS, IL-10 and IL-6 content and IL-10/TNF-α ratio in retroperitoneal, IL-10 and TNF-α content in gonadal, and IL-6 content in mesenteric adipose tissues [51] improves the results of treatment of maternal gestational diabetes [61] reduces neonatal complications [61] can decreases the number of malformations in fetuses after exposure to cyclophosphamide, but too high dose increases the toxicity of cyclophosphamide [62]

2. Rhodiola

2.1. Characteristic and Immunomodulatory Properties

Genus *Rhodiola* (family *Crassulaceae*) consists of 200 species, out of which over 20 species have medicinal properties. *Rhodiola* extracts contain phenylethanoid salidroside and tyrosol, phenolic acids (i.e., chlorogenic, ferulic, ellagic, and p-coumaric), and flavonoids (i.e., fisetin, naringenin, kaempferol, epicatechin, luteolin, quercetin, epigallocatechin, and (+)-catechin) [63–65]. They have been used in traditional Asian and European medicine such as tonics, adaptogens, antidepressants, and anti-inflammatory compounds [66]. The extracts from these plants also have anticancer, antibacterial, and immunomodulatory properties [67–70]. *Rhodiola* extracts, given for seven days to mice infected with *Pseudomonas aeruginosa*, decrease the infection. These mice have a higher number and higher metabolic activity of blood leukocytes [71]. *Rhodiola* extracts also have a direct antiviral and antibacterial effect against hepatitis C virus (HCV) and *Mycobacterium tuberculosis* [72,73]. At present, there are several clinical therapies available, which use *Rhodiola* plants to stimulate the immune system [74]. One of the well-characterized plant species from the *Rhodiola* genus which was supplemented in pregnancy and lactation is *Rhodiola kirilowii*, which was supplemented as lyophilized water extract (RKW) or 50% hydro-alcoholic extract (RKW-A) in the pregnancy and lactation period in mice (about 42 days of supplementation).

2.2. Effects on Mothers

Supplementation of mice during pregnancy and lactation with water extract (RKW) or 50% hydro-alcoholic extract (RKW-A) of *Rhodiola kirilowii* (concentration 20 mg extract/kg body weight) had no effect on the average body weight as compared to the control group (receiving sterile water). There were no differences in the mean weight and mass index of selected organs: liver, kidneys, spleen, brain, and eyeballs, between the study groups. Macroscopic assessment of organs also did not reveal any changes in their structure. The morphological elements of blood: WBC (number of white blood cells/mm^3), RBC (number of red blood cells/mm^3), HGB (hemoglobin, g/dL), HCT (hematocrit, %), MCH (mean corpuscular hemoglobin, pg), MCHC (mean hemoglobin concentration, g/dL), RDW (red blood cell distribution width, %), PLT (platelet count /mm^3), and MPV (mean platelet volume, fL), did not differ between the control group and the groups receiving extracts from *Rhodiola kirilowii*. There were no differences in the population of cells belonging to the adaptive immunity system, T cells (CD3+, CD4+, CD8+) and B cells (CD19+), in the blood. However, some small changes in the composition and functioning of innate immunity cells were noticed. Mice fed with RKW extracts showed a lower percentage of cells with a respiratory burst in granulocytes (PhagoBurst test) [28]. In contrast, supplementation with RKW-A extract caused an increase in the percentage of granulocytes and monocytes in the blood with the respiratory burst. Other components of non-specific immunity have not changed (including the number and percentage of NK (natural killer) cells and the percentage of phagocytic cells). There were no changes in the concentration of selected cytokines in the serum: Th1 (IL-2, TNF-α, INF-γ), Th2 (IL-4, IL-6, IL-10), and Th17 (IL-17a) [30].

Despite the lack of differences in the weight and mass index of the spleen in mothers fed with *Rhodiola kirilowii* extracts, significant changes in spleen morphology and structure were observed. Spleens from mothers fed during pregnancy and the lactation water or hydroalcoholic extracts from *Rhodiola kirilowii* contained a significantly lower number of cells per gram of organ [29]. In the cytometric study, a significant reduction in the percentage of lymphocytes was associated with an increase in the percentage of monocytes and granulocytes in the spleen only in the group receiving a 50% hydro-alcoholic extract of *Rhodiola kirilowii*. However, no significant changes in the percentage of the innate (CD335+) and adaptive (CD3+, CD4+, CD8+, CD19+) cell populations between the study groups were observed. Analysis of the total number of cell populations per gram of organ showed no difference in the number of CD3+ and CD8+ cells between groups. However, we found that both extracts reduced the number of CD4+ and CD19+ cells. In addition, water extract significantly reduced the total number of NK cells (CD335+) [31]. The observed changes in the number of cells in the spleen suggest that treatment caused a certain degree of impairment of the adaptive immune response. Therefore, we decided to examine the spleen cells' (mainly T and B cells) proliferation response to mitogens stimulations (ex vivo studies). We found that there were no significant differences in the proliferative activity of splenocytes stimulated with lipopolysaccharide (LPS), phytohemagglutinin (PHA), or concanavalin A (ConA). This means that the functionality of these cells, despite the lower number in the spleen, has been preserved. However, the observed, unfavorable reduction in the number of splenocytes is a disturbing sign, which should be taken into account in the long-term administration of extracts from *Rhodiola kirilowii* to pregnant women [29,30].

The RKW-A group had a higher concentration of VEGF (vascular endothelial growth factor) and bFGF (basic fibroblast growth factor) than the control group. These trends were associated with decreased proliferation of endothelial cells (HECa10) after the supplementation of medium with the serum isolated from mothers fed during pregnancy and lactation with (RKW-A). However, the RKW group showed increased migration of HECa10 cells [30]. The obtained results led to the conclusion that supplementation of hydro-alcoholic extracts of *Rhodiola kirilowii* may cause modulation of angiogenesis processes in developing fetuses. A similar effect was observed in previous studies in which RKW-A extract inhibited tumor angiogenesis and the RKW had no effect [63].

In conclusion, slight changes in adaptive immunity (blood) and in the number of splenocytes with a lack of side effects on the range of morphological blood parameters of mother mice should be considered as a positive effect of supplementation, with such a long period of use. Usually, plant-derived immunomodulatory drugs are used for no more than 2–3 weeks. This is due to the fact that prolonged administration of immunostimulants may cause lack of stimulation, and in extreme situations, deregulations of the immune system, as with what was seen in aquaculture [75]. Authors suggested that for successful use of immunostimulators, not only appropriate timing of administration, but also dosage and period of administration are necessary.

2.3. *Effects on Offspring*

The animal mass analysis did not show a significant difference between the offspring from the control group and the group supplemented with water extract of *Rhodiola kirilowii*. The mean weight of offspring whose mothers were fed with 50% hydro-alcoholic extract was about 7% lower than in the control group ($p < 0.01$). There were no significant differences in peripheral blood morphometric parameters (WBC, RBC, HCT, MCH, MCHC, RDW, RDW-a, PLT, and MPV) between the control group and the groups receiving *Rhodiola kirilowii* extracts. There was a slight, but significant, increase in hemoglobin concentration (about 0.6 mg/dL) in the group supplemented with *Rhodiola kirilowii* water extract [32].

The analysis of selected components of the adaptive and innate immune system in the blood and spleens of offspring, whose mothers were fed during pregnancy and lactation extracts from *Rhodiola kirilowii*, showed significant differences. A significant decrease in the mean percentage of lymphocytes (approximately 6%, $p < 0.05$) in peripheral blood and an increase in the mean percentage of granulocytes (approximately 20%, $p < 0.05$) were observed in the RKW group (a similar trend was observed in the RKW-A group, however, it was not statistically significant). The analysis of the lymphocyte population showed a significant decrease in the percentage of CD3+ cells (RKW-14%, $p = 0.0434$, RKW-A-10%, $p = 0.0337$) and CD4+ (15%, $p = 0.0184$ and 13%, $p = 0.0116$, respectively). In addition, a lower percentage of CD8+ cells and a higher percentage of NK cells (CD335+) were observed in the RKW group. There were no changes in the percentage of B cells (CD19+) and the percentage of regulatory T cells (CD4+, CD25+, FoxP3+) and CD4+, CD25+ cells between the examined groups [32].

A significant decrease in the percentage of CD4+ in the peripheral blood may indicate a certain impairment of adaptive immunity, which may lead to the disorders in the stimulation of CD19+ cells and the production of specific antibodies. In part, these results were confirmed in the SRBC (sheep red blood cells) test (immunization of mice with sheep red blood cells), in which much lower levels of anti-SRBC antibodies were observed in the serum of mice whose mothers were fed during pregnancy and lactation with RKW-A [33]. The explanation of the lower immune response after RKW-A supplementation may also be associated with an increased concentration of IL-10 in the serum. This cytokine has anti-inflammatory activity and inhibits the synthesis of other pro-inflammatory cytokines that are necessary to activate the immune system in response to antigens. No such changes were observed for water extract (RKW) [33].

Both extracts of *Rhodiola kirilowii* consumed during pregnancy and lactation by mothers stimulated the phagocytosis process in their offspring. There was an increase in the phagocytosis of opsonized *E. coli* bacteria and the intensity of the oxygen burst after stimulation with *E. coli* and zymosan [32]. Interestingly, in the RKW group, there was a significant reduction in serum IL-17a concentration [33]. IL-17a is a cytokine responsible inter alia for supporting phagocytosis of extracellular bacteria. It seems that the observed situation may be related to the activation of granulocytes by polyphenolic compounds present in the extracts, which in turn leads to a reduction of IL-17a secretion (immune system is not "over-activated"). The lack of additional stimulation by IL-17a could also lead to a decrease in the population of phagocytic monocytes and oxygen burst after zymosan stimulation in the RKW group [33].

Spleens of mice fed with *Rhodiola kirilowii* extracts did not differ in mass and mass index (spleen weight/mouse weight) and cellularity compared to the spleens obtained from the control group. There were no significant differences in the morphology of the spleens. In the cytometric study of spleen cells, no significant differences in the percentage of CD3+, CD4+, CD8+, CD19+, and CD335+ cells were noticed [32]. Histological analysis showed no significant difference in the number and location of CD4+ cells, but a significant difference in tissue localization and the number of CD8+ cells. These cells were found not only in usual locations within the spleen but also in the perivascular lymphatic sheath (PALS), the follicular zone of B cells, and in the red pulp. In addition, there was a much higher number of CD8+ cells in the central part of the spleen [34]. This may indicate increased mobility of these cells and thus increased ability to respond to antiviral responses. Supplementation of mothers with extracts from *Rhodiola kirilowii* during pregnancy and lactation also influenced cell proliferation in response to mitogen supplementation: lipopolysaccharide (LPS), phytohaemagglutinin (PHA), and concanavalin A (ConA). A decrease in cell proliferation rate was observed in the RKW-A group after the supplementation of LPS and PHA when compared to the control group. There was a reduction of proliferation rate in the RKW-A group after stimulation with ConA when compared to the RKW group [32]. The presented data indicated attenuation of the ability of adaptive immunity in the hydro-alcoholic *Rhodiola kirilowii* group.

Changes in the percentage of blood cells associated with adaptive immune response (mainly CD3+) suggested a possible negative effect on the maturation of these cells in the thymus in the offspring. The mean thymus weight and the thymic index did not differ between the groups. There were no significant differences in the morphology of the thymus between groups. There were also no abnormalities in the structure of lobules, medulla, cortex ratio, and epithelial cell content. No thymic hypertrophy or atrophy was detected. The offspring of mice whose mothers were fed during pregnancy and lactation RKW and RKW-A extracts had a significantly lower number of apoptotic cells (marker M30) than the control group. However, there was no significant difference in the number of cells synthesizing IL-7 [35]. The obtained data led to the conclusion that extracts from *Rhodiola kirilowii* prolonged the function of thymus cells in the offspring, which may be important for overcoming the infection.

Moreover, Lewicki et al. (2017) [76] found that there were no significant differences in the mass index and macroscopic structure of the kidneys between the examined groups. A higher percentage of individuals with serum creatinine above 0.65 mg % was found in the RKW and RKW-A groups. In addition, the offspring of mothers from RKW-A group had slightly increased urea concentration and decreased cystatin C concentration. These data suggested some abnormalities in the kidneys.

In the RKW-A group, a higher number of tufts per mm^2 was observed and their smaller diameter may indicate their atrophy. These changes may have been caused directly by the active substances in the extracts from *Rhodiola kirilowii* present in the maternal sera, and/or indirectly by affecting the secretion of proangiogenic factors. The differences were observed in the concentration of polyphenols in mice-mothers supplemented with RKW or RKW-A (mainly catechin and salidroside), a lower concentration of VEGF in the sera of the offspring from the RKW-A group [30]. These data indicate that hydro-alcoholic extract should not be long-term supplemented to pregnant women.

3. Echinacea

3.1. Characteristic and Immunomodulatory Properties

Echinacea is a plant belonging to the species from the *Asteraceae* family [77]. There are three species of *Echinacea* with medicinal properties, including *Echinacea purpurea*, *Echinacea pallida*, and *Echinacea angustifolia* [78]. *Echinacea* extracts contained alkamides, ketoalkenes, caffeic acid derivatives, polysaccharides, glycoproteins, and caftaric acid, which are responsible for the medical activity of the plant.

Echinacea-based drugs contribute to a shortening of the various types of infections and colds [79,80]. This is due to the active ingredients such as polysaccharides, alkaloids, coffee acid derivatives [81], and proteoglycans that have immunomodulatory, antiviral, antioxidant, and anti-inflammatory properties [78]. Polysaccharides, especially arabinogalactans, activate macrophages and have a cytotoxic effect against cancer cells [82,83]. During this process, various biological products are formed [84], including nitric oxide, which has a defensive function in the immune system [85]. Bacterial infections contribute to the formation of the inflammatory mediators, which in turn leads to the increase of the nitric oxide levels [86]. This compound is very harmful to healthy cells [87,88]. Studies have shown that the alcohol extracts of the *Echinacea purpurea*, *Echinacea pallida*, and *Echinacea angustifolia* significantly reduce the production of nitric oxide [86]. The extract also increased the number of non-activated macrophage cells that are the first to defend the body against infections [86]. The active ingredients present in *Echinacea* also show antioxidant activity [89–92]. Such components include the alkamids that have an antioxidant effect on the coffee acid derivatives [92].

3.2. Effects on Mothers

Dabboul et al. (2016) conducted a study to check the reproductive and immune parameters of pregnant rabbits during *Echinacea pallida* diet supplementation [36]. The studies were performed on 100 pregnant rabbits at the age of 21 weeks and supplemented with 3 g/day of *Echinacea pallida* for 4 weeks. The tests were carried out on days 0, 14, and 28 of the experiment. The effect of this plant on blood morphology parameters of mothers: red blood cells (n/mm^3), hemoglobin (g/dL), hematocrit (%), mean corpuscular volume (fL), mean corpuscular hemoglobin (pg), mean hemoglobin concentration (g/dL), red blood cell distribution width (%), platelet count (n/mm^3), mean thrombocyte volume (PCT,%), mean platelet volume (fL), platelet distribution width (%), number of white blood cells (n/mm3), lymphocytes (%), monocytes (%), neutrophils (%), eosinophils (%), and basophils (%) has not been observed.

The concentration of total protein (g/dL), glutamic oxoloacetic transaminase (UI/L), blood urea nitrogen (mg/dL), albumin (g/dL), urea (mg/dL), and cholesterol (mg/dL) were also analyzed. The serum protein was determined using semi-automatic agarose gel electrophoresis. Blood and immune parameters were determined in three periods (day 0, day 14, and day 28) and were subjected to statistical analysis using the GLM thematic model. In the case of reproductive parameters, the analysis was carried out for the specific *Echinacea* test and the control sample using the Student's *t*-test. The results of the study showed that *Echinacea* supplementation does not affect hematological and reproductive parameters. Also, in the case of immune parameters, there were no significant differences between the test and control groups.

In another study carried out by Maass et al. (2005), dried *Echinacea purpurea* was introduced in the diet of sows and its effect on the results of plasma enzymes, blood, lymphocyte proliferation, antibodies, and immunoglobulin content in colostrum were checked [37]. The experiments were carried out with the use of various concentrations of *Echinacea* in the diet during different periods of pregnancy and lactation. The period of *Echinacea* supplementation from days 85–110 of pregnancy and in the 4th, 6th, and 9th week of lactation was considered. The study was carried out on 36 sows from the 85th day of pregnancy to the 28th day of lactation. Animals were divided into three experimental groups by weight. The diet during pregnancy and lactation was supplemented by 0%, 1.2%, or 3.6% and 0%, 0.5%, or 1.5% *Echinacea*. Due to the lack of data for pigs, the dose of *Echinacea* was given based on human recommendations (16.5 mg of freshly squeezed juice/kg). Blood analysis was performed on day 85 of pregnancy as well as on day 1 and 28 of lactation. The colostrum was collected manually from 1 to 6 hours after delivery.

Body mass, body temperature, health status, crude protein (6.37 *Kjeldahl-N), immunoglobulins, hematological, and clinic–chemical parameters (alkaline phosphatase, alanine, and aspartate, and gamma-glutamyltransferase aminotransferase) were analyzed using acquired samples. No influence of *Echinacea* on the enzyme results (alkaline phosphatase (U/L), alanine aminotransferase (U/L), aspartate aminotransferase (U/L), gamma-glutamyl transferase (U/L)) was observed. The level of crude protein in colostrum was lower in the *Echinacea* supplemented group. There was no statistical difference in the levels of leukocytes (10^9/L), erythrocytes (10^{12}/L), lymphocytes (%), granulocytes, neutrophils (%), eosinophils (%), basophils (%), or monocytes (%) between the study (*Echinacea* supplemented) and control group. Also, similar results were obtained in a group of breeding pigs. The experiment included two phases of *Echinacea* supplementation (1–3 weeks and 7–9 weeks) and an intermediate phase without supplementation (4–6 weeks). The experiment aimed to investigate the immune effect and the production of antibodies during vaccination of pigs. A differential vaccine was given, which was administered at week 1 and week 5 of the experiment. IgG1 immunoglobulin in colostrum was determined using ELISA technique. From the obtained data, such as the hematological analysis and the varied number of blood cells, supplementation had no effect. The level of antibodies in the plasma showed a significant effect of *Echinacea* in relation to all antibodies, which caused a significantly higher immune response in the control group. The health of the animals was also good.

Chow et al. (2006) focused on studying the effects of *Echinacea* on immunity and spontaneous miscarriages. The study was conducted in mice in which *Echinacea* was fed from the beginning to the 10th, 11th, 12th, 13th, and 14th days of pregnancy [38]. The mother's spleen and bone marrow were collected for examination. The effect of *Echinacea* on hematopoietic cells in the spleen and bone marrow was determined using the Student's *t*-test. The significant differences were found in the results obtained from the immune system analysis in the third trimester in the spleen of pregnant mice. The parameters and number of spleen lymphocytes and nucleated erythroid cells were decreased in *Echinacea*-fed mice. The bone marrow parameters were not influenced by the *Echinacea* supplementation. The results also indicated that miscarriages are more likely to happen in the early stages of pregnancy (10–11 days) in the *Echinacea*-fed mice. Based on these results, it was decided not to suggest the consumption of *Echinacea* in the early stages of pregnancy in women. On the other hand, the results of clinical trials conducted by Heitman et al. (2016) did not show adverse effects of *Echinacea* supplementation of mothers during pregnancy [41].

3.3. *Effects on Offspring*

Despite the large number of papers which confirmed the immunomodulatory effect of *Echinacea* spp. and a lot of products on the market containing *Echinacea*, there is still a little evidence of offspring safety after uses of the herb in pregnancy and lactation. In 2007, Barcz et al. investigated the effect of alcoholic extracts of *Echinacea* purpurea given to pregnant mice on angiogenic activity and tissue VEGF and bFGF production of their fetuses. Eight pregnant females, from the 1st to the 18th day of pregnancy, were given a 0.06 g solution of *Echinacea* purpurea from different formulations (three mothers were given Esberitox, another three were Echinapur, while two mothers were fed Immunalforte). On day 18, the females were sacrificed, and the fetuses were used for the angiogenesis test. It was found that two *Echinacea* drugs lowered the number of embryos in litter and significantly diminished the vascular endothelial growth factor (VEGF) and the basic fibroblast growth factor (bFGF) content of embryos tissue [39]. The effect of mothers' supplementation in pregnancy and lactation of *Echinacea pallida* on the health of their offspring was also studied by Kovitvadhi et al. (2016) [40]. The authors supplemented sows with *Echinacea* from days 85–110 of pregnancy and in the 4th, 6th, and 9th week of lactation. Offspring from those mothers exhibited an increased phagocytic in blood activity and a higher bacterial diversity compared to other groups. There was no statistically significant difference in animal growth, blood parameters, and humoral immune response against vaccination or against the rabbit hemorrhagic disease virus.

The data from the human studies revealed no effect of *Echinacea* treatment in pregnancy and lactation in mothers on the health of their offspring. The Gallo et al. (2000) study also showed no effect of consuming *Echinacea* during pregnancy on the increased risk of malformations [42]. Also, Perri et al. (2006), in a prospective cohort study, concluded that *Echinacea* is non-teratogenic when used during pregnancy and lactation. The conclusions were based on a lack of evidence that maternal *Echinacea* consumption varied affected major or minor birth defects, differences in pregnancy outcome, delivery method, maternal weight gain, gestational age, infant birth weight, or fetal distress. It should be noted that daily dosage was varied, however, *Echinacea* supplementation was usually used by mothers for up to 7 days [43]. In a cohort study, Heitmann et al. (2016) evaluated the impact of prenatal exposure to *Echinacea* and the consequences of its use on malformations and adverse pregnancy outcomes. Based on the analysis of questionnaires completed by pregnant women at 17 and 30 weeks of pregnancy, 6 months after birth, and information on pregnancy results from the Norwegian birth register, there was no increased risk of malformations or adverse delivery results, such as premature delivery [41].

4. Ginseng

4.1. Characteristic and Immunomodulatory Properties

Ginseng belongs to angiosperms, the *Araliaceae* family, *Panax L.* genus. There are thirteen ginseng species, the most popular of which are *Panax ginseng* C.A. Meyer, *Panax quinquefolium* L., *Panax japonicus* C.A. Meyer. For thousands of years, it has been used in East Asia as a medicinal plant due to the active substances found in the root. These are polysaccharides, flavonoids, fatty acids, peptides, and saponins [93].

The main active substances in the ginseng root are ginsenosides. These are chemical compounds that belong to saponins. Due to the structure, there are three main groups: the protopanaxadiol group, the oleanane group, and the protopanaxatriol group [94]. Ginsenosides have been shown to have anti-inflammatory properties, mainly by inhibiting the production of TNF-α in a mouse macrophage cell line RAW264.7, that was exposed to lipopolysaccharide stimulation [95]. Lee et al. (2005) showed that 20-*O*-beta-D-glucopyranosyl-20 (*S*)-protopanaxadiol inhibits TPA-induced expression of COX-2, which in turn may contribute to antitumor activity [96]. Also, Ginsenoside-Re can inhibit the interaction between LPS and TLR4 (toll-like receptor 4) [97]. Other important active substances of ginseng root are polyphenols and polysaccharides [98]. Byeon et al. (2012) have shown that ginseng derived polysaccharides can be used as an immunostimulant via TLR2 (toll-like receptor 2), which mediates the activation of macrophages [99]. Also, TLR2 mediated functional activation of macrophages can be boosted by wortmannin-targeted enzymes. Ginseng polysaccharides also have immunomodulatory, anticancer, and antidiabetic effects [100].

4.2. General Effect of Ginseng

For thousands of years, ginseng root has been used as an immuno-stimulating plant. With the development of science, further properties and mechanisms of ginseng's actions have been discovered.

The administration of the ginseng extract has a positive effect on the spinal cord injury and thus has a neuroprotective effect [101]. However, it has been proven that the use of ginseng extract during pregnancy may have a teratogenic effect. According to research by Khalid et al. (2008), a high dose of the extract may also lead to the development of bone defects [102].

The literature describes many mechanisms of action of ginseng on the immune system. Kim et al. (2009) found that ginsan, ginseng-derived polysaccharide, has immunomodulatory effects on dendritic cells. They showed that ginsan stimulates dendritic cells by inducing their maturation. Ginsan stimulates secretion of cytokines from dendritic cells, increases the proliferation of allogeneic CD4 + lymphocytes, and enhances the expression of CD86 on the surface of dendritic cells [103]. Shin et al. (2002) have shown that ginseng acidic polysaccharides enhance the phagocytic activity of macrophages, stimulates cytokine secretion, and leads to the increased CD14 expression [104]. It has also been proven that ginseng increases the activity of NK cells [105]. Ginseng has been shown to protect mice against sepsis caused by *Staphylococcus aureus* by decreasing the secretion of inflammatory cytokines TNF-α, IL-1β, IL-6, IFN-γ, IL-12, and IL-18 [106]. Chan et al. (2011) focused on bird flu H9N2. They showed that ginsenosides (protopanaxatriol and ginsenoside Re) have protective properties against the H9N2 virus. Protopanaxatriol reduced the expression of IP10 (interferon gamma-induced protein 10), while the second ginsenoside reduces the DNA damage caused by the virus (H9N2-induced inflammation and apoptosis) [107].

4.3. *Effects on Mothers*

The effects of substances derived from ginseng on pregnant women are not yet fully understood. Xi et al. (2017) investigated the effect of supplementation of polysaccharides derived from ginseng root in a pregnant sow. The extract was given to sows from the 90th day of pregnancy to the 28th day after the birth of the progeny. There was no effect of ginseng supplementation on the total number of piglets, live piglets, weak piglets, and birth weight of piglets, which means that the herb had not affected the reproduction process. Moreover, ginseng treatment in pregnancy and lactation caused a significant increase in the total immunoglobulin G concentration in milk and serum of sows, which was associated with elevated levels of cytokines: IL-2, IL-6, TNF-α, and IFN-γ [44]. Taken together, the results present evidence that ginseng supplemented in pregnancy and lactation modulates the adaptive immunity of mothers.

Also, the positive effect of ginseng supplementation on the function immune system was reported by Concha et al. (1996). Authors investigated ginseng immunomodulatory effects isolated from peripheral blood or milk lymphocyte in an in vitro study. They showed that ginseng has a stimulating effect on both groups of isolated lymphocytes after pokeweed mitogen stimulation [45]. The same scholars have shown, a few years later, that subcutaneous injections of extract from the root of panax ginseng CA Meyer at a dose of 8 mg/kg body weight per day for 6 days can stimulate the innate immunity in cows with staphylococcus aureus infection. In ginseng-treated groups, the numbers of S. aureus-infected quarters and milk somatic cell counts tended to decrease. Moreover, the phagocytosis and oxidative burst activity of blood neutrophils isolated from cows treated with ginseng were significantly increased one week after injection, as well as the number of monocytes in blood [46]. These findings suggested that not only adaptive, but also innate immunity, may be affected after ginseng treatment in pregnant and lactating mothers.

4.4. *Effects on Offspring*

The supplementation of ginseng extract in the sow's diet may have a beneficial effect on the development of immunity in newborns [44]. This is not only associated with passive immunity delivered to infants by milk (the higher ability of the mother's immune system for the elimination of pathogens) but also with modulation in an immune response in newborns. Maternal supplementation of ginseng significantly increased IL-2 (an important part of organism response to microbial infection) and TNF-α (phagocytosis stimulant) concentration in the piglets' serum.

Ginseng supplementation in pregnancy or the lactation period also plays a protective role against some negative factors. Administration of ginseng extract during pregnancy exposed to prenatal stress reduces the incidence of schizophrenia in the offspring [47]. According to the studies of Saadeldin et al. (2018), administration of an aqueous ginseng extract to pregnant females during exposure to phthalates and bisphenol A alleviates the toxic effects of these compounds in offspring [48]. Wanderly et al. (2013) studied if giving pregnant rats a ginseng extract could reverse the increase in testosterone production induced by dexamethasone. The extract was administered to females from 10 to 20 days of pregnancy by gavage, while dexamethasone was administered by injections from the 14th day to the 21st day of pregnancy. Adult male offspring were sacrificed, and blood, testis, and prostate were removed for further ex vivo examinations and morphological analysis. Plasma was obtained from the blood and the testosterone concentration was tested. The study showed that the ginseng extract is able to reverse the negative effect of dexamethasone on the synthesis of testosterone in Leydig cells [49].

The use of ginseng in pregnancy, however, has some limitations. The study by Belanger et al. (2016) showed that ginseng extracts have a negative effect on pregnancy in mice. Also, in vitro direct exposure to the ginseng extract reduced development in a concentration responsive manner [50].

5. Camellia

5.1. *Characteristic and Immunomodulatory Properties*

Camellia sinensis (black tea) [108] and *Camellia sinensis, Theaceae* (green tea) [109] are two of the most popular botanical plants. They are cultivated in over 30 countries, especially in tropical areas [53]. Infusions from tea are consumed in different countries, but its consumption is most popular in East Asia [110]. The main active ingredients of tea are polyphenols, more specifically catechins: epigallocatechin, epicatechin, and epicatechin gallate [111–113], which are characterized by antioxidant properties [112,114]. The most biologically active catechins are epigalocatechingallate [108].

Green tea can modulate macrophages and dendritic cells [115,116], as well as immunomodulatory properties of the immune system [117]. Tea can stimulate immunity by stimulating the secretion of antibodies [118,119]. It also acts as an antioxidant and has anticancer activity [120]. Black tea has a positive effect on the cardiovascular system [121]. Due to the limited data regarding the impact of tea consumption on pregnancy, caution is recommended [122]. High concentrations of black tea extract may be toxic during pregnancy [123].

5.2. *Effects on Mothers*

Losinskas-Hachul et al. (2018) [51] investigated the effect of green tea intake (400 mg/kg of body weight/day) by rat-mothers from the first day of pregnancy until the end of lactation on maternal and offspring metabolism. They showed that the intake of the extract by the mother increases the ratio of IL-10/TNF-α and IL-1β in mesenteric adipose tissue and causes a decrease in catalase activity in the liver. It has been proven that the intake of green tea extract during the lactation period inhibits the penetration of macrophages and increases the expression of AMPK (5′AMP-activated protein kinase), which affects the secretion of insulin [52]. A high dose of black tea extract (100 mg/kg of body weight/day) may contribute to changes in blood and kidneys of pregnant rats. The study by Dey et al. (2017) showed significant alterations in urinary calcium, creatinine, and urea during the prenatal period, while exhibited proteinuria, ketonuria, and histology showed nephrotoxicity during the postnatal period. The herb also affected concentrations of proinflammatory cytokines and decreased anti-inflammatory cytokines compared to the control group [53]. Moreover, the supplementation of black tea extract causes a decrease of hemoglobin concentration and loss of the biconcave structure of erythrocytes. It was also shown that the extract from black tea increases WBC levels in the mother′s blood and induced significant changes in the histology of liver and serum enzymes [54].

Kayiran et al. (2013) examined whether black tea consumed during pregnancy affects the oxidative/antioxidant status of breast milk. The mother′s milk was analyzed for lipid peroxidation based on malondialdehyde (MDA) levels and reduced glutathione levels (GSH). The study did not show a correlation between the amount of tea consumed and the level of MDA and GSH, which suggests that breast milk is insensitive to the antioxidants present in tea [124].

Deficiency of folic acid increases the risk of neural tube defects in the prenatal period. It has been shown that the levels of folic acid in serum is much lower in pregnant women who consumed more caffeine and tannins (in the form of coffee and oolong tea). According to Otake et al. (2018), pregnant women should minimize the consumption of drinks containing caffeine [55].

Epigallocatechin gallate (EGCG), a natural compound of green tea, has been shown to increase the efficacy of oral nifedipine treatment in severe pregnancy-induced preeclampsia [56]. On the other hand, excessive drinking tea during pregnancy may be associated with an increased risk of pre-eclampsia. Tea components affect this risk through a number of likely mechanisms, for example, as pathways associated with the modulation of angiogenic factors or with oxidative stress [57].

In the Jochum et al. (2017) study, pregnant women were given 300 ml of black tea and the content of flavonoids in milk was evaluated. It was shown that flavonoids (catechin, epicatechin) cannot be detected in milk samples, and the consumption of tea alone did not affect the total antioxidant capacity of breast milk [125].

5.3. *Effects on Offspring*

It has been shown that the consumption of green tea extract in pregnancy affects offspring's health. The consumption of Japanese and Chinese tea during pregnancy is also associated with an increased risk of premature birth [58]. Yang et al. (2018) showed that drinking tea during pregnancy is a risk factor for low birth weight of offspring [59]. Camelia supplementation of mothers in the pregnancy or lactation period exhibits also health benefits. According to the research by Hachul et al. (2018), the mother's intake of green tea extract exerts a protective action on the progeny that is on a high-fat diet. The extract protects against dyslipidemia, glucose intolerance, and fat accumulation. However, the mother's intake of this extract has a pro-inflammatory effect on the adipose tissue of progeny that is not on a high-fat diet [60]. Also, Losinskas-Hachul et al. (2018) [51] observed this relationship in their rat study. The pump that fed rats the green tea extract was shown to decrease the retroperitoneal adipose tissue relative weight and SOD activity, but increased adiponectin, LPS, IL-10, IL-6 contentl and IL-10/TNF-α ratio in retroperitoneal, IL-10, and TNF-α content in gonadal, and IL-6 content in mesenteric adipose tissues. These changes indicated that the consumption of green tea extracts altered the inflammatory status of 28 day old offspring. Moreover, epigallocatechin 3-gallate supplementation improved the results of treatment of maternal and maternal gestational diabetes. It affects the reduction of neonatal complications, i.e., low birth weight and hypoglycemia, and alleviates the mother's diabetic symptoms [61].

Tea extract showed also a protective role after exposure of compounds which have a negative influence on health. It has been showed that a moderate dose of green tea extract can decrease the number of malformations in fetuses after exposure to a teratogen, such as cyclophosphamide. However, too high a dose increases the toxicity of cyclophosphamide [62].

Due to the limited amount of research on the consumption of tea by pregnant and lactating women and the popularity of tea, further research is necessary.

6. Limitations in Medicinal Herbs Usage

There is no denying the fact that the use of medicinal herbs has its limitations and risks. Plant extracts may contain hundreds of compounds that have specific pharmacologic effects that may be synergistic or antagonistic [126]. Ginseng extract showed contradictory effects in animals, such as histamine and antihistamine-like actions, hypertensive and hypotensive effects, and stimulatory or depressant activity on the central nervous system [127,128]. The synergistic effects of the plant compounds have been shown in Cinchona, which has almost 30 alkaloids [129]. Four of those, cinchonine, l-isomer cinchonidine, quinine, and d-isomer quinidine, have antiplasmodial activity [130].

However, Druilhe et al. (1988) showed that the mixture of alkaloids is two to ten times more effective in vitro than any of the alkaloids used separately [131]. Differences in the bioactivity of extracts of the same plant may result from differences in the composition and concentration of active compounds. However, studies investigating substance that differentiates the extracts often do not lead to the discovery of the active substance responsible for the biological effect, such as in the case of Rhodiola and epigallocatechin [132]. Therefore, it is possible that the positive effects of medicinal herbs are based on the complex relationship between pharmacologic effects of the herb's compounds, and usage of the single compound would not have any significant therapeutic effects.

Also, it is unpractical to isolate and assess every active ingredient from the herbal extract, since the resources required would be huge [133]. Isolation and investigation of every active compound in a plant extract would be laborious and might not render any meaningful results due to synergistic effects between plant compounds.

As another limitation of medicinal herbs usage, one has to consider geographical differences and potential contamination of the extract resulting from the culture, collection, and storage of the herbs [134]. Variation in the secondary metabolites content between plants may be caused by the region of origin, season, cultivar, and nitrogen availability [135,136]. For example, Marrassini et al. (2018) showed that total polyphenols, flavonoids, and tannins content in Urera aurantiaca obtained from two different regions of the same country is significantly different [137].

Therefore, since a simple medication must be a single substance with a proven therapeutic effect, it may never be possible to register any medical herb as a drug, and another unified approach must be implemented for the registration and pharmacovigilance of medicinal herbs.

7. Conclusions

The results presented here suggest that some of the immunomodulators, supplemented in pregnancy and lactation, may affect offspring health. Therefore, before the recommendation to use plant supplementation in the maternal diet to enhance immune system function, the safety of its use should be determined in tests performed on in vivo models. Ideally, if the mechanism of action of these compounds was determined, or the isolation of the substance responsible for the positive biological effect of the plant was achieved. Unfortunately, there is still insufficient knowledge in this topic, which can explain the lack of studies on the effects of medicinal herbs supplementation on the health of pregnant women and their offspring in the database of the national institutes of health (www.clinicaltrials.gov).

Author Contributions: Conceptualization: A.L., S.L. Investigation: A.L., K.R., A.K., Ł.S., A.J., R.Z.; Original draft preparation: A.L., K.R., A.K., Ł.S., R.Z.; Developed search terms and eligibility criteria: A.L., A.J.; Supervision: R.Z. and S.L.; critical evaluation: S.L.; Review and editing—all authors.

References

1. Hecht, A. Drug safety labeling for doctors. *FDA Consum.* **1979**, *13*, 12–13. [PubMed]
2. Skopińska-Różewska, E.; Mościcka-Wesołowska, M.; Wasiutyński, A.; Małdyk, J.; Malejczyk, M.; Pazdur, J. Lymphatic system of mice born from mothers treated with ampicillin or cloxacillin during gestation. *Arch. Immunol. Ther. Exp.* **1986**, *34*, 203–208.
3. Jedrychowski, W.; Gałaś, A.; Whyatt, R.; Perera, F. The prenatal use of antibiotics and the development of allergic disease in one year old infants. A preliminary study. *Int. J. Occup. Med. Environ. Health* **2006**, *19*, 70–76. [CrossRef] [PubMed]
4. Jin, M.; Li, Q.; Gu, Y.; Wan, B.; Huang, J.; Xu, X.; Huang, R.; Zhang, Y. Leonurine suppresses neuroinflammation through promoting oligodendrocyte maturation. *J. Cell Mol. Med.* **2019**, *23*, 1470–1485. [CrossRef]

5. Soutar, D.A.; Doucette, C.D.; Liwski, R.S.; Hoskin, D.W. Piperine, a Pungent Alkaloid from Black Pepper, Inhibits B Lymphocyte Activation and Effector Functions. *Phytother. Res.* **2017**, *31*, 466–474. [CrossRef]
6. Sang, X.-X.; Wang, R.-L.; Zhang, C.-E.; Liu, S.-J.; Shen, H.-H.; Guo, Y.-M.; Zhang, Y.-M.; Niu, M.; Wang, J.-B.; Bai, Z.-F.; et al. Sophocarpine Protects Mice from ConA-Induced Hepatitis via Inhibition of the IFN-Gamma/STAT1 Pathway. *Front. Pharmacol.* **2017**, *8*, 140. [CrossRef]
7. Song, J.-Y.; Han, S.-K.; Son, E.-H.; Pyo, S.-N.; Yun, Y.-S.; Yi, S.-Y. Induction of secretory and tumoricidal activities in peritoneal macrophages by ginsan. *Int. Immunopharmacol.* **2002**, *2*, 857–865. [CrossRef]
8. Jiménez-Arellanes, A.; Luna-Herrera, J.; Cornejo-Garrido, J.; López-García, S.; Castro-Mussot, M.E.; Meckes-Fischer, M.; Mata-Espinosa, D.; Marquina, B.; Torres, J.; Hernández-Pando, R. Ursolic and oleanolic acids as antimicrobial and immunomodulatory compounds for tuberculosis treatment. *BMC Complement. Altern. Med.* **2013**, *13*, 258. [CrossRef] [PubMed]
9. Ayeka, P.A.; Bian, Y.; Githaiga, P.M.; Zhao, Y. The immunomodulatory activities of licorice polysaccharides (Glycyrrhiza uralensis Fisch.) in CT 26 tumor-bearing mice. *BMC Complement. Altern. Med.* **2017**, *17*, 536. [CrossRef] [PubMed]
10. Zheng, R.; Jie, S.; Hanchuan, D.; Moucheng, W. Characterization and immunomodulating activities of polysaccharide from Lentinus edodes. *Int. Immunopharmacol.* **2005**, *5*, 811–820. [CrossRef] [PubMed]
11. Bhat, B.A.; Dhar, K.L.; Puri, S.C.; Qurishi, M.A.; Khajuria, A.; Gupta, A.; Qazi, G.N. Isolation, characterization and biological evaluation of datura lactones as potential immunomodulators. *Bioorg. Med. Chem.* **2005**, *13*, 6672–6677. [CrossRef]
12. Chung, J.W.; Choi, R.J.; Seo, E.-K.; Nam, J.-W.; Dong, M.-S.; Shin, E.M.; Guo, L.Y.; Kim, Y.S. Anti-inflammatory effects of (Z)-ligustilide through suppression of mitogen-activated protein kinases and nuclear factor-κB activation pathways. *Arch. Pharm. Res.* **2012**, *35*, 723–732. [CrossRef] [PubMed]
13. Hu, J.-Z.; Huang, J.-H.; Xiao, Z.-M.; Li, J.-H.; Li, X.-M.; Lu, H.-B. Tetramethylpyrazine accelerates the function recovery of traumatic spinal cord in rat model by attenuating inflammation. *J. Neurol. Sci.* **2013**, *324*, 94–99. [CrossRef]
14. Jantan, I.; Ahmad, W.; Bukhari, S.N.A. Corrigendum: Plant-derived immunomodulators: An insight on their preclinical evaluation and clinical trials. *Front. Plant Sci.* **2018**, *9*, 1178. [CrossRef]
15. Riva, A.; Ronchi, M.; Petrangolini, G.; Bosisio, S.; Allegrini, P. Improved Oral Absorption of Quercetin from Quercetin Phytosome®, a New Delivery System Based on Food Grade Lecithin. *Eur. J. Drug Metab. Pharmacokinet.* **2019**, *44*, 169–177. [CrossRef]
16. Tyagi, N.; Song, Y.H.; De, R. Recent progress on biocompatible nanocarrier-based genistein delivery systems in cancer therapy. *J. Drug Target* **2019**, *27*, 394–407. [CrossRef] [PubMed]
17. Zhai, Z.; Liu, Y.; Wu, L.; Senchina, D.S.; Wurtele, E.S.; Murphy, P.A.; Kohut, M.L.; Cunnick, J.E. Enhancement of innate and adaptive immune functions by multiple *Echinacea* species. *J. Med. Food* **2007**, *10*, 423–434. [CrossRef] [PubMed]
18. Orhan, D.D.; Ozçelik, B.; Ozgen, S.; Ergun, F. Antibacterial, antifungal, and antiviral activities of some flavonoids. *Microbiol. Res.* **2010**, *165*, 496–504. [CrossRef] [PubMed]
19. Pérez-Cano, F.J.; Massot-Cladera, M.; Rodríguez-Lagunas, M.J.; Castell, M. Flavonoids Affect Host-Microbiota Crosstalk through TLR Modulation. *Antioxid* **2014**, *3*, 649–670. [CrossRef]
20. Serafini, M.; Peluso, I.; Raguzzini, A. Flavonoids as anti-inflammatory agents. *Proc. Nutr. Soc.* **2010**, *69*, 273–278. [CrossRef]
21. Leyva-López, N.; Gutierrez-Grijalva, E.P.; Ambriz-Perez, D.L.; Heredia, J.B. Flavonoids as Cytokine Modulators: A Possible Therapy for Inflammation-Related Diseases. *Int. J. Mol. Sci.* **2016**, *17*, 921. [CrossRef]
22. Mirossay, L.; Varinská, L.; Mojžiš, J. Antiangiogenic Effect of Flavonoids and Chalcones: An Update. *Int. J. Mol. Sci.* **2017**, *19*, 27. [CrossRef]
23. Skopiński, P.; Skopińska-Różewska, E.; Sommer, E.; Chorostowska-Wynimko, J.; Rogala, E.; Cendrowska, I.; Chrystowska, D.; Filewska, M.; Białas-Chromiec, B.; Bany, J. Chocolate feeding of pregnant mice influences length of limbs of their progeny. *Pol. J. Vet. Sci.* **2003**, *6*, 57–59. [PubMed]
24. Skopiński, P.; Szaflik, J.; Duda-Król, B.; Nartowska, J.; Sommer, E.; Chorostowska-Wynimko, J.; Demkow, U.; Skopinska-Rózewska, E. Suppression of angiogenic activity of sera from diabetic patients with non-proliferative retinopathy by compounds of herbal origin and sulindac sulfone. *Int. J. Mol. Med.* **2004**, *14*, 707–711. [CrossRef] [PubMed]

25. Skopińska-Różewska, E.; Balan, B.J.; Sommer, E.; Chorostowska-Wynimko, J.; Bany, J.; Wasiutynski, A.; Siwicki, A.K. The influence of chocolate feeding of pregnant mice on the immunological response of their progeny. *Pol. J. Food Nutr. Sci.* **2004**, *54*, 67–70.
26. Chorostowska-Wynimko, J.; Skopińska-Różewska, E.; Sommer, E.; Rogala, E.; Skopiński, P.; Wojtasik, E. Multiple effects of theobromine on fetus development and postnatal status of the immune system. *Int. J. Tissue React.* **2004**, *26*, 53–60. [PubMed]
27. Patera, J.; Chorostowska-Wynimko, J.; Słodkowska, J.; Borowska, A.; Skopiński, P.; Sommer, E.; Wasiutyński, A.; Skopińska-Różewska, E. Morphometric and functional abnormalities of kidneys in the progeny of mice fed chocolate during pregnancy and lactation. *Folia Histochem. Cytobiol.* **2006**, *44*, 207–211.
28. Lewicki, S.; Skopińska-Różewska, E.; Lewicka, A.; Zdanowski, R. Long-term supplementation of Rhodiola kirilowii extracts during pregnancy and lactation does not affect mother health status. *J. Matern. Fetal Neonatal. Med.* **2019**, *32*, 838–844. [CrossRef]
29. Lewicki, S.; Stankiewicz, W.; Skopińska-Różewska, E.; Wilczak, J.; Leśniak, M.; Suska, M.; Siwicki, A.K.; Skopiński, P.; Zdanowski, R. Spleen content of selected polyphenols, splenocytes morphology and function in mice fed Rhodiola kirilowii extracts during pregnancy and lactation. *Pol. J. Vet. Sci.* **2015**, *18*, 847–855. [CrossRef]
30. Zdanowski, R.; Skopińska-Różewska, E.; Wilczak, J.; Borecka, A.; Lewicka, A.; Lewicki, S. Different effects of feeding pregnant and lactating mice Rhodiola kirilowii aqueous and hydro-alcoholic extracts on their serum angiogenic activity and content of selected polyphenols. *Cent. Eur. J. Immunol.* **2017**, *42*, 17–23. [CrossRef] [PubMed]
31. Lewicki, S.; Skopińska-Różewska, E.; Zdanowski, R. The decrease in number of splenic lymphocytes in mice fed Rhodiola kirilowii during pregnancy and lactation concerns mainly CD19+ and CD4+ cells. *Cent. Eur. J. Immunol.* **2017**, *42*, 331–335. [CrossRef] [PubMed]
32. Lewicki, S.; Skopińska-Różewska, E.; Brewczyńska, A.; Zdanowski, R. Administration of Rhodiola kirilowii Extracts during Mouse Pregnancy and Lactation Stimulates Innate but Not Adaptive Immunity of the Offspring. *J. Immunol. Res.* **2017**, *2017*, 8081642. [CrossRef] [PubMed]
33. Lewicki, S.; Bałan, B.J.; Skopińska-Różewska, E.; Zdanowski, R.; Stelmasiak, M.; Szymański, Ł.; Stankiewicz, W. Modulatory effects of feeding pregnant and lactating mice Rhodiola kirilowii extracts on the immune system of offspring. *Exp. Ther. Med.* **2016**, *12*, 3450–3458. [CrossRef] [PubMed]
34. Lewicki, S.; Orłowski, P.; Krzyżowska, M.; Kiepura, A.; Skopińska-Różewska, E.; Zdanowski, R. The effect of feeding mice during gestation and nursing with Rhodiola kirilowii extracts or epigallocatechin on CD4 and CD8 cells number and distribution in the spleen of their progeny. *Cent. Eur. J. Immunol.* **2017**, *42*, 10–16. [CrossRef] [PubMed]
35. Bień, K.; Lewicki, S.; Zdanowski, R.; Skopińska-Różewska, E.; Krzyżowska, M. Feeding Pregnant and Lactating Mice Rhodiola kirilowii Extracts helps to Preserve Thymus Function of their Adult Progeny. *Pol. J. Vet. Sci.* **2016**, *19*, 581–587. [CrossRef] [PubMed]
36. Dabbou, S.; Rotolo, L.; Kovitvadhi, A.; Bergagna, S.; Dezzutto, D.; Barbero, R.; Rubiolo, P.; Schiavone, A.; De Marco, M.; Helal, A.N.; et al. Rabbit dietary supplementation with pale purple coneflower. 1. Effects on the reproductive performance and immune parameters of does. *Animal* **2016**, *10*, 1101–1109. [CrossRef] [PubMed]
37. Maass, N.; Bauer, J.; Paulicks, B.R.; Böhmer, B.M.; Roth-Maier, D.A. Efficiency of *Echinacea* purpurea on performance and immune status in pigs. *J. Anim. Physiol. Anim. Nutr.* **2005**, *89*, 244–252. [CrossRef] [PubMed]
38. Chow, G.; Johns, T.; Miller, S.C. Dietary *Echinacea* purpurea during murine pregnancy: Effect on maternal hemopoiesis and fetal growth. *Biol. Neonatol.* **2006**, *89*, 133–138. [CrossRef] [PubMed]
39. Barcz, E.; Sommer, E.; Nartowska, J.; Balan, B.; Chorostowska-Wynimko, J.; Skopińska-Rózewska, E. Influence of *Echinacea* purpurea intake during pregnancy on fetal growth and tissue angiogenic activity. *Folia Histochem. Cytobiol.* **2007**, *45* (Suppl. 1), S35–S39.
40. Kovitvadhi, A.; Gai, F.; Dabbou, S.; Ferrocino, I.; Rotolo, L.; Falzone, M.; Vignolini, C.; Gennero, M.S.; Bergagna, S.; Dezzutto, D.; et al. Rabbit dietary supplementation with pale purple coneflower. 2. Effects on the performances, bacterial community, blood parameters and immunity of growing rabbits. *Animal* **2016**, *10*, 1110–1117. [CrossRef] [PubMed]

41. Heitmann, K.; Havnen, G.C.; Holst, L.; Nordeng, H. Pregnancy outcomes after prenatal exposure to *Echinacea*: The Norwegian Mother and Child Cohort Study. *Eur. J. Clin. Pharmacol.* **2016**, *72*, 623–630. [CrossRef] [PubMed]
42. Gallo, M.; Sarkar, M.; Au, W.; Pietrzak, K.; Comas, B.; Smith, M.; Jaeger, T.V.; Einarson, A.; Koren, G. Pregnancy outcome following gestational exposure to *Echinacea*: A prospective controlled study. *Arch. Intern. Med.* **2000**, *160*, 3141–3143. [CrossRef]
43. Perri, D.; Dugoua, J.-J.; Mills, E.; Koren, G. Safety and efficacy of *Echinacea* (*Echinacea* angustafolia, e. purpurea and e. pallida) during pregnancy and lactation. *Can. J. Clin. Pharm.* **2006**, *13*, e262–e267.
44. Xi, Q.-Y.; Jiang, Y.; Zhao, S.; Zeng, B.; Wang, F.; Wang, L.-N.; Jiang, Q.-Y.; Zhang, Y.-L. Effect of ginseng polysaccharides on the immunity and growth of piglets by dietary supplementation during late pregnancy and lactating sows. *Anim. Sci. J.* **2017**, *88*, 863–872. [CrossRef] [PubMed]
45. Concha, C.; Hu, S.; Holmberg, O. The proliferative responses of cow stripping milk and blood lymphocytes to pokeweed mitogen and ginseng in vitro. *Vet. Res.* **1996**, *27*, 107–115. [PubMed]
46. Hu, S.; Concha, C.; Johannisson, A.; Meglia, G.; Waller, K.P. Effect of subcutaneous injection of ginseng on cows with subclinical Staphylococcus aureus mastitis. *J. Vet. Med. B Infect. Dis. Vet. Public Health* **2001**, *48*, 519–528. [CrossRef] [PubMed]
47. Kim, Y.O.; Lee, H.-Y.; Won, H.; Nah, S.-S.; Lee, H.-Y.; Kim, H.-K.; Kwon, J.-T.; Kim, H.-J. Influence of Panax ginseng on the offspring of adult rats exposed to prenatal stress. *Int. J. Mol. Med.* **2015**, *35*, 103–109. [CrossRef] [PubMed]
48. Saadeldin, I.M.; Hussein, M.A.; Suleiman, A.H.; Abohassan, M.G.; Ahmed, M.M.; Moustafa, A.A.; Moumen, A.F.; Abdel-Aziz Swelum, A. Ameliorative effect of ginseng extract on phthalate and bisphenol A reprotoxicity during pregnancy in rats. *Environ. Sci. Pollut. Res. Int.* **2018**, *25*, 21205–21215. [CrossRef] [PubMed]
49. Wanderley, M.I.; Saraiva, K.L.A.; César Vieira, J.S.B.; Peixoto, C.A.; Udrisar, D.P. Foetal exposure to Panax ginseng extract reverts the effects of prenatal dexamethasone in the synthesis of testosterone by Leydig cells of the adult rat. *Int. J. Exp. Pathol.* **2013**, *94*, 230–240. [CrossRef] [PubMed]
50. Belanger, D.; Calder, M.D.; Gianetto-Berruti, A.; Lui, E.M.; Watson, A.J.; Feyles, V. Effects of American Ginseng on Preimplantation Development and Pregnancy in Mice. *Am. J. Chin. Med.* **2016**, *44*, 981–995. [CrossRef]
51. Hachul, A.C.L.; Boldarine, V.T.; Neto, N.I.P.; Moreno, M.F.; Carvalho, P.O.; Sawaya, A.C.H.F.; Ribeiro, E.B.; do Nascimento, C.M.O.; Oyama, L.M. Effect of the consumption of green tea extract during pregnancy and lactation on metabolism of mothers and 28d-old offspring. *Sci. Rep.* **2018**, *8*, 1869. [CrossRef]
52. Matsumoto, E.; Kataoka, S.; Mukai, Y.; Sato, M.; Sato, S. Green tea extract intake during lactation modified cardiac macrophage infiltration and AMP-activated protein kinase phosphorylation in weanling rats from undernourished mother during gestation and lactation. *J. Dev. Orig. Health Dis.* **2017**, *8*, 178–187. [CrossRef]
53. Dey, A.; Gomes, A.; Dasgupta, S.C. Black Tea (Camellia sinensis) Extract Induced Prenatal and Postnatal Toxicity in Experimental Albino rats. *Pharm. Mag.* **2017**, *13*, S769–S774.
54. Dey, A.; Gomes, A.; Dasgupta, S.C. Black Tea (Camellia sinensis) Extract Induced Changes in Blood and Liver Parameters on Pregnant and Lactating Experimental Albino Rats. *Proc. Zool. Soc.* **2019**, *72*, 25–31. [CrossRef]
55. Otake, M.; Sakurai, K.; Watanabe, M.; Mori, C. Association Between Serum Folate Levels and Caffeinated Beverage Consumption in Pregnant Women in Chiba: The Japan Environment and Children's Study. *J. Epidemiol.* **2018**, *28*, 414–419. [CrossRef] [PubMed]
56. Shi, D.-D.; Guo, J.-J.; Zhou, L.; Wang, N. Epigallocatechin gallate enhances treatment efficacy of oral nifedipine against pregnancy-induced severe pre-eclampsia: A double-blind, randomized and placebo-controlled clinical study. *J. Clin. Pharm. Ther.* **2018**, *43*, 21–25. [CrossRef]
57. Wei, S.-Q.; Xu, H.; Xiong, X.; Luo, Z.-C.; Audibert, F.; Fraser, W.D. Tea consumption during pregnancy and the risk of pre-eclampsia. *Int. J. Gynaecol Obstet.* **2009**, *105*, 123–126. [CrossRef]
58. Okubo, H.; Miyake, Y.; Tanaka, K.; Sasaki, S.; Hirota, Y. Maternal total caffeine intake, mainly from Japanese and Chinese tea, during pregnancy was associated with risk of preterm birth: The Osaka Maternal and Child Health Study. *Nutr. Res.* **2015**, *35*, 309–316. [CrossRef]
59. Yang, J.; Chen, M.J.; Wang, X.X.; Sun, X.; Wang, X.; Wang, X.R.; Xia, Y.K. Association between maternal tea consumption in pregnancy and birth outcomes. *Chin. J. Prev. Med.* **2018**, *52*, 1013–1017.

60. Hachul, A.C.L.; Boldarine, V.T.; Neto, N.I.P.; Moreno, M.F.; Ribeiro, E.B.; do Nascimento, C.M.O.; Oyama, L.M. Maternal consumption of green tea extract during pregnancy and lactation alters offspring's metabolism in rats. *PLoS ONE* **2018**, *13*, e0199969. [CrossRef] [PubMed]
61. Zhang, H.; Su, S.; Yu, X.; Li, Y. Dietary epigallocatechin 3-gallate supplement improves maternal and neonatal treatment outcome of gestational diabetes mellitus: A double-blind randomised controlled trial. *J. Hum. Nutr. Diet.* **2017**, *30*, 753–758. [CrossRef] [PubMed]
62. Logsdon, A.L.; Herring, B.J.; Lockard, J.E.; Miller, B.M.; Kim, H.; Hood, R.D.; Bailey, M.M. Exposure to green tea extract alters the incidence of specific cyclophosphamide-induced malformations. *Birth Defects Res. B Dev. Reprod. Toxicol.* **2012**, *95*, 231–237. [CrossRef] [PubMed]
63. Zdanowski, R.; Skopińska-Różewska, E.; Wasiutyński, A.; Skopiński, P.; Siwicki, A.K.; Sobiczewska, E.; Lewicki, S.; Buchwald, W.; Kocik, J.; Stankiewicz, W. The effect of Rhodiola kirilowii extracts on tumor-induced angiogenesis in mice. *Cent. Eur. J. Immunol.* **2012**, *37*, 131–139.
64. Grace, M.H.; Yousef, G.G.; Kurmukov, A.G.; Raskin, I.; Lila, M.A. Phytochemical Characterization of an Adaptogenic Preparation from Rhodiola heterodonta. *Nat. Prod. Commun.* **2009**, *4*, 1053–1058. [CrossRef] [PubMed]
65. Zhou, J.-T.; Li, C.-Y.; Wang, C.-H.; Wang, Y.-F.; Wang, X.-D.; Wang, H.-T.; Zhu, Y.; Jiang, M.-M.; Gao, X.-M. Phenolic Compounds from the Roots of Rhodiola crenulata and Their Antioxidant and Inducing IFN-γ Production Activities. *Molecules* **2015**, *20*, 13725–13739. [CrossRef] [PubMed]
66. Grech-Baran, M.; Pietrosiuk, A.; Sykłowska-Baranek, K.; Giebułtowicz, J. Activity of tyrosol glucosyltransferase in Rhodiola kirilowii transgenic root cultures. *Planta Med.* **2012**, *78*, PI228. [CrossRef]
67. Mishra, K.P.; Ganju, L.; Singh, S.B. Anti-cellular and immunomodulatory potential of aqueous extract of Rhodiola imbricata rhizome. *Immunopharmacol. Immunotoxicol.* **2012**, *34*, 513–518. [CrossRef]
68. Cui, J.-L.; Guo, T.-T.; Ren, Z.-X.; Zhang, N.-S.; Wang, M.-L. Diversity and antioxidant activity of culturable endophytic fungi from alpine plants of Rhodiola crenulata, R. angusta, and R. sachalinensis. *PLoS ONE* **2015**, *10*, e0118204. [CrossRef]
69. Wójcik, R.; Siwicki, A.K.; Skopińska-Różewska, E.; Wasiutyński, A.; Sommer, E.; Furmanowa, M. The effect of Chinese medicinal herb Rhodiola kirilowii extracts on cellular immunity in mice and rats. *Pol. J. Vet. Sci.* **2009**, *12*, 399–405.
70. Zdanowski, R.; Lewicki, S.; Skopińska-Różewska, E.; Buchwald, W.; Mrozikiewicz, P.M.; Stankiewicz, W. Alcohol- and water-based extracts obtained from Rhodiola rosea affect differently the number and metabolic activity of circulating granulocytes in Balb/c mice. *Ann. Agric. Environ. Med.* **2014**, *21*, 120–123.
71. Bany, J.; Zdanowska, D.; Skopińska-Różewska, E.; Sommer, E.; Siwicki, A.K.; Wasiutyński, A. The effect of Rhodiola rosea extracts on the bacterial infection in mice. *Cent. Eur. J. Immunol.* **2009**, *34*, 35–37.
72. Zuo, G.; Li, Z.; Chen, L.; Xu, X. Activity of compounds from Chinese herbal medicine Rhodiola kirilowii (Regel) Maxim against HCV NS3 serine protease. *Antivir. Res.* **2007**, *76*, 86–92. [CrossRef] [PubMed]
73. Wong, Y.-C.; Zhao, M.; Zong, Y.-Y.; Chan, C.-Y.; Che, C.-T. Chemical constituents and anti-tuberculosis activity of root of Rhodiola kirilowii. *China J. Chin. Mater. Med.* **2008**, *33*, 1561–1565.
74. Khanna, K.; Mishra, K.P.; Ganju, L.; Singh, S.B. Golden root: A wholesome treat of immunity. *Biomed. Pharmacother.* **2017**, *87*, 496–502. [CrossRef] [PubMed]
75. Barman, D.; Nen, P.; Mandal, S.C.; Kumar, V. Immunostimulants for Aquaculture Health Management. *J. Mar. Sci. Res. Dev.* **2013**, *3*, 134. [CrossRef]
76. Lewicki, S.; Skopińska-Różewska, E.; Bałan, B.J.; Kalicki, B.; Patera, J.; Wilczak, J.; Wasiutyński, A.; Zdanowski, R. Morphofunctional Renal Alterations in Progeny of Mice Fed Rhodiola kirilowii Extracts or Epigallocatechin During Pregnancy and Lactation. *J. Med. Food* **2017**, *20*, 86–92. [CrossRef] [PubMed]
77. Blumenthal, M.; Farnsworth, N.R. *Echinacea* angustifolia in rhinovirus infections. *N. Engl. J. Med.* **2005**, *353*, 1971–1972. [PubMed]
78. Barnes, J.; Anderson, L.A.; Gibbons, S.; Phillipson, J.D. *Echinacea* species (*Echinacea* angustifolia (DC.) Hell., *Echinacea* pallida (Nutt.) Nutt., *Echinacea* purpurea (L.) Moench): A review of their chemistry, pharmacology and clinical properties. *J. Pharm. Pharmacol.* **2005**, *57*, 929–954. [CrossRef] [PubMed]
79. Schoop, R.; Klein, P.; Suter, A.; Johnston, S.L. *Echinacea* in the prevention of induced rhinovirus colds: A meta-analysis. *Clin. Ther.* **2006**, *28*, 174–183. [CrossRef]
80. Shah, S.A.; Sander, S.; White, C.M.; Rinaldi, M.; Coleman, C.I. Evaluation of *Echinacea* for the prevention and treatment of the common cold: A meta-analysis. *Lancet Infect. Dis.* **2007**, *7*, 473–480. [CrossRef]

81. Cheminat, A.; Zawatzky, R.; Becker, H.; Brouillard, R. Caffeoyl conjugates from *Echinacea* species: Structures and biological activity. *Phytochemistry* **1988**, *27*, 2787–2794. [CrossRef]
82. Melchart, D.; Clemm, C.; Weber, B.; Draczynski, T.; Worku, F.; Linde, K.; Weidenhammer, W.; Wagner, H.; Saller, R. Polysaccharides isolated from *Echinacea* purpurea herba cell cultures to counteract undesired effects of chemotherapy—A pilot study. *Phytother. Res.* **2002**, *16*, 138–142. [CrossRef] [PubMed]
83. Luettig, B.; Steinmüller, C.; Gifford, G.E.; Wagner, H.; Lohmann-Matthes, M.L. Macrophage activation by the polysaccharide arabinogalactan isolated from plant cell cultures of *Echinacea* purpurea. *J. Natl. Cancer Inst.* **1989**, *81*, 669–675. [CrossRef] [PubMed]
84. Forman, H.J.; Torres, M. Redox signaling in macrophages. *Mol. Asp. Med.* **2001**, *22*, 189–216. [CrossRef]
85. Hobbs, A.J.; Higgs, A.; Moncada, S. Inhibition of nitric oxide synthase as a potential therapeutic target. *Annu. Rev. Pharmacol. Toxicol.* **1999**, *39*, 191–220. [CrossRef] [PubMed]
86. Zhai, Z.; Haney, D.; Wu, L.; Solco, A.; Murphy, P.A.; Wurtele, E.S.; Kohut, M.L.; Cunnick, J.E. Alcohol extracts of *Echinacea* inhibit production of nitric oxide and tumor necrosis factor-alpha by macrophages in vitro. *Food Agric. Immunol.* **2007**, *18*, 221–236. [CrossRef] [PubMed]
87. Brüne, B.; Götz, C.; Meßmer, U.K.; Sandau, K.; Hirvonen, M.-R.; Lapetina, E.G. Superoxide Formation and Macrophage Resistance to Nitric Oxide-mediated Apoptosis. *J. Biol. Chem.* **1997**, *272*, 7253–7258. [CrossRef] [PubMed]
88. Chang, C.Y.; Tucci, M.; Baker, R.C. Lipopolysaccharide-stimulated nitric oxide production and inhibition of cell proliferation is antagonized by ethanol in a clonal macrophage cell line. *Alcohol* **2000**, *20*, 37–43. [CrossRef]
89. Facino, R.M.; Carini, M.; Aldini, G.; Saibene, L.; Pietta, P.; Mauri, P. Echinacoside and caffeoyl conjugates protect collagen from free radical-induced degradation: A potential use of *Echinacea* extracts in the prevention of skin photodamage. *Planta Med.* **1995**, *61*, 510–514. [CrossRef]
90. Hu, C.; Kitts, D.D. Studies on the antioxidant activity of *Echinacea* root extract. *J. Agric. Food Chem.* **2000**, *48*, 1466–1472. [CrossRef]
91. Pellati, F.; Benvenuti, S.; Magro, L.; Melegari, M.; Soragni, F. Analysis of phenolic compounds and radical scavenging activity of *Echinacea* spp. *J. Pharm. Biomed. Anal.* **2004**, *35*, 289–301. [CrossRef]
92. Dalby-Brown, L.; Barsett, H.; Landbo, A.-K.R.; Meyer, A.S.; Mølgaard, P. Synergistic antioxidative effects of alkamides, caffeic acid derivatives, and polysaccharide fractions from *Echinacea* purpurea on in vitro oxidation of human low-density lipoproteins. *J. Agric. Food Chem.* **2005**, *53*, 9413–9423. [CrossRef] [PubMed]
93. Choi, K. Botanical characteristics, pharmacological effects and medicinal components of Korean Panax ginseng C A Meyer. *Acta Pharmacol. Sin.* **2008**, *29*, 1109–1118. [CrossRef] [PubMed]
94. Baek, S.-H.; Bae, O.-N.; Park, J.H. Recent methodology in ginseng analysis. *J. Ginseng Res.* **2012**, *36*, 119–134. [CrossRef] [PubMed]
95. Rhule, A.; Navarro, S.; Smith, J.R.; Shepherd, D.M. Panax notoginseng attenuates LPS-induced pro-inflammatory mediators in RAW264.7 cells. *J. Ethnopharmacol.* **2006**, *106*, 121–128. [CrossRef] [PubMed]
96. Lee, J.-Y.; Shin, J.-W.; Chun, K.-S.; Park, K.-K.; Chung, W.-Y.; Bang, Y.-J.; Sung, J.-H.; Surh, Y.-J. Antitumor promotional effects of a novel intestinal bacterial metabolite (IH-901) derived from the protopanaxadiol-type ginsenosides in mouse skin. *Carcinogenesis* **2005**, *26*, 359–367. [CrossRef] [PubMed]
97. Lee, I.-A.; Hyam, S.R.; Jang, S.-E.; Han, M.J.; Kim, D.-H. Ginsenoside Re ameliorates inflammation by inhibiting the binding of lipopolysaccharide to TLR4 on macrophages. *J. Agric. Food Chem.* **2012**, *60*, 9595–9602. [CrossRef] [PubMed]
98. Kim, S.-J.; Murthy, H.N.; Hahn, E.-J.; Lee, H.L.; Paek, K.-Y. Parameters affecting the extraction of ginsenosides from the adventitious roots of ginseng (Panax ginseng C.A. Meyer). *Sep. Purif. Technol.* **2007**, *56*, 401–406. [CrossRef]
99. Byeon, S.E.; Lee, J.; Kim, J.H.; Yang, W.S.; Kwak, Y.-S.; Kim, S.Y.; Choung, E.S.; Rhee, M.H.; Cho, J.Y. Molecular mechanism of macrophage activation by red ginseng acidic polysaccharide from Korean red ginseng. *Mediat. Inflamm.* **2012**, *2012*, 732860. [CrossRef] [PubMed]
100. Baek, S.-H.; Lee, J.G.; Park, S.Y.; Bae, O.N.; Kim, D.-H.; Park, J.H. Pectic polysaccharides from Panax ginseng as the antirotavirus principals in ginseng. *Biomacromolecules* **2010**, *11*, 2044–2052. [CrossRef] [PubMed]
101. Kim, Y.O.; Kim, Y.; Lee, K.; Na, S.W.; Hong, S.P.; Valan Arasu, M.; Yoon, Y.W.; Kim, J. Panax ginseng Improves Functional Recovery after Contusive Spinal Cord Injury by Regulating the Inflammatory Response in Rats: An In Vivo Study. *Evid. Based Complement. Altern. Med.* **2015**, *2015*, 817096. [CrossRef] [PubMed]

102. Khalid, S.; Tahir, M.; Shoro, A.A. Ginseng Induced Fetal Skeletal Malformations. 2008. Available online: http://www.pjmhsonline.com/ginseng_induced_fetal_skeletal_m.htm (accessed on 29 June 2019).
103. Kim, M.-H.; Byon, Y.-Y.; Ko, E.-J.; Song, J.-Y.; Yun, Y.-S.; Shin, T.; Joo, H.-G. Immunomodulatory activity of ginsan, a polysaccharide of panax ginseng, on dendritic cells. *Korean J. Physiol. Pharmacol.* **2009**, *13*, 169–173. [CrossRef] [PubMed]
104. Shin, J.-Y.; Song, J.-Y.; Yun, Y.-S.; Yang, H.-O.; Rhee, D.-K.; Pyo, S. Immunostimulating effects of acidic polysaccharides extract of Panax ginseng on macrophage function. *Immunopharmacol. Immunotoxicol.* **2002**, *24*, 469–482. [CrossRef] [PubMed]
105. Jie, Y.H.; Cammisuli, S.; Baggiolini, M. Immunomodulatory effects of Panax Ginseng C.A. Meyer in the mouse. *Agents Actions* **1984**, *15*, 386–391. [CrossRef] [PubMed]
106. Ahn, J.-Y.; Song, J.-Y.; Yun, Y.-S.; Jeong, G.; Choi, I.-S. Protection of Staphylococcus aureus-infected septic mice by suppression of early acute inflammation and enhanced antimicrobial activity by ginsan. *FEMS Immunol. Med. Microbiol.* **2006**, *46*, 187–197. [CrossRef] [PubMed]
107. Chan, L.Y.; Kwok, H.H.; Chan, R.W.Y.; Peiris, M.J.S.; Mak, N.K.; Wong, R.N.S.; Chan, M.C.W.; Yue, P.Y.K. Dual functions of ginsenosides in protecting human endothelial cells against influenza H9N2-induced inflammation and apoptosis. *J. Ethnopharmacol.* **2011**, *137*, 1542–1546. [CrossRef] [PubMed]
108. Chattopadhyay, C.; Chakrabarti, N.; Chatterjee, M.; Mukherjee, S.; Sarkar, K.; Chaudhuri, A.R. Black tea (Camellia sinensis) decoction shows immunomodulatory properties on an experimental animal model and in human peripheral mononuclear cells. *Pharmacogn. Res.* **2012**, *4*, 15–21. [CrossRef] [PubMed]
109. Kuo, C.-L.; Chen, T.-S.; Liou, S.-Y.; Hsieh, C.-C. Immunomodulatory effects of EGCG fraction of green tea extract in innate and adaptive immunity via T regulatory cells in murine model. *Immunopharmacol. Immunotoxicol.* **2014**, *36*, 364–370. [CrossRef] [PubMed]
110. McKay, D.L.; Blumberg, J.B. The role of tea in human health: An update. *J. Am. Coll. Nutr.* **2002**, *21*, 1–13. [CrossRef] [PubMed]
111. Chen, Z.; Zhu, Q.Y.; Tsang, D.; Huang, Y. Degradation of green tea catechins in tea drinks. *J. Agric. Food Chem.* **2001**, *49*, 477–482. [CrossRef]
112. Chen, N.; Bezzina, R.; Hinch, E.; Lewandowski, P.A.; Cameron-Smith, D.; Mathai, M.L.; Jois, M.; Sinclair, A.J.; Begg, D.P.; Wark, J.D.; et al. Green tea, black tea, and epigallocatechin modify body composition, improve glucose tolerance, and differentially alter metabolic gene expression in rats fed a high-fat diet. *Nutr. Res.* **2009**, *29*, 784–793. [CrossRef] [PubMed]
113. Graham, H.N. Green tea composition, consumption, and polyphenol chemistry. *Prev. Med.* **1992**, *21*, 334–350. [CrossRef]
114. Anderson, R.A.; Polansky, M.M. Tea enhances insulin activity. *J. Agric. Food Chem.* **2002**, *50*, 7182–7186. [CrossRef] [PubMed]
115. Kawai, K.; Tsuno, N.H.; Kitayama, J.; Okaji, Y.; Yazawa, K.; Asakage, M.; Hori, N.; Watanabe, T.; Takahashi, K.; Nagawa, H. Epigallocatechin gallate attenuates adhesion and migration of CD8+ T cells by binding to CD11b. *J. Allergy Clin. Immunol.* **2004**, *113*, 1211–1217. [CrossRef] [PubMed]
116. Williamson, M.P.; McCormick, T.G.; Nance, C.L.; Shearer, W.T. Epigallocatechin gallate, the main polyphenol in green tea, binds to the T-cell receptor, CD4: Potential for HIV-1 therapy. *J. Allergy Clin. Immunol.* **2006**, *118*, 1369–1374. [CrossRef] [PubMed]
117. Tripathi, S.; Bruch, D.; Gatto, L.A.; Kittur, D.S. Green tea extract prolongs allograft survival as an adjunctive therapy along with low dose cyclosporine A. *J. Surg. Res.* **2009**, *154*, 85–90. [CrossRef] [PubMed]
118. Hamer, M. The beneficial effects of tea on immune function and inflammation: A review of evidence from in vitro, animal, and human research. *Nutr. Res.* **2007**, *27*, 373–379. [CrossRef]
119. Donà, M.; Dell'Aica, I.; Calabrese, F.; Benelli, R.; Morini, M.; Albini, A.; Garbisa, S. Neutrophil restraint by green tea: Inhibition of inflammation, associated angiogenesis, and pulmonary fibrosis. *J. Immunol.* **2003**, *170*, 4335–4341. [CrossRef] [PubMed]
120. Frei, B.; Higdon, J.V. Antioxidant activity of tea polyphenols in vivo: Evidence from animal studies. *J. Nutr.* **2003**, *133*, 3275S–3284S. [CrossRef] [PubMed]
121. Datta, P.; Sarkar, A.; Biswas, A.K.; Gomes, A. Anti arthritic activity of aqueous extract of Indian black tea in experimental and clinical study. *Orient. Pharm. Exp. Med.* **2012**, *12*, 265–271. [CrossRef]

122. Isbrucker, R.A.; Edwards, J.A.; Wolz, E.; Davidovich, A.; Bausch, J. Safety studies on epigallocatechin gallate (EGCG) preparations. Part 3: Teratogenicity and reproductive toxicity studies in rats. *Food Chem. Toxicol.* **2006**, *44*, 651–661. [CrossRef] [PubMed]
123. Wang, D.; Meng, J.; Xu, K.; Xiao, R.; Xu, M.; Liu, Y.; Zhao, Y.; Yao, P.; Yan, H.; Liu, L. Evaluation of oral subchronic toxicity of Pu-erh green tea (camellia sinensis var. assamica) extract in Sprague Dawley rats. *J. Ethnopharmacol.* **2012**, *142*, 836–844. [CrossRef] [PubMed]
124. Kayiran, S.M.; Ince, D.A.; Aldemir, D.; Gurakan, B. Investigating the effect of black tea consumption during pregnancy on the oxidant/antioxidant status of breastmilk. *Breastfeed. Med.* **2013**, *8*, 187–190. [CrossRef] [PubMed]
125. Jochum, F.; Alteheld, B.; Meinardus, P.; Dahlinger, N.; Nomayo, A.; Stehle, P. Mothers' Consumption of Soy Drink But Not Black Tea Increases the Flavonoid Content of Term Breast Milk: A Pilot Randomized, Controlled Intervention Study. *Ann. Nutr. Metab.* **2017**, *70*, 147–153. [CrossRef] [PubMed]
126. Chong, S.K.; Oberholzer, V.G. Ginseng–is there a use in clinical medicine? *Postgrad Med. J.* **1988**, *64*, 841–846. [CrossRef] [PubMed]
127. Takagi, K.; Saito, H.; Tsuchiya, M. Pharmacological studies of Panax Ginseng root: Pharmacological properties of a crude saponin fraction. *Jpn. J. Pharmacol.* **1972**, *22*, 339–346. [CrossRef] [PubMed]
128. Kim, H.J.; Kim, P.; Shin, C.Y. A comprehensive review of the therapeutic and pharmacological effects of ginseng and ginsenosides in central nervous system. *J. Ginseng Res.* **2013**, *37*, 8–29. [CrossRef] [PubMed]
129. Kacprzak, K.M. Chemistry and Biology of Cinchona Alkaloids. In *Natural Products*; Ramawat, K.G., Mérillon, J.-M., Eds.; Springer: Berlin/Heidelberg, Germany, 2013; pp. 605–641. ISBN 978-3-642-22143-9.
130. Karle, J.M.; Bhattacharjee, A.K. Stereoelectronic features of the cinchona alkaloids determine their differential antimalarial activity. *Bioorg. Med. Chem.* **1999**, *7*, 1769–1774. [CrossRef]
131. Druilhe, P.; Brandicourt, O.; Chongsuphajaisiddhi, T.; Berthe, J. Activity of a combination of three cinchona bark alkaloids against Plasmodium falciparum in vitro. *Antimicrob. Agents Chemother.* **1988**, *32*, 250–254. [CrossRef]
132. Bałan, B.J.; Skopińska-Różewska, E.; Skopiński, P.; Zdanowski, R.; Leśniak, M.; Kiepura, A.; Lewicki, S. Morphometric abnormalities in the spleen of the progeny of mice fed epigallocatechin during gestation and nursing. *Pol. J. Vet. Sci.* **2017**, *20*, 5–12. [CrossRef]
133. World Health Organization (Ed.) *National Policy on Traditional Medicine and Regulation of Herbal Medicines: Report of a WHO Global Survey*; World Health Organization: Geneva, Switzerland, 2005; ISBN 978-92-4-159323-6.
134. Chan, K. Some aspects of toxic contaminants in herbal medicines. *Chemosphere* **2003**, *52*, 1361–1371. [CrossRef]
135. Bouterfas, K.; Mehdadi, Z.; Elaoufi, M.M.; Latreche, A.; Benchiha, W. Antioxidant activity and total phenolic and flavonoids content variations of leaves extracts of white Horehound (Marrubium vulgare Linné) from three geographical origins. *Ann. Pharm. Fr.* **2016**, *74*, 453–462. [CrossRef] [PubMed]
136. Arnold, T.; Tanner, C.; Hatch, W. Phenotypic variation in polyphenolic content of the tropical brown alga Lobophora variegata as a function of nitrogen availability. *Mar. Ecol. Prog. Ser.* **1995**, *123*, 177–183. [CrossRef]
137. Marrassini, C.; Peralta, I.; Anesini, C. Comparative study of the polyphenol content-related anti-inflammatory and antioxidant activities of two Urera aurantiaca specimens from different geographical areas. *Chin. Med.* **2018**, *13*, 22. [CrossRef] [PubMed]

5

Energy Intake Requirements in Pregnancy

Jasper Most [1], Sheila Dervis [2], Francois Haman [2], Kristi B Adamo [2] and Leanne M Redman [1,*]

1 Pennington Biomedical Research Center, Baton Rouge, LA 70808, USA
2 School of Human Kinetics, University of Ottawa, Ottawa, ON K1N 6N5, Canada
* Correspondence: leanne.redman@pbrc.edu

Abstract: Energy intake requirements in pregnancy match the demands of resting metabolism, physical activity, and tissue growth. Energy balance in pregnancy is, therefore, defined as energy intake equal to energy expenditure plus energy storage. A detailed understanding of these components and their changes throughout gestation can inform energy intake recommendations for minimizing the risk of poor pregnancy outcomes. Energy expenditure is the sum of resting and physical activity-related expenditure. Resting metabolic rate increases during pregnancy as a result of increased body mass, pregnancy-associated physiological changes, i.e., cardiac output, and the growing fetus. Physical activity is extremely variable between women and may change over the course of pregnancy. The requirement for energy storage depends on maternal pregravid body size. For optimal pregnancy outcomes, women with low body weight require more fat mass accumulation than women with obesity, who do not require to accumulate fat mass at all. Given the high energy density of fat mass, these differences affect energy intake requirements for a healthy pregnancy greatly. In contrast, the energy stored in fetal and placental tissues is comparable between all women and have small impact on energy requirements. Different prediction equations have been developed to quantify energy intake requirements and we provide a brief review of the strengths and weaknesses and discuss their application for healthy management of weight gain in pregnant women.

Keywords: pregnancy; energy expenditure; energy intake; physical activity; metabolic rate; fetal development

---

1. Introduction

Pregnancy is a determining period of future health for women and children. For the mother, poor pregnancy outcomes including excess gestational weight gain, gestational diabetes, hypertension and preeclampsia, or having a cesarean section increase the risk for future obesity, type 2 diabetes and cardiovascular diseases [1,2]. An infant born to a mother who experienced poor pregnancy outcomes is at increased risk for preterm birth, macrosomia and growth restriction, catch-up growth, adiposity and insulin resistance [3–5]. This increased risk for metabolic disease is not only limited to infancy or childhood, but is carried into adulthood [6,7].

One of the key factors for achieving optimal pregnancy outcomes is energy balance or the relationship between energy intake, energy expenditure and energy storage in maternal and fetal tissues. The energy intake requirement for a pregnant woman reflects the amount of energy needed to support maternal and fetal metabolism (energy expenditure) and fetal growth and accumulation of energy depots during pregnancy (energy storage). Individual energy requirements depend on numerous factors such as maternal pregravid body size, physical activity, and the physiological demands of pregnancy in each trimester.

Between 1980 and 2010, various groups studied the energy requirements of pregnant women (Table 1). However, these studies come with limitations which are seldom considered when translating the findings into energy requirement recommendations. First, except for one study [8], the energy costs of weight gain are estimated based on all women studied. As such, women with excess weight gain likely cause an overestimation of the energy intake requirements because they deposited more energy than necessary, and their larger body size caused larger energy expenditure. Second, only one study estimated energy costs for recommended weight gain [8], but classification of both maternal pregravid body mass index (BMI) and recommendations for weight gain in pregnancy have since been revised. Third, women with obesity are significantly underrepresented. In 2014, the prevalence of obesity in women of childbearing age was 37% [9], whereas only three women with obesity have been enrolled in energy requirement studies in total [10]. Similarly, the prevalence of obesity is even larger among women of ethnic minorities (African American 57%, Hispanics 43%), yet the vast majority of women studied were Caucasian. These are important considerations for the assessment of energy requirements because both obesity and race have well-established effects on energy expenditure. The observation that offspring of African-American mothers are already prone to obesity suggests that energy metabolism may not only be differently regulated between races, but that this differential regulation is transmitted from one generation to the next, independent of environmental factors or lifestyle. Lastly, the main determinant of energy expenditure is body weight and thus, due to weight gain, energy expenditure increases during pregnancy. An accurate estimation of the energy costs that are a result of the increase in body weight as compared to the increased metabolic rate per body mass, or due to the fetus requires appropriate adjustment for the increase in weight gain. Herein, we review the energy intake requirements specific to the components of energy expenditure, including resting metabolic rate, fetal development, and physical activity. We also provide an estimate of the energy required to gain the appropriate amount of fat mass that relates to the recommended weight gain.

Table 1. Subject Characteristics of Cohorts in Energy Requirement Studies of Pregnancy.

First Author	Measurement Time Points	Cohort Size	Ethnicity	Age	BMI	Excess GWG
	Weeks Gestation	N	White, AA, Other			
Butte, UW [10]	0, 22, 36	17	15, 0, 2	31 ± 4	18.9 ± 0.8	18%
Butte, NW [10]	0, 22, 36	34	24, 4, 5	30 ± 3	22.1 ± 1.5	35%
Butte, OV/OB [10]	0, 22, 36	12	9, 2, 1	31 ± 5	28.8 ± 2.6	100%
Forsum[1] [11]	0, 17, 30	22		29 ± 4	22.3 ± 3.1	
Forsum[2] [11]	0, 36	19		28 ± 4	22.1 ± 3.4	
Goldberg [12]	0, 6, 12, 18, 24, 30, 36	12	12, 0, 0	29 ± 3	23.0 ± 3.3	
Kopp [13]	0, 9, 25, 35	10		29 ± 5	23.1 ± 2.1	10%
Lof [14]	0, 14, 34	23		30 ± 4	24.2 ± 4.8	
Most [15]	15, 36	54	28, 22, 4	28 ± 5	35.8 ± 5.0	67%

Age and BMI (body mass index) are presented as mean ± SD at enrollment. AA: African-American, Others: Hispanic, Asian, Biracial, 'Other', Excess GWG: gestational weight gain exceeding the guidelines at the time (1990), UW: underweight, NW: normal weight, OV: overweight, OB: obesity, Forsum[1] and Forsum[2] indicate the two different cohorts in the study: both measured before pregnancy, but at different times during gestation; Butte reported data per BMI class: 'UW' indicates underweight: BMI ≤ 19.8 kg/m^2, 'NW' indicates normal weight: BMI 19.8–26 kg/m^2, and 'OV/OB' indicates overweight/obesity: BMI ≥ 26 kg/m^2.

To assist women and healthcare providers in achieving healthy rates of gestational weight gain, prediction models have been developed to estimate energy intake requirements. In the final Section 5 of this review, we discuss the accuracy, strengths and limitations of these prediction models and propose future directions for studies that are needed to better understand the high prevalence of excess gestational weight gain among pregnant women.

2. Overview of Energy Intake Requirements of Healthy Pregnancy

2.1. Definition of Energy Requirements

Energy intake requirements are defined as dietary intake that is essential for an individual to sustain optimal health outcomes [16]. In a non-pregnant population, this is generally weight maintenance. In that case, the goal is to achieve long-term energy balance, by maintaining an energy intake that approximates energy expenditure. Total daily energy expenditure (TDEE) is the sum of energy expended to support the resting metabolic rate (RMR), diet-induced thermogenesis and physical activity. RMR accounts for 60–80% of TDEE and is dependent on body mass, sex, age and race. Diet-induced thermogenesis or the energy expended in response to the digestion and processing of food accounts for 10% of TDEE. Lastly, activity-related energy expenditure, the most variable component, includes energy expended during activity associated with daily living and structured bouts of exercise. The quality of the diet and type of activity may affect the determinants of energy balance, but these interactions are not discussed.

2.2. Energy Requirements in Pregnancy

Energy intake requirements in pregnancy are defined as dietary intake necessary to support optimal development of maternal tissues as well as to support fetal growth and development [1]. Therefore, requirements encompass energy intake that not only balances maternal and fetal energy expenditure but also provides additional energy for fetal growth, as well as the growth of maternal tissues such as fat mass, breast tissue, uterus and placenta. Thus, energy intake requirements in pregnancy are not aimed at weight maintenance, but for appropriate rates of weight gain, which in turn, minimizes the risks of adverse outcomes in the mother and her offspring.

For women of normal weight (body mass index 18.5 to 24.9 kg/m^2), the recommended amount of weight gain during pregnancy is 11.5 to 16 kg, according to the 2009 Institute of Medicine guidelines [1]. Within this range of weight gain, the risk for non-elective cesarean delivery, postpartum weight retention, preterm birth, small- or large-for-gestational-age birth, and childhood obesity is minimized. The weight gain recommendations are inversely proportional to maternal body mass index at conception and, therefore, allow for more weight gain for women classified as underweight (12.5–18 kg) and less weight gain for women who are classified as overweight (7–11.5 kg) and with obesity (5–9 kg). For women with obesity, the weight gain recommendations have recently been challenged. Acknowledging limitations of available data [17–19], the Institute of Medicine was unable to suggest weight gain recommendations by obesity class [1]. Since then epidemiological studies propose that optimal pregnancy outcomes in women with severe obesity (body mass index $\geq$ 35 kg/m^2) are achieved if weight gain is restricted to less than 5 kg or weight is maintained across pregnancy [20–26].

3. Energy Requirements for Expenditure

3.1. Total Energy Expenditure

3.1.1. Appropriate Adjustment of Energy Expenditure Data

As in non-pregnant populations, there is a linear association between energy expenditure and body size in pregnant women such that energy expenditure is higher in heavier women, see Figure 1 [10,27,28]. To be able to assess metabolic or behavioral differences or adaptations in energy expenditure between women, energy expenditure needs to be compared independent of body weight and this requires appropriate statistical adjustment of the raw (or absolute) data [27]. The consensus among energy metabolism experts is that the relationship between energy expenditure and body weight (or body composition) is best characterized by a linear regression with an intercept greater than 0 ($EE = a + b \times BW$ or $EE = a + b \times FFM + c \times FM$), and not by a simple ratio ($EE = b \times BW$). A ratio assumes that the intercept of the relationship between energy expenditure and weight (or body composition) is equal to 0, see Figure 1A. Using a linear regression rather than a ratio to describe the relationship between body weight and energy expenditure reduces the coefficients 'b' for body weight (regression: 11.97, ratio: 21.56), improves the fit of the regression line (regression $R^2 = 0.66$, ratio $R^2 = 0.22$), and eliminates systematic bias for the estimation of individual variability, see Figure 1B,C. Using a ratio, women with lower body weight will be falsely characterized as having high energy expenditure ('Residual'), and vice versa, women with more body weight will be falsely characterized as having low energy expenditure.

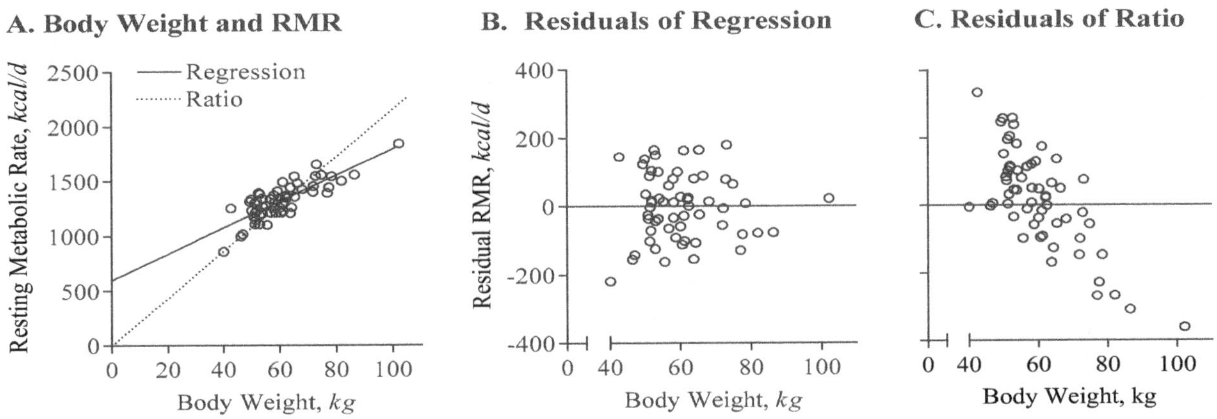

Figure 1. Appropriate adjustment of energy-expenditure data. (**A**) The association between body weight and resting metabolic rate is characterized by linear regression (solid line, RMR[*kcal/d*] = 598 + 11.97 × BW[*kg*], $R^2 = 0.66$) and ratio (pointed line, RMR[*kcal/d*] = 21.56 × BW[*kg*], $R^2 = 0.22$); of note, logarithmic or polynomial approximations do not improve the prediction of RMR (for both, $R^2 = 0.67$). (**B**) Residual resting metabolic rate (RMR), calculated as measured RMR minus predicted RMR; based on the regression equation in (**A**); the residuals show no structural over- or underestimate based on body weight. (**C**) Residual RMR, based on the ratio equation; women with increased body weight have significant lower residual RMR, and would be considered as having a low adjusted metabolic rate.

3.1.2. Measurement by Doubly Labeled Water

Ideally, TDEE is objectively measured in free-living conditions by doubly labeled water [29]. The principle behind doubly labeled water is to indirectly assess carbon dioxide production from the differential dilution rates of deuterium (^2H) and oxygen-18 isotope (^{18}O) after a prescribed dose of the isotope-cocktail is ingested. After ingestion of the water, deuterium dilutes into the body water pool and is excreted from the body via urine, sweat and water vapor in breath. In contrast, the oxygen isotope is excreted not only through the loss of water but also as carbon dioxide. Thus, the difference in dilution rates of ^2H and ^{18}O is proportional to carbon dioxide production. Then, estimation of TDEE from carbon dioxide production requires an assumption or quantification of the oxygen consumption, which can be inferred by measurement or estimation of the respiratory quotient (EE[*kcal/d*] = VCO_2 [*L/d*] × (1.1 + 3.9/RQ)) [29]. In most cases, the respiratory quotient or the ratio of carbon dioxide production to oxygen consumption will not be measured throughout the doubly labeled water period, and thus, requires assumptions. The best estimate for the respiratory quotient, which describes the macronutrient composition of the energy expenditure, is the food quotient, which describes the macronutrient composition of the energy intake. In most (pregnant and non-pregnant) studies, a respiratory quotient equivalent to a standard western-style diet of 0.86 is used (35–40% energy from fat) [30]. In 12 h overnight measurements of the energy expenditure, we observed no significant deviation from this commonly used value (unpublished).

The use of doubly labeled water to estimate TDEE is limited to a period of 7–14 days. Measurements of energy expenditure throughout pregnancy, therefore, require repeated, independent assessments of TDEE at the beginning and end of the assessment period of interest. The mean energy expenditure throughout pregnancy can then be calculated by the trapezoid method [31–35]. A limitation of this approach is the assumption of linearity between TDEE measurements. More frequent measurements of body weight and activity throughout this period, which is more feasible than TDEE, increase specificity, e.g., towards trimester-specific requirements.

3.1.3. First Trimester

Groups have performed cross-sectional comparisons of TDEE between pregnant and non-pregnant women [36–39]; however, these are outside of the scope of the current review. In Figure 2, we show published, time-series data of TDEE throughout pregnancy. On average, TDEE increases by approximately 15 kcal per day per week or by 420 kcal per day from pre-pregnancy to delivery. Prospective measurements of TDEE prior to pregnancy and in the first trimester have been reported in four studies of non-obese women [10–12,14]. One study included women with obesity (n = 3), but they were combined with overweight women [10]; another did not report changes in body weight during pregnancy [13]. On average, TDEE does not change during the first trimester, at an average increase in body weight of 3.2 kg [10–12,14]. Based on reported average changes in body mass and composition in these studies, we estimated the changes in TDEE after adjustment for changes in body mass. Using the linear regression equation of TDEE proposed by Gilmore and Butte et al. [31] that estimates TDEE from fat-free mass, fat mass and age ($TDEE_{pred}[kcal/d] = 1528 + 29.4 \times FFM[kg] + 13.6 \times FM[kg] - 21 \times age[years]$), body-weight-adjusted TDEE declines by 55 kcal/d from pre-pregnancy until 13 weeks of gestation across all studies. The components of TDEE that contribute to this decline could be of metabolic and/or behavioral origin, which we will discuss in the following sections.

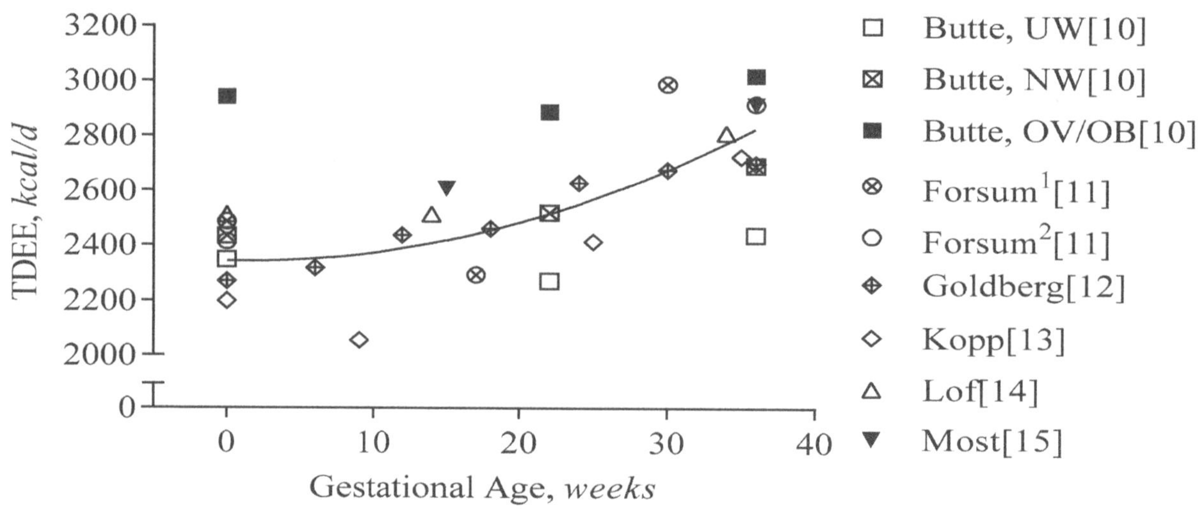

Figure 2. Total Daily Energy Expenditure during Gestation. Total daily energy expenditure (TDEE) is presented per study and gestational age (GA). The regression line represents the average increase during gestation ($TDEE[kcal/d] = 2343 - 1 \times GA[weeks] + 0.4 \times GA^2[weeks]$, $R^2 = 0.62$). Forsum[1] and Forsum[2] indicate the two different cohorts in the study: both measured before pregnancy, but at different times during gestation; Butte reported the changes in TDEE per BMI class: 'UW' indicates underweight: BMI ≤ 19.8 kg/m^2, 'NW' indicates normal weight: BMI 19.8–26 kg/m^2, and 'OV/OB' indicates overweight/obesity: BMI ≥ 26 kg/m^2.

3.1.4. Second and Third Trimester

Only half a dozen studies have obtained prospective measurements of TDEE during the second and third trimester of pregnancy using doubly labeled water [10–15]. On average, TDEE increased by 18 kcal/d/week or ~420 kcal/d from week 13 to 36, at an average increase in body weight of 10.3 kg [10–15]. After adjusting for the change in body weight, the increase in TDEE was 170 kcal/d from early to late pregnancy (13 to 36 weeks). Using individual data from 112 women [10,15], we estimated that after adjustment for body weight change, the increase in TDEE was only ~75 kcal/d; 110 kcal/d in non-obese women and 45 kcal/d in women with obesity.

Based on these findings, energy expenditures from the second to the third trimester, are linearly related to weight gain with an estimated 45–170 kcal/d increase. Aside from metabolic and/or behavioral adaptations to pregnancy by the mother, the additional increase in TDEE also reflects the contribution of the fetus, since fetal metabolic rate has a disproportionately high energy expenditure to mass (100 kcal/d/kg body weight vs. ~25 kcal/d/kg in adults) [40,41]. The metabolic contribution of the placenta to TDEE is poorly understood but is likely an additional contributing factor. Therefore, to understand the individual determinants of energy requirements in pregnancy, it is important to assess the components of TDEE separately.

3.2. Basal Metabolism

3.2.1. Measurement by Indirect Calorimetry

Differentiation of the metabolic and behavioral adaptations to pregnancy requires the assessment of individual components of TDEE, i.e., resting metabolic rate (RMR), diet-induced thermogenesis and activity-related energy expenditure. The largest component of TDEE is RMR, which accounts for 60–80% of daily energy requirements [10–12,14,28]. In majority of studies, RMR is measured by indirect calorimetry using a bedside ventilated hood system. In contrast to using doubly labeled water, oxygen consumption and carbon dioxide production are directly measured. The measurement of RMR occurs during fasting conditions over 30–60 min and extrapolated to 24 h. The RMR measurements have a high degree of accuracy, estimated at 3% [42], by test-retest reliability studies.

3.2.2. First Trimester

As with TDEE, only a few studies have assessed RMR before pregnancy and in early pregnancy. In Figure 3, we present data from studies with prospective assessments of RMR and TDEE. On average, RMR increased by 60 kcal/d during the first trimester (pre-pregnancy until week 13 [10–12,14] weeks gestation), and by 20 kcal/d after adjustment for the increase in body weight. A comparable increase in RMR (+30 kcal/d) was observed using individual data obtained by Butte and colleagues [10]. Thus, aside from changes in energy expenditure due to body weight, metabolic rate increases to a small extent, likely due to increased cardiac output [43] and/or hormonal changes, e.g., progesterone, human chorionic gonadotropin [44].

3.2.3. Second and Third Trimester

During the second and third trimester, RMR increases by 390 kcal/d (or 17 kcal/d/week). Considering the change in body weight, the increase in RMR across studies was predicted at 170 kcal/d [31]. Thus >50% of the increase in RMR (215 kcal/d) is not explained by body weight but by the increased metabolic cost of pregnancy [10–12,14] that includes increased cardiac output [43], increased work of breathing [45], fetal activity, metabolic rate of fetal tissues [40].

3.3. Physical Activity/Exercise

Physical activity throughout pregnancy is crucial for healthy gestation, despite the increased physiological demands placed on the body [46–48]. Accordingly, many specialized guidelines and recommendations have been established [49–53] to promote women to accrue sufficient activity throughout gestation. These guidelines recommend at least 150 min of moderate physical activity every week. In support of these physical activity guidelines, meta-analyses [46–48] report that habitual exercise reduces the risks of excessive gestational weight gain by 32%, gestational diabetes by 38%, hypertension by 39%, moderate depression by 67% and of macrosomia by 39%. Despite the concomitant benefits of following physical activity guidelines during pregnancy, presently, less than 50% of women adhere to the guidelines [54–58].

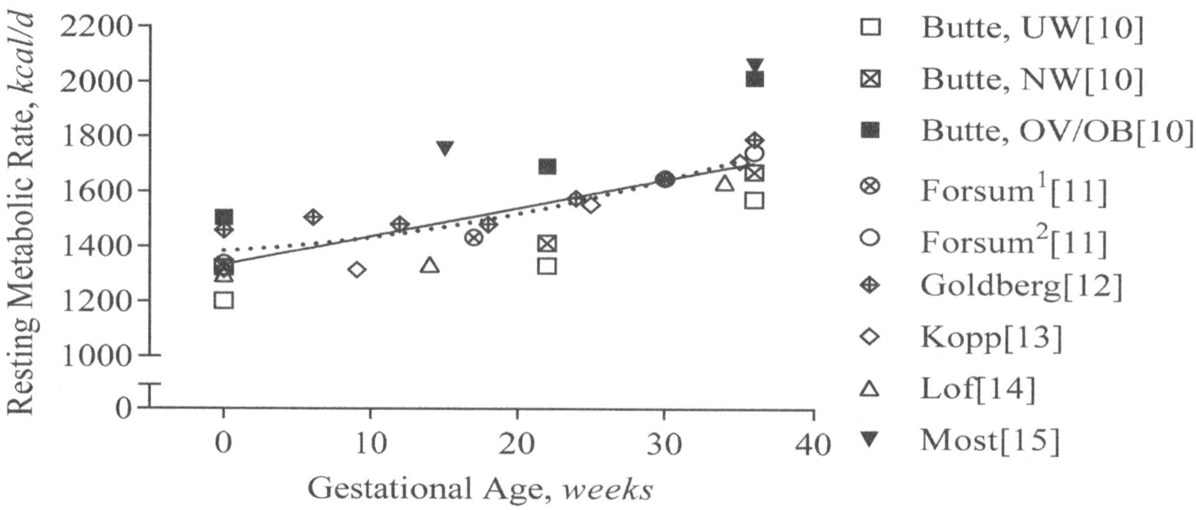

Figure 3. Resting Metabolic Rate during Gestation. Resting metabolic rate is presented per study and gestational age (GA). The regression line represents the average increase in the resting metabolic rate during gestation (RMR[*kcal/d*] = 1334 + 10.3 × GA[*weeks*], $R^2 = 0.55$, using non-linear regression (pointed line) did not improve the prediction, $R^2 = 0.57$). Forsum[1] and Forsum[2] indicate the two different cohorts in the study: both measured before pregnancy, but at different times during gestation; Butte reported the changes in RMR per BMI class: 'UW' indicates underweight: BMI ≤ 19.8 kg/m^2, 'NW' indicates normal weight: BMI 19.8–26 kg/m^2, and 'OV/OB' indicates overweight/obesity: BMI ≥ 26 kg/m^2.

3.3.1. Measurement of Physical Activity

Physical activity can be quantified through measurement of the energy expenditure related to physical activity or through measurement of body movement. Using available calorimetry data, the easiest manner of quantifying activity-related energy expenditure is by subtracting metabolic rate and diet-induced thermogenesis (10% of TDEE) from total daily energy expenditure (activity-related EE = TDEE − 0.1x TDEE − RMR). Because body size not only affects RMR but also activity-related energy expenditure, the most widely used adjustment is determined by assessing the physical activity level (PAL), calculated as TDEE divided by RMR (PAL = TDEE/RMR). Of note, PAL may underestimate physical activity levels due to the increased RMR during pregnancy, but validation studies have yet to be performed. To assess the inter-individual variability within a cohort or over time, activity-related energy expenditure can also be assessed as the residual of the linear regression, TDEE = a + b × RMR; this value is positive for subjects with higher physical activity than average and is negative for subjects with lower physical activity than average independent of metabolic body size. Because residual activity-related energy expenditure is adjusted for the RMR, this value is directly proportional to the amount of physical activity. Calorimetric assessments of activity-related energy expenditure are limited by their relatively high costs and are, therefore, limited to small cohorts.

Devices that objectively measure physical activity such as accelerometers (i.e., Actigraph, Actical, RT3, FitBit) are widely used in scientific studies, and by the public to overcome the limitations associated with calorimetric measurements. Accelerometry assesses the magnitude and duration of movement and gravitational forces of activity to yield outcome variables such as time-stamped activity counts, duration and intensity. An advantageous feature that some accelerometers possess (e.g., Actical) is the inclusion of a pedometer or step counter, which are shown to be valuable objective tools for assessing physical activity interventions in pregnant women [59–61]. Accelerometers can be combined with heart rate monitors to obtain a more objective measure of intensity, relative to an individual's fitness level [62,63]. To obtain a calorimetric estimate of physical activity (or total energy expenditure), accelerometry-variables are imputed into proprietary equations that predict, but do not measure, energy expenditure from body weight, height, and age of an individual.

Lastly, the easiest, cheapest and most established method for the evaluation of the level of physical activity include physical activity questionnaires, physical activity recall records and diaries. Specifically, during pregnancy, the 'gold standard' Physical Activity Questionnaire (PPAQ) is a widely accepted tool to assess the level of physical activity [64]. This self-administered questionnaire requires that participants report time spent in 32 different categories of activities including household/caregiving (13 activities), occupational (5 activities), sports/exercise (8 activities), transportation (3 activities), and in-activities (3 activities) [64]. Limitations of self-report methods include their low accuracy and reliability [65–67], as demonstrated by a significant overestimation of physical activity compared to accelerometers [65,68–70].

3.3.2. First Trimester

In Figure 4, we provide the physical activity level data of the calorimetry studies of pregnancy. During the first trimester, physical activity declined minimally in energy-requirement studies (−60 kcal/d, −2%, −0.08 PAL). Early in pregnancy, physical-activity-related energy expenditure accounted for 26–39% of energy expenditure in non-obese women [10–12,14] and for 23% in women with obesity [28].

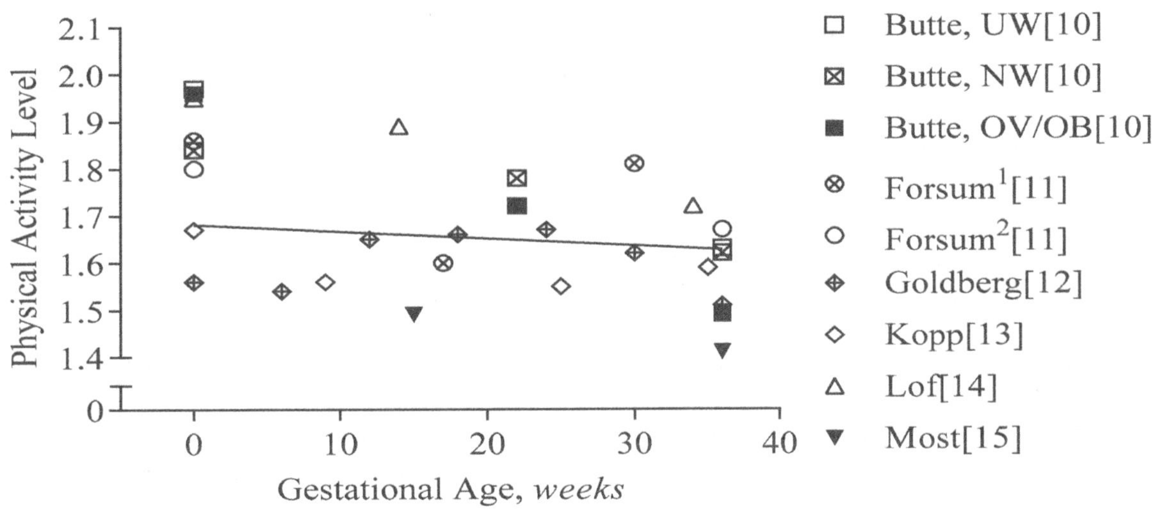

Figure 4. Physical activity level during gestation. Physical activity level is presented per study and gestational age (GA). The regression line represents the average decline in the physical activity level during gestation (PAL = 1.68 − 0.0015 × GA[*weeks*], R^2 = 0.02). Forsum[1] and Forsum[2] indicate the two different cohorts in the study: both measured before pregnancy, but at different times during gestation; Butte reported the changes in PAL per BMI class: 'UW' indicates underweight: BMI ≤ 19.8 kg/m^2, 'NW' indicates normal weight: BMI 19.8–26 kg/m^2, and 'OV/OB' indicates overweight/obesity: BMI ≥ 26 kg/m^2.

3.3.3. Second and Third Trimester

During the second and third trimesters, physical-activity-related energy expenditure decreased further by 3% (PAL, −0.12) [10–12,14]. Importantly, there is a significant variation between the studies; some report an increase in PAL of 0.37 [11], and others a decrease of −0.38 in women with overweight and obesity [10]; in a cohort of women who were exclusively obese (n = 54), PAL declined by 0.12 [15].

The variability in changes in activity is confirmed by studies using accelerometry. Some data show a decrease in physical activity level [55,71], while others reported no change [55,72,73]. The discrepancy in the literature may also relate to inconsistent methods of measurement, i.e., self-reported questionnaires vs. different various objective measures. Among a wide variety of demographic variables that may account for differences in physically active and inactive pregnant women, education and socio-economic status are consistently reported as predictors [54,74]. Therefore, while health care professionals should be encouraging all women to adopt an active lifestyle adherent to the recommendations of ≥150 min per week, they need to be cognizant of a woman's demographic and socio-economic status and ensure their guidance is relevant and feasible.

4. Energy Cost for Weight Gain

4.1. Determination of Appropriate Weight Gain and Composition

In addition to the energy intake requirements needed to balance energy expenditure, total energy intake requirements also encompass energy deposition which during pregnancy includes maternal fat accumulation and fetal growth. The amount and composition of healthy weight gain are highly variable between women, particularly by BMI class [8]. Large epidemiological studies have assessed the range of gestational weight gain for each BMI class that are associated with the lowest risk for adverse pregnancy outcomes [17–19]. Based on these studies, the recommendations for appropriate weight gain are inversely related to pregravid BMI [1]. Translating these weight gain goals into energy intake requirements involves an understanding of weight gain composition because the components, i.e., fat mass and fat-free mass, have different contributions to the total weight gain and have different energy densities.

The differences in recommended weight gain have been attributed to the variance in fat mass accumulation, but not fat-free mass [8,15,75,76]. Thus, recommendations for higher weight gain, e.g., in underweight or normal weight as compared to overweight and obese women, imply that more fat mass is accumulated while the variability in fat-free mass is smaller, and from the perspective of energy content, less significant.

In most pregnancy studies, the density of fat-free mass is assumed to be 771 kcal/kg and the density of fat mass 9500 kcal/kg [10,31,34,35]. Thus, the determination of energy intake requirements for pregnancy is developed through the energy balance equation as:

$$\text{EIR}\ [kcal/d] = \text{TDEE} + (771[kcal/kg] \times \text{dFFM}[kg] + 9500\ [kcal/kg] \times \text{dFM}[kg])$$

in which EIR is the estimated energy intake requirement, TDEE is the average total energy expenditure during pregnancy, and dFM and dFFM are the changes in fat and fat-free mass during pregnancy.

4.2. Measurement of Body Composition in Pregnancy

The measurement of changes in body composition during pregnancy is challenging (time-constraints) and costly, thus limited to small cohorts. Available methods include air displacement plethysmography, isotope dilution, skinfold thickness measurement, bioimpedance, and magnetic resonance imaging, which we have recently reviewed for their applications in pregnancy [77]. While all methods can be used in pregnancy, the trade-off between cost, time and precision determines the best choice. The most important consideration for the use of all methods in pregnancy is the adjustment for an increase in fat-free mass hydration during pregnancy. Based on classic data by van Raaij et al. [78], we have developed a prediction equation to estimate fat-free mass hydration dependent on gestational age that allows standardization of methods across studies:

$$\text{Hydration FFM}\ [L/kg] = 0.724 + 0.00008484 \times \text{GA}[weeks] + 0.00001435 \times \text{GA}[weeks]^2$$

where FFM is fat-free mass and GA is gestational age; $R^2 = 0.998$, $p < 0.001$, and

$$\text{Density FFM}\ [kg/L] = 1.1 - 0.00002988 \times \text{GA}[weeks] - 0.00000731 \times \text{GA}[weeks]^2$$

where FFM is fat-free mass and GA is gestational age; $R^2 = 0.999$, $p < 0.001$.

4.3. First Trimester

Independent of BMI class, the weight gain recommendations during the first trimester are 0.5 to 2.0 kg for all women [1]. To date, no study has assessed the composition of early pregnancy weight gain, specifically for women that adhered to this recommendation. Using a conservative estimate for the energy density of overall weight gain (7400 kcal/kg) [79], the energy requirements for weight gain in early pregnancy are ~3,700–14,800 kcal, or 40–165 kcal/d over 13 weeks.

4.4. Second and Third Trimester

The accumulation of fat-free mass during the third and second trimester is ~7–8 kg and comparable between women of different BMI classes [8,10,77]. Assuming an energy density of 771 kcal/kg fat-free mass, the energy required to support this fat-free mass accumulation is 5000–6000 kcal or 30–35 kcal per day, while studies report ~4,000–12,000 kcal [80,81] or 20–60 kcal/d. Considering the low energy density of fat-free mass, the variability in fat-free mass accumulation does not strongly impact energy requirements. In contrast, the variability in fat mass accumulation largely affects the energy requirements for weight gain in pregnancy.

Several studies have assessed the energy requirements for weight and fat mass gain during the second and third trimesters, yet few studies have determined these requirements specific to women who gained the recommended amount of weight. Based on Lederman et al. [8], pregnant women with a normal weight and recommended weight gain (BMI 19.8–26 kg/m^2 and 11.5–16 kg, respectively) accumulated ~4 kg of fat mass between 14 and 37 weeks gestation. The energy intake requirements to support this energy deposition in fat is ~240 kcal/d over 22.7 weeks (i.e., 4 kg $\times$ 9500 kcal $\times$ kg^{-1}/159 d = 240 kcal/d). For underweight or overweight women, gains in fat mass were 6.0 and 2.8 kg, and the respective energy intake requirements were 360 kcal/d and 165 kcal/d. For women with obesity, we have recently shown that recommended weight gain is achieved with an average 2.5 kg loss of fat mass (15 to 36 weeks of gestation) [15]. Therefore, instead of women with obesity depositing energy, 160 kcal/d of energy are mobilized from fat mass in the second and third trimester, and can, therefore, be subtracted from energy intake requirements. Given that 160 kcal/d is mobilized from fat tissue, while the accumulation of fat-free mass only requires 20–60 kcal/d, the factor of energy storage in the energy balance equation is negative and thus energy intake in pregnant women with obesity should be lower than energy expenditure.

5. Models that Estimate Energy Intake Requirements

Experimental reports evaluating energy intake requirements have been an essential tool to educate women and clinicians on the optimal energy intake during pregnancy. The Institute of Medicine, using available data at the time published 'Equations to Estimate Energy Requirement for Pregnant Women' (p. 316) [1]. The equation is based on the requirements of non-pregnant women (EIR = 354 − 6.91 × age [*years*] + PA × 9.36 × BW [*kg*] + 726 × height [*m*], in which EIR are estimated energy requirements, PA is physical activity (1.00 for PAL < 1.4, 1.12 for $1.4 \leq$ PAL ≤ 1.59, 1.27 for $1.6 \leq$ PAL ≤ 1.89, and 1.45 for $1.9 \leq$ PAL ≤ 2.5), and BW is body weight. Importantly, by including physical activity as a variable, this model accounts for individual differences in the level and changes in activity. Energy costs for weight gain are assumed to be constant (180 kcal/d).

A dynamic model for the estimation of energy requirements for optimal weight gain has been developed to better acknowledge the different contributions of fat and fat-free mass in different BMI classes [34]. This model based on the most comprehensive studies of energy requirements in women without obesity [10,12,13], estimates the energy requirements to achieve the recommended rate for weight gain. The TDEE in this model is estimated using maternal age, body weight, and height, but not physical activity.

Importantly, both the Institute of Medicine and the model by Thomas and colleagues, have included all available data to develop an energy requirement prediction, and, therefore, have included data of women with excess and inadequate weight gain. Future models can, thus, be improved by restricting models to those women with appropriate weight gain only.

5.1. First Trimester

For the recommended weight gain of 0.5–2 kg in the first trimester [1], the Institute of Medicine and American College of Obstetricians and Gynecologists recommended women maintain pregravid energy intake throughout the first trimester because the energy costs for weight gain are considered minimal [1,82].

The energy intake requirement model suggests that all women should consume an additional 100–200 kcal/d to support first-trimester weight gain, assuming that physical activity does not decline during the first trimester [10,34]. For women with obesity, we have recently shown that the model significantly overestimates energy requirements by 400 kcal/d due to unaccounted lower levels of physical activity as compared to the non-obese cohorts, on which the model is based [28].

Similar to the Institute of Medicine, we estimate the energy requirements to be 50–150 kcal/d. An average decline in physical activity (PAL, −0.08 or −5%, or 60 kcal/d) may compensate those energy costs, but this compensation may differ greatly between individuals.

5.2. Second and Third Trimester

The Institute of Medicine estimates the energy requirements during the second and third trimester to be 340 kcal/d and 452 kcal/d, respectively [83]. The estimate is calculated as the sum of the increased energy expenditure over pregnancy (8 kcal/d/week) and the costs of energy deposition (180 kcal/d). The increase in energy expenditure is consistent with our estimates, whereas the proposed energy cost for deposition neglects BMI-specific weight gain recommendations. In 2016, the American College of Obstetricians and Gynecologists have, thus, adjusted their recommendations by acknowledging that 'if you were overweight or obese, you may need fewer extra calories' [82], without specific guidance.

The energy intake requirements model by Thomas et al. [34] estimated surplus energy requirements to be only 400–600 kcal/d for underweight and normal-weight women, and 220–350 kcal per day for overweight or obese pregnant women [34]. Because our estimates are based on the same data, they agree for underweight, normal-weight and overweight women. However, the model was developed from women without obesity or with obesity coupled with excess gestational weight gain, and, therefore, for women with obesity, the model overestimates fat mass gains and thus energy requirements [15].

During the second and third trimester, we estimate that the energy requirements for expenditure increase by 15 kcal/d per week, half of which is explained by the increase in body weight and half by increased metabolic rate largely due to cardiac output and fetal metabolism. The energy requirements for recommended weight gain differ by BMI class and range between 360 kcal/d for underweight women, to −165 kcal/d for women with obesity, with the variation explained by fat mass accumulation [8,77] at a constant fat-free mass accumulation equivalent of ~50 kcal/d.

6. Limitations and Practical Considerations

6.1. First Trimester

In clinical practice and research settings, it is challenging to quantify changes occurring in the first trimester. Such an assessment requires a measurement prior to pregnancy and, ideally, close to conception. In most studies, pre-pregnancy weights are estimated or abstracted from charts, which lacks the control required to define energy requirements accurately. Moreover, access to weight data only precludes interpretation of changes in body composition. Given the importance of the changes during the first trimester, innovative study designs need to be developed to overcome this barrier.

6.2. *Variability in Energy Expenditure*

Based on findings by Ravussin et al. in the late 1980s [84], studies have investigated whether variability in the RMR would increase the risk of increased fat accumulation. Indeed, multiple studies [27,85–87] support this hypothesis, showing that women with low RMR, that is residual RMR adjusted for body weight or fat-free mass, gained more weight than women with higher adjusted RMR. However, these studies adjusted energy expenditure using ratios, which prohibits them from reliable conclusions. Nevertheless, in a re-analysis of the data generated by Butte (1994), we confirmed the hypothesis of excess weight gain in women with lower adjusted RMR, who were not obese [27]; however, we did not observe this in women with obesity [15]. The origin of these differences in RMR remains to be determined since body mass and composition explain only ~70% of its variation [28].

One of the determinants of energy expenditure is race. As in non-pregnant cohorts [88], RMR in pregnant African-American women is lower than in Caucasian women (−80 kcal/d or −5%) [33]. This difference does not change over time and, therefore, adjusting energy intake recommendations early in pregnancy is likely sufficient to consider the lower energy requirements of African-American women during pregnancy.

We have reported that TDEE adjusted for body composition is ~600 kcal/d lower in women with obesity [28] as compared to women without obesity [10,27,31]. Obesity status itself, after adjustment for body weight, does not seem to affect RMR [28]. The difference in TDEE likely relates to differences in physical activity, the timing of energy expenditure measurements and ethnicity of the cohorts. Indeed, women with obesity were less active than women without obesity (PAL, 1.5 vs. 1.8) [28]; energy expenditure in the cohort with obesity was measured ~8 weeks earlier than in the cohort without obesity (8 weeks × 15 kcal/week = 120 kcal/d) [10,31,77]; and 50% of women in the obese cohort were African-American women, who have significantly lower energy expenditure (−8%) [33].

6.3. *Communication of Recommendations*

The communication of energy intake recommendations must be improved. Studies show that only one in four women feels appropriately informed on weight gain or energy intake goals suitable for pregnancy [89]. Aside from the notion that some form of communication has to be initiated, qualitative studies are needed to inform how such information should be best communicated to patients. For example, based on our recent study in women with obesity, the same energy intake target can be expressed differently; e.g., 2700 kcal/d, 17 kcal/d/kg body weight, the diet should be equivalent to early pregnancy energy expenditure, or eat ~5% less during pregnancy. Possible ways of communicating these results to patients (pregnant women) that may be received and perceived differently are 'try and follow the energy intake requirement estimates using this equation/model' [1,34], 'try to maintain your usual diet throughout pregnancy', or 'try to eat 5% fewer calories than you are expending'. Importantly, such recommendations need to consider potential declines in physical activity. More work is needed to establish best practices for knowledge translation and dissemination of this information. How to best inform and guide women to make appropriate decisions and choices while pregnant is an active field of research.

7. Summary

In summary, energy intake requirements during the first trimester are minimally different from requirements before pregnancy (Table 2). Therefore, the Institute of Medicine model adopted from non-pregnancy provides valid estimates of energy requirements to match energy expenditure. During the second and third trimester, the development of the fetus and pregnancy-associated changes in the mother occur, i.e., increased blood volume, cardiac output, increase energy requirements by ~390 kcal/d, with small variations between women of differing body sizes. We estimate that 50% of this increase is proportional to the increase in body mass, and 50% is due to the increased metabolic costs of pregnancy and metabolic rate of the fetus. However, the energy requirements for weight gain differ significantly.

We estimate that to achieve the recommendations for healthy gestational weight gain [83], underweight women store 360 kcal/d as fat tissue, normal-weight women store ~240 kcal/d, overweight women store 165 kcal/d, and women with obesity do not store energy at all, but instead mobilize 160 kcal/d from adipose tissue energy stores.

Table 2. Summary of changes in body mass, composition and energy expenditure, proportional and independent of body weight changes.

	Tri-Mester	Body Weight	Fat-Free Mass	Fat Mass	TDEE	TDEE, Pred	TDEE, Res	RMR	RMR, Pred	RMR, Res
Non-Obesity										
Forsum1	1	2.1	0.2	1.9	−146	26	−172	73	25	48
Goldberg	1	1.7	0.2	1.5	181	22	159	26	21	5
Butte, UW	1	4.6	2.1	2.5	−45	91	−136	76	67	9
Butte, NW	1	3.4	1.7	1.7	51	68	−18	53	50	3
Butte, OV/OB	1	5.0	1.9	3.1	−31	93	−124	111	71	41
Lof	1	2.3	0.9	1.4	2	41	−39	33	32	1
Average	1	3.2	1.2	2.0	2	57	−55	62	44	18
Non-Obesity										
Forsum1	2 and 3	11.5	10.4	1.1	1226	312	914	381	199	181
Goldberg	2 and 3	8.0	5.9	2.0	252	193	59	298	129	168
Butte, UW	2 and 3	8.7	7.1	1.6	274	221	54	399	145	254
Butte, NW	2 and 3	11.7	8.9	2.8	284	290	−5	427	192	235
Butte, OV/OB	2 and 3	13.1	9.7	3.5	219	323	−104	531	215	316
Lof	2 and 3	10.8	7.5	3.3	341	256	85	349	173	176
Average		10.6	8.2	2.4	433	266	167	397	176	222
Obesity										
Most	2 and 3	8.5	8.2	0.3	335	237	98	335	150	185

Changes in kilograms and kcal per day. TDEE: Total daily energy expenditure, Pred: predicted, changes proportional to changes in body weight, Res: Residual, changes independent of changes in body weight, RMR: resting metabolic rate. Forsum1 indicate the two different cohorts in the study: both measured before pregnancy, but at different times during gestation; Butte reported the changes in PAL per BMI class: 'UW' indicates underweight: BMI ≤ 19.8 kg/m^2, 'NW' indicates normal weight: BMI 19.8–26 kg/m^2, and 'OV/OB' indicates overweight/obesity: BMI ≥ 26 kg/m^2.

Current methods to assess energy intake requirements are limited in their prediction of energy expenditure and energy storage. Specifically, body composition and physical activity data during the first trimester are scarce. Given the importance of the first trimester for placental and fetal development [90], more studies are required to better inform patients and clinicians how to achieve healthier pregnancies. Particularly in women with obesity, energy expenditure (i.e., physical activity) and energy deposition are overestimated and thus would allow women to consume an amount of energy that would result in excess gestational weight gain. The level of physical activity is the most variable component of energy expenditure and requires consideration on an individual level. Commercially available accelerometers or built-in devices in mobile phones may assist women to maintain or increase their level of physical activity during pregnancy; currently, less than 50% of women meet the recommendations by leading institutions dedicated to promoting a healthy pregnancy. Adherence to recommendations related to energy intake and energy expenditure (physical activity) are key factors that will assist women in maintaining an appropriate energy balance thereby supporting the needs of pregnancy and the growing fetus.

Author Contributions: Conceptualization, J.M, K.B.A., L.M.R.; methodology, J.M., S.D.; software, J.M.; validation, K.B.A., F.H., L.M.R.; formal analysis, J.M.; investigation, J.M., S.D., F.H., K.B.A., L.M.R.; K.B.A., L.M.R.; data curation, J.M.; writing—original draft preparation, J.M., S.D.; writing—review and editing, L.M.R.; visualization, J.M.; supervision, K.B.A., L.M.R; project administration, K.B.A, L.M.R.; funding acquisition, K.B.A., L.M.R.

Acknowledgments: We would like to acknowledge Drs Nancy Butte and Anne Gilmore for their work on energy requirements in women without obesity, and for providing us with individual data of this study.

References

1. Institute of Medicine (US) and National Research Council (US) Committee to Reexamine IOM Pregnancy Weight Guidelines. Determining optimal weight gain. In *Weight Gain during Pregnancy: Reexamining the Guidelines*; Rasmussen, K.M., Yaktine, A.L., Eds.; National Academies Press: Washington, DC, USA, 2009.
2. Kominiarek, M.A.; Peaceman, A.M. Gestational weight gain. *Am. J. Obstet. Gynecol.* **2017**, *217*, 642–651. [CrossRef] [PubMed]
3. Laitinen, J.; Jaaskelainen, A.; Hartikainen, A.L.; Sovio, U.; Vaarasmaki, M.; Pouta, A.; Kaakinen, M.; Jarvelin, M.R. Maternal weight gain during the first half of pregnancy and offspring obesity at 16 years: A prospective cohort study. *BJOG* **2012**, *119*, 716–723. [CrossRef] [PubMed]
4. Catalano, P.M.; Farrell, K.; Thomas, A.; Huston-Presley, L.; Mencin, P.; de Mouzon, S.H.; Amini, S.B. Perinatal risk factors for childhood obesity and metabolic dysregulation. *Am. J. Clin. Nutr.* **2009**, *90*, 1303–1313. [CrossRef] [PubMed]
5. Sridhar, S.B.; Darbinian, J.; Ehrlich, S.F.; Markman, M.A.; Gunderson, E.P.; Ferrara, A.; Hedderson, M.M. Maternal gestational weight gain and offspring risk for childhood overweight or obesity. *Am. J. Obstet. Gynecol.* **2014**, *211*, 259.e1–259.e8. [CrossRef] [PubMed]
6. Reynolds, R.M.; Allan, K.M.; Raja, E.A.; Bhattacharya, S.; McNeill, G.; Hannaford, P.C.; Sarwar, N.; Lee, A.J.; Bhattacharya, S.; Norman, J.E. Maternal obesity during pregnancy and premature mortality from cardiovascular event in adult offspring: Follow-up of 1 323 275 person years. *BMJ* **2013**, *347*, f4539. [CrossRef] [PubMed]
7. Mamun, A.A.; Kinarivala, M.; O'Callaghan, M.J.; Williams, G.M.; Najman, J.M.; Callaway, L.K. Associations of excess weight gain during pregnancy with long-term maternal overweight and obesity: Evidence from 21 y postpartum follow-up. *Am. J. Clin. Nutr.* **2010**, *91*, 1336–1341. [CrossRef] [PubMed]
8. Lederman, S.A.; Paxton, A.; Heymsfield, S.B.; Wang, J.; Thornton, J.; Pierson, R.N., Jr. Body fat and water changes during pregnancy in women with different body weight and weight gain. *Obstet. Gynecol.* **1997**, *90*, 483–488. [CrossRef]
9. Flegal, K.M.; Kruszon-Moran, D.; Carroll, M.D.; Fryar, C.D.; Ogden, C.L. Trends in obesity among adults in the united states, 2005 to 2014. *JAMA* **2016**, *315*, 2284–2291. [CrossRef]
10. Butte, N.F.; Wong, W.W.; Treuth, M.S.; Ellis, K.J.; O'Brian Smith, E. Energy requirements during pregnancy based on total energy expenditure and energy deposition. *Am. J. Clin. Nutr.* **2004**, *79*, 1078–1087. [CrossRef]
11. Forsum, E.; Kabir, N.; Sadurskis, A.; Westerterp, K. Total energy expenditure of healthy swedish women during pregnancy and lactation. *Am. J. Clin. Nutr.* **1992**, *56*, 334–342. [CrossRef]
12. Goldberg, G.R.; Prentice, A.M.; Coward, W.A.; Davies, H.L.; Murgatroyd, P.R.; Wensing, C.; Black, A.E.; Harding, M.; Sawyer, M. Longitudinal assessment of energy expenditure in pregnancy by the doubly labeled water method. *Am. J. Clin. Nutr.* **1993**, *57*, 494–505. [CrossRef] [PubMed]
13. Kopp-Hoolihan, L.E.; van Loan, M.D.; Wong, W.W.; King, J.C. Longitudinal assessment of energy balance in well-nourished, pregnant women. *Am. J. Clin. Nutr.* **1999**, *69*, 697–704. [CrossRef] [PubMed]
14. Lof, M.; Forsum, E. Activity pattern and energy expenditure due to physical activity before and during pregnancy in healthy swedish women. *Br. J. Nutr.* **2006**, *95*, 296–302. [CrossRef] [PubMed]
15. Most, J.; St Amant, M.; Hsia, D.; Altazan, A.; Thomas, D.; Gilmore, A.; Vallo, P.; Beyl, R.; Ravussin, E.; Redman, L. Evidence-based recommendations for energy intake in pregnant women with obesity. *J. Clin. Invest.* **2019**, *130*. [CrossRef] [PubMed]
16. Institute of Medicine. Energy. In *Dietary Reference Intake for Energy, Carbohydrate, Fiber, Fat, Fatty Acids, Cholesterol, Protein, and Amino Acids*; The National Academies Press: Washington, DC, USA, 2005; pp. 107–264.
17. Bracero, L.A.; Byrne, D.W. Optimal maternal weight gain during singleton pregnancy. *Gynecol. Obstet. Investig.* **1998**, *46*, 9–16. [CrossRef] [PubMed]
18. Cedergren, M.I. Optimal gestational weight gain for body mass index categories. *Obstet. Gynecol.* **2007**, *110*, 759–764. [CrossRef] [PubMed]
19. Nohr, E.A.; Vaeth, M.; Baker, J.L.; Sorensen, T.; Olsen, J.; Rasmussen, K.M. Combined associations of prepregnancy body mass index and gestational weight gain with the outcome of pregnancy. *Am. J. Clin. Nutr.* **2008**, *87*, 1750–1759. [CrossRef]
20. Blomberg, M. Maternal and neonatal outcomes among obese women with weight gain below the new institute of medicine recommendations. *Obstet. Gynecol.* **2011**, *117*, 1065–1070. [CrossRef]

21. Bodnar, L.M.; Pugh, S.J.; Lash, T.L.; Hutcheon, J.A.; Himes, K.P.; Parisi, S.M.; Abrams, B. Low gestational weight gain and risk of adverse perinatal outcomes in obese and severely obese women. *Epidemiology* **2016**, *27*, 894–902. [CrossRef]
22. Bodnar, L.M.; Siminerio, L.L.; Himes, K.P.; Hutcheon, J.A.; Lash, T.L.; Parisi, S.M.; Abrams, B. Maternal obesity and gestational weight gain are risk factors for infant death. *Obesity* **2016**, *24*, 490–498. [CrossRef]
23. Faucher, M.A.; Barger, M.K. Gestational weight gain in obese women by class of obesity and select maternal/newborn outcomes: A systematic review. *Women Birth* **2015**, *28*, e70–e79. [CrossRef] [PubMed]
24. Robillard, P.Y.; Dekker, G.; Boukerrou, M.; Le Moullec, N.; Hulsey, T.C. Relationship between pre-pregnancy maternal bmi and optimal weight gain in singleton pregnancies. *Heliyon* **2018**, *4*, e00615. [CrossRef] [PubMed]
25. Durie, D.E.; Thornburg, L.L.; Glantz, J.C. Effect of second-trimester and third-trimester rate of gestational weight gain on maternal and neonatal outcomes. *Obstet. Gynecol.* **2011**, *118*, 569–575. [CrossRef] [PubMed]
26. Santos, S.; Eekhout, I.; Voerman, E.; Gaillard, R.; Barros, H.; Charles, M.A.; Chatzi, L.; Chevrier, C.; Chrousos, G.P.; Corpeleijn, E.; et al. Gestational weight gain charts for different body mass index groups for women in europe, north america, and oceania. *BMC Med.* **2018**, *16*, 201. [CrossRef] [PubMed]
27. Most, J.; Redman, L.M. Does energy expenditure influence body fat accumulation in pregnancy? *Am. J. Obstet. Gynecol.* **2019**, *220*, 119–120. [CrossRef] [PubMed]
28. Most, J.; Vallo, P.M.; Gilmore, L.A.; St Amant, M.; Hsia, D.S.; Altazan, A.D.; Beyl, R.A.; Ravussin, E.; Redman, L.M. Energy expenditure in pregnant women with obesity does not support energy intake recommendations. *Obesity* **2018**, *26*, 992–999. [CrossRef] [PubMed]
29. International Atomic Energy Agency. *Assessment of Body Composition and Total Energy Expenditure in Humans Using Stable Isotope Techniques*; IAEA: Vienna, Austria, 2009.
30. Black, A.E.; Prentice, A.M.; Coward, W.A. Use of food quotients to predict respiratory quotients for the doubly-labelled water method of measuring energy expenditure. *Hum. Nutr. Clin. Nutr.* **1986**, *40*, 381–391. [PubMed]
31. Gilmore, L.A.; Butte, N.F.; Ravussin, E.; Han, H.; Burton, J.H.; Redman, L.M. Energy intake and energy expenditure for determining excess weight gain in pregnant women. *Obstet. Gynecol.* **2016**, *127*, 884–892. [CrossRef] [PubMed]
32. Gilmore, L.A.; Ravussin, E.; Bray, G.A.; Han, H.; Redman, L.M. An objective estimate of energy intake during weight gain using the intake-balance method. *Am. J. Clin. Nutr.* **2014**, *100*, 806–812. [CrossRef] [PubMed]
33. Most, J.; Gilmore, L.A.; Altazan, A.D.; St Amant, M.; Beyl, R.A.; Ravussin, E.; Redman, L.M. Propensity for adverse pregnancy outcomes in african-american women may be explained by low energy expenditure in early pregnancy. *Am. J. Clin. Nutr.* **2018**, *107*, 957–964. [CrossRef]
34. Thomas, D.M.; Navarro-Barrientos, J.E.; Rivera, D.E.; Heymsfield, S.B.; Bredlau, C.; Redman, L.M.; Martin, C.K.; Lederman, S.A.; Linda, M.C.; Butte, N.F. Dynamic energy-balance model predicting gestational weight gain. *Am. J. Clin. Nutr.* **2012**, *95*, 115–122. [CrossRef] [PubMed]
35. Most, J.; Broskey, N.T.; Altazan, A.D.; Beyl, R.A.; St Amant, M.; Hsia, D.S.; Ravussin, E.; Redman, L.M. Is energy balance in pregnancy involved in the etiology of gestational diabetes in women with obesity? *Cell Metab.* **2019**, *29*, 231–233. [CrossRef] [PubMed]
36. Heini, A.; Schutz, Y.; Diaz, E.; Prentice, A.M.; Whitehead, R.G.; Jequier, E. Free-living energy expenditure measured by two independent techniques in pregnant and nonpregnant gambian women. *Am. J. Physiol.* **1991**, *261*, E9–E17. [CrossRef] [PubMed]
37. Singh, J.; Prentice, A.M.; Diaz, E.; Coward, W.A.; Ashford, J.; Sawyer, M.; Whitehead, R.G. Energy expenditure of gambian women during peak agricultural activity measured by the doubly-labelled water method. *Br. J. Nutr.* **1989**, *62*, 315–329. [CrossRef] [PubMed]
38. Lof, M. Physical activity pattern and activity energy expenditure in healthy pregnant and non-pregnant swedish women. *Eur. J. Clin. Nutr.* **2011**, *65*, 1295–1301. [CrossRef] [PubMed]
39. Gradmark, A.; Pomeroy, J.; Renstrom, F.; Steiginga, S.; Persson, M.; Wright, A.; Bluck, L.; Domellof, M.; Kahn, S.E.; Mogren, I.; et al. Physical activity, sedentary behaviors, and estimated insulin sensitivity and secretion in pregnant and non-pregnant women. *BMC Pregnancy Childbirth* **2011**, *11*, 44. [CrossRef] [PubMed]
40. Diem, K. Metabolisme basal. In *Tables Scientifiques*; Geigy, J.R.S.A., Ed.; Departement Pharmaceutique: Basel, Switzerland, 1963; Volume 6, pp. 637–643.

41. Sparks, J.W.; Girard, J.R.; Battaglia, F.C. An estimate of the caloric requirements of the human fetus. *Neonatology* **1980**, *38*, 113–119. [CrossRef] [PubMed]
42. Lam, Y.Y.; Ravussin, E. Analysis of energy metabolism in humans: A review of methodologies. *Mol. Metab.* **2016**, *5*, 1057–1071. [CrossRef] [PubMed]
43. Meah, V.L.; Cockcroft, J.R.; Backx, K.; Shave, R.; Stohr, E.J. Cardiac output and related haemodynamics during pregnancy: A series of meta-analyses. *Heart* **2016**, *102*, 518–526. [CrossRef] [PubMed]
44. Napso, T.; Yong, H.E.J.; Lopez-Tello, J.; Sferruzzi-Perri, A.N. The role of placental hormones in mediating maternal adaptations to support pregnancy and lactation. *Front. Physiol.* **2018**, *9*, 1091. [CrossRef]
45. Mottola, M.F. Physical activity and maternal obesity: Cardiovascular adaptations, exercise recommendations, and pregnancy outcomes. *Nutr. Rev.* **2013**, *71* (Suppl. 1), S31–S36. [CrossRef]
46. Ferraro, Z.M.; Contador, F.; Tawfiq, A.; Adamo, K.B.; Gaudet, L. Gestational weight gain and medical outcomes of pregnancy. *Obstet. Med.* **2015**, *8*, 133–137. [CrossRef] [PubMed]
47. Davenport, M.H.; Sobierajski, F.; Mottola, M.F.; Skow, R.J.; Meah, V.L.; Poitras, V.J.; Gray, C.E.; Jaramillo Garcia, A.; Barrowman, N.; Riske, L.; et al. Glucose responses to acute and chronic exercise during pregnancy: A systematic review and meta-analysis. *Br. J. Sports Med.* **2018**, *52*, 1357–1366. [CrossRef] [PubMed]
48. Ruchat, S.M.; Mottola, M.F.; Skow, R.J.; Nagpal, T.S.; Meah, V.L.; James, M.; Riske, L.; Sobierajski, F.; Kathol, A.J.; Marchand, A.A.; et al. Effectiveness of exercise interventions in the prevention of excessive gestational weight gain and postpartum weight retention: A systematic review and meta-analysis. *Br. J. Sports Med.* **2018**, *52*, 1347–1356. [CrossRef] [PubMed]
49. Pate, R.R.; Pratt, M.; Blair, S.N.; Haskell, W.L.; Macera, C.A.; Bouchard, C.; Buchner, D.; Ettinger, W.; Heath, G.W.; King, A.C.; et al. Physical activity and public health. A recommendation from the centers for disease control and prevention and the american college of sports medicine. *JAMA* **1995**, *273*, 402–407. [CrossRef] [PubMed]
50. Ferguson, B. Acsm's guidelines for exercise testing and prescription 9th ed. 2014. *J. Can. Chiropr. Assoc.* **2014**, *58*, 328.
51. Lauer, E.E.; Jackson, A.W.; Martin, S.B.; Morrow, J.R., Jr. Meeting usdhhs physical activity guidelines and health outcomes. *Int. J. Exerc. Sci.* **2017**, *10*, 121–127. [PubMed]
52. Davenport, M.H.; Ruchat, S.M.; Mottola, M.F.; Davies, G.A.; Poitras, V.J.; Gray, C.E.; Garcia, A.J.; Barrowman, N.; Adamo, K.B.; Duggan, M.; et al. 2019 canadian guideline for physical activity throughout pregnancy: Methodology. *J. Obstet. Gynaecol. Can.* **2018**, *40*, 1468–1483. [CrossRef] [PubMed]
53. Mottola, M.F.; Davenport, M.H.; Ruchat, S.-M.; Davies, G.A.; Poitras, V.J.; Gray, C.E.; Jaramillo Garcia, A.; Barrowman, N.; Adamo, K.B.; Duggan, M.; et al. 2019 canadian guideline for physical activity throughout pregnancy. *Br. J. Sports Med.* **2018**, *52*, 1339. [CrossRef] [PubMed]
54. Ribeiro Santos, P.C.; Abreu, S.; Moreira, C.; Lopes, D.; Santos, R.; Alves, O.; Silva, P.; Montenegro, N.; Mota, J. Impact of compliance with different guidelines on physical activity during pregnancy and perceived barriers to leisure physical activity. *J. Sports Sci.* **2014**, *32*, 1398–1408. [CrossRef]
55. Hesketh, K.R.; Evenson, K.R. Prevalence of us pregnant women meeting 2015 acog physical activity guidelines. *Am. J. Prev. Med.* **2016**, *51*, e87–e89. [CrossRef] [PubMed]
56. Di Fabio, D.R.; Blomme, C.K.; Smith, K.M.; Welk, G.J.; Campbell, C.G. Adherence to physical activity guidelines in mid-pregnancy does not reduce sedentary time: An observational study. *Int. J. Behav. Nutr. Phys. Act.* **2015**, *12*, 27. [CrossRef] [PubMed]
57. Hayman, M.; Short, C.; Reaburn, P. An investigation into the exercise behaviours of regionally based australian pregnant women. *J. Sci. Med. Sport* **2016**, *19*, 664–668. [CrossRef] [PubMed]
58. Smith, K.M.; Campbell, C.G. Physical activity during pregnancy: Impact of applying different physical activity guidelines. *J. Pregnancy* **2013**, *2013*, 165617. [CrossRef] [PubMed]
59. Renault, K.M.; Norgaard, K.; Nilas, L.; Carlsen, E.M.; Cortes, D.; Pryds, O.; Secher, N.J. The treatment of obese pregnant women (top) study: A randomized controlled trial of the effect of physical activity intervention assessed by pedometer with or without dietary intervention in obese pregnant women. *Am. J. Obstet. Gynecol.* **2014**, *210*, 134.e1–134.e9. [CrossRef] [PubMed]
60. Medek, H.; Halldorsson, T.; Gunnarsdottir, I.; Geirsson, R.T. Physical activity of relatively high intensity in mid-pregnancy predicts lower glucose tolerance levels. *Acta Obstet. Gynecol. Scand.* **2016**, *95*, 1055–1062. [CrossRef] [PubMed]

61. Renault, K.M.; Carlsen, E.M.; Haedersdal, S.; Nilas, L.; Secher, N.J.; Eugen-Olsen, J.; Cortes, D.; Olsen, S.F.; Halldorsson, T.I.; Norgaard, K. Impact of lifestyle intervention for obese women during pregnancy on maternal metabolic and inflammatory markers. *Int. J. Obes.* **2017**, *41*, 598–605. [CrossRef]
62. Kraal, J.J.; Sartor, F.; Papini, G.; Stut, W.; Peek, N.; Kemps, H.M.; Bonomi, A.G. Energy expenditure estimation in beta-blocker-medicated cardiac patients by combining heart rate and body movement data. *Eur. J. Prev. Cardiol.* **2016**, *23*, 1734–1742. [CrossRef]
63. Kim, D.; Cho, J.; Oh, H.; Chee, Y.; Kim, I. The estimation method of physical activity energy expenditure considering heart rate variability. In Proceedings of the 2009 36th Annual Computers in Cardiology Conference (CinC), Park City, UT, USA, 13–16 September 2009; pp. 413–416.
64. Chasan-Taber, L.; Schmidt, M.D.; Roberts, D.E.; Hosmer, D.; Markenson, G.; Freedson, P.S. Development and validation of a pregnancy physical activity questionnaire. *Med. Sci. Sports Exerc.* **2004**, *36*, 1750–1760. [CrossRef]
65. Ara, I.; Aparicio-Ugarriza, R.; Morales-Barco, D.; Nascimento de Souza, W.; Mata, E.; Gonzalez-Gross, M. Physical activity assessment in the general population; validated self-report methods. *Nutr. Hosp.* **2015**, *31* (Suppl. 3), 211–218.
66. Bell, R.; Tennant, P.W.; McParlin, C.; Pearce, M.S.; Adamson, A.J.; Rankin, J.; Robson, S.C. Measuring physical activity in pregnancy: A comparison of accelerometry and self-completion questionnaires in overweight and obese women. *Eur. J. Obstet. Gynecol. Reprod. Biol.* **2013**, *170*, 90–95. [CrossRef] [PubMed]
67. Harrison, C.L.; Thompson, R.G.; Teede, H.J.; Lombard, C.B. Measuring physical activity during pregnancy. *Int. J. Behav. Nutr. Phys. Act.* **2011**, *8*, 19. [CrossRef] [PubMed]
68. Brett, K.E.; Wilson, S.; Ferraro, Z.M.; Adamo, K.B. Self-report pregnancy physical activity questionnaire overestimates physical activity. *Can. J. Public Health* **2015**, *106*, e297–e302. [CrossRef] [PubMed]
69. Lemmens, P.M.C.; Sartor, F.; Cox, L.G.E.; den Boer, S.V.; Westerink, J. Evaluation of an activity monitor for use in pregnancy to help reduce excessive gestational weight gain. *BMC Pregnancy Childbirth* **2018**, *18*, 312. [CrossRef] [PubMed]
70. Conway, M.R.; Marshall, M.R.; Schlaff, R.A.; Pfeiffer, K.A.; Pivarnik, J.M. Physical activity device reliability and validity during pregnancy and postpartum. *Med. Sci. Sports Exerc.* **2018**, *50*, 617–623. [CrossRef] [PubMed]
71. Mudd, L.M.; Evenson, K.R. Review of impacts of physical activity on maternal metabolic health during pregnancy. *Curr. Diabetes Rep.* **2015**, *15*, 6. [CrossRef] [PubMed]
72. Acog Committee Opinion. Exercise during pregnancy and the postpartum period. *Int. J. Gynaecol. Obstet.* **2002**, *77*, 79–81. [CrossRef]
73. Horns, P.N.; Ratcliffe, L.P.; Leggett, J.C.; Swanson, M.S. Pregnancy outcomes among active and sedentary primiparous women. *J. Obstet. Gynecol. Neonatal Nurs.* **1996**, *25*, 49–54. [CrossRef]
74. Gaston, A.; Cramp, A. Exercise during pregnancy: A review of patterns and determinants. *J. Sci. Med. Sport* **2011**, *14*, 299–305. [CrossRef]
75. Butte, N.F.; Ellis, K.J.; Wong, W.W.; Hopkinson, J.M.; Smith, E.O. Composition of gestational weight gain impacts maternal fat retention and infant birth weight. *Am. J. Obstet. Gynecol.* **2003**, *189*, 1423–1432. [CrossRef]
76. Berggren, E.K.; Groh-Wargo, S.; Presley, L.; Hauguel-de Mouzon, S.; Catalano, P.M. Maternal fat, but not lean, mass is increased among overweight/obese women with excess gestational weight gain. *Am. J. Obstet. Gynecol.* **2016**, *214*, e741–e745. [CrossRef] [PubMed]
77. Most, J.; Marlatt, K.L.; Altazan, A.D.; Redman, L.M. Advances in assessing body composition during pregnancy. *Eur. J. Clin. Nutr.* **2018**, *72*, 645–656. [CrossRef] [PubMed]
78. van Raaij, J.M.; Peek, M.E.; Vermaat-Miedema, S.H.; Schonk, C.M.; Hautvast, J.G. New equations for estimating body fat mass in pregnancy from body density or total body water. *Am. J. Clin. Nutr.* **1988**, *48*, 24–29. [CrossRef] [PubMed]
79. Tataranni, P.A.; Harper, I.T.; Snitker, S.; Del Parigi, A.; Vozarova, B.; Bunt, J.; Bogardus, C.; Ravussin, E. Body weight gain in free-living pima indians: Effect of energy intake vs. expenditure. *Int. J. Obes. Relat. Metab. Disord.* **2003**, *27*, 1578–1583. [CrossRef] [PubMed]
80. Butte, N.F.; King, J.C. Energy requirements during pregnancy and lactation. *Public Health Nutr.* **2005**, *8*, 1010–1027. [CrossRef] [PubMed]

81. Durnin, J.V. Energy requirements of pregnancy. *Diabetes* **1991**, *40* (Suppl. 2), 152–156. [CrossRef]
82. American College of Obstetricians and Gynecologists. Nutrition in pregnancy. In *Your Pregnancy and Childbirth: Month to Month*, 6th ed.; ACOG: Washington, DC, USA, 2016; pp. 313–327.
83. IOM (Institute of Medicine); NRC (National Research Council). *Weight Gain during Pregnancy: Reexamining the Guidelines*; The National Academies Press: Washington, DC, USA, 2009.
84. Ravussin, E.; Lillioja, S.; Knowler, W.C.; Christin, L.; Freymond, D.; Abbott, W.G.; Boyce, V.; Howard, B.V.; Bogardus, C. Reduced rate of energy expenditure as a risk factor for body-weight gain. *N. Engl. J. Med.* **1988**, *318*, 467–472. [CrossRef] [PubMed]
85. Berggren, E.K.; O'Tierney-Ginn, P.; Lewis, S.; Presley, L.; De-Mouzon, S.H.; Catalano, P.M. Variations in resting energy expenditure: Impact on gestational weight gain. *Am. J. Obstet. Gynecol.* **2017**, *217*, 445.e1–445.e6. [CrossRef] [PubMed]
86. Lof, M.; Olausson, H.; Bostrom, K.; Janerot-Sjoberg, B.; Sohlstrom, A.; Forsum, E. Changes in basal metabolic rate during pregnancy in relation to changes in body weight and composition, cardiac output, insulin-like growth factor I, and thyroid hormones and in relation to fetal growth. *Am. J. Clin. Nutr.* **2005**, *81*, 678–685. [CrossRef]
87. Meng, Y.; Groth, S.W.; Stewart, P.; Smith, J.A. An exploration of the determinants of gestational weight gain in african american women: Genetic factors and energy expenditure. *Biol. Res. Nurs.* **2018**, *20*, 118–125. [CrossRef]
88. Katzmarzyk, P.T.; Most, J.; Redman, L.M.; Rood, J.; Ravussin, E. Energy expenditure and substrate oxidation in white and african american young adults without obesity. *Eur. J. Clin. Nutr.* **2018**, *72*, 920–922. [CrossRef] [PubMed]
89. Deputy, N.P.; Sharma, A.J.; Kim, S.Y.; Olson, C.K. Achieving appropriate gestational weight gain: The role of healthcare provider advice. *J. Womens Health* **2018**, *27*, 552–560. [CrossRef] [PubMed]
90. Stephenson, J.; Heslehurst, N.; Hall, J.; Schoenaker, D.; Hutchinson, J.; Cade, J.E.; Poston, L.; Barrett, G.; Crozier, S.R.; Barker, M.; et al. Before the beginning: Nutrition and lifestyle in the preconception period and its importance for future health. *Lancet* **2018**, *391*, 1830–1841. [CrossRef]

6

Can a Simple Dietary Screening in Early Pregnancy Identify Dietary Habits Associated with Gestational Diabetes?

Laufey Hrolfsdottir [1,2,*], Ingibjorg Gunnarsdottir [1], Bryndis Eva Birgisdottir [1], Ingibjorg Th Hreidarsdottir [3], Alexander Kr. Smarason [2], Hildur Hardardottir [3,4] and Thorhallur I. Halldorsson [1,5]

1 Unit for Nutrition Research, Landspitali University Hospital and Faculty of Food Science and Nutrition, University of Iceland, Eiríksgata 29 101 Reykjavik, Iceland
2 Institution of Health Science Research, University of Akureyri and Akureyri Hospital, Eyrarlandsvegi, 600 Akureyri, Iceland
3 Department of Obstetrics and Gynecology, Landspitali University Hospital, Hringbraut, 101 Reykjavík, Iceland
4 Faculty of Medicine, University of Iceland, Vatnsmýrarvegi 16, 101 Reykjavík, Iceland
5 Centre for Fetal Programming, Department of Epidemiology Research, Statens Serum Institut, Artillerivej 5, 2300 Copenhagen, Denmark
* Correspondence: laufeyh@sak.is

Abstract: Gestational diabetes mellitus (GDM) is predominantly a lifestyle disease, with diet being an important modifiable risk factor. A major obstacle for the prevention in clinical practice is the complexity of assessing diet. In a cohort of 1651 Icelandic women, this study examined whether a short 40-item dietary screening questionnaire administered in the 1st trimester could identify dietary habits associated with GDM. The dietary variables were aggregated into predefined binary factors reflecting inadequate or optimal intake and stepwise backward elimination was used to identify a reduced set of factors that best predicted GDM. Those binary factors were then aggregated into a risk score (range: 0–7), that was mostly characterised by frequent consumption of soft drinks, sweets, cookies, ice creams and processed meat. The women with poor dietary habits (score ≥ 5, $n = 302$), had a higher risk of GDM (RR = 1.38; 95%CI = 3, 85) compared with women with a more optimal diet (score ≤ 2, $n = 407$). In parallel, a pilot ($n = 100$) intervention was conducted among overweight and obese women examining the effect of internet-based personalized feedback on diet quality. Simple feedback was given in accordance with the answers provided in the screening questionnaire in 1st trimester. At the endpoint, the improvements in diet quality were observed by, as an example, soft drink consumption being reduced by ~1 L/week on average in the intervention group compared to the controls. Our results suggest that a simple dietary screening tool administered in the 1st trimester could identify dietary habits associated with GMD. This tool should be easy to use in a clinical setting, and with simple individualized feedback, improvements in diet may be achieved.

Keywords: dietary habits; maternal nutrition; gestational diabetes; food frequency questionnaire; dietary screening

---

1. Introduction

Gestational diabetes mellitus (GDM) is a major pregnancy complication, defined as glucose intolerance with onset during pregnancy. The prevalence of GDM in European countries ranges from 2 to 22% with a median of 6% [1]. GDM has been associated with several adverse outcomes [2], including offspring macrosomia [3] and the mothers' increased risk of the development of type 2 diabetes postpartum [4]. Longitudinal studies also suggest that offspring of mothers diagnosed with GDM are more prone to metabolic abnormalities later in life [5].

High pre-pregnancy BMI is one of the strongest risk factors for GDM and it is commonly used to identify pregnant women at risk for further monitoring [6]. The use of BMI to identify women at GDM risk does, however, have its limitations as high BMI alone is by no means an indicator for unhealthy dietary habits or a lifestyle that may influence GDM risk. Improvements in weight are also difficult to achieve in the short term and during pregnancy, other modifiable risk factors, such as diet, must be prioritised.

Recent observational studies indicate that unhealthy dietary habits before [7,8] and during pregnancy [9–12] are associated with a higher risk of GDM. Despite the observational nature, the link between poor carbohydrate and fat quality observed in these studies is both biologically plausible and in line with the established risk factors for type 2 diabetes [13]. However, an important limitation for targeting dietary habits of pregnant women is that the dietary assessment methods, developed for research purposes, are time-consuming and difficult to use in maternal care [14]. The complexity of diet is also challenging in terms of focusing efforts. To bypass this challenge, previous intervention studies have often focused on adherence to relatively strict dietary regimes aimed at achieving major changes [15–17]. These strategies have generally resulted in limited compliance and unclear benefits, highlighting the need to explore more targeted and flexible approaches.

The aim of this study was to examine if a short dietary screening questionnaire administered in weeks 11–14 of gestation could be used to identify unhealthy dietary habits associated with GMD and, in parallel, to investigate if a simple personalized web-based feedback tool could result in improvement in dietary habits in pregnancy.

2. Materials and Methods

This study was based on two studies of different designs that recruited pregnant women in Iceland from 2015 to 2017. In a cohort setting, this study examined, in a set of 1651 women, the association between dietary habits recorded in early pregnancy and the risk of GDM. In parallel, a pilot (n = 100) intervention study was conducted to test to what extent dietary changes could be achieved in the study population. In terms of the prevention and use in a clinical setting, an association between dietary habits and pregnancy complications such as GDM is limited on its own, unless there are indications that changes in those dietary factors can be modified using low intensity and cost-effective measures. This is the logic behind conducting these studies and to combine them in one paper.

2.1. The Cohort Study

The PREWICE cohort (PREgnant Women of ICEland) has been described elsewhere [18]. All women (n = 2734) with singleton pregnancies who attended a routine early ultrasound (11–14 week of gestation) at the prenatal diagnostic unit at Landspitali University Hospital in Reykjavik, South Iceland between 1 October, 2015 to 31 September, 2016, were invited to take part in the study. In total, 2113 women, (~50% of all births in Iceland during the study period) agreed to participate, whereof 417 (~20%) had missing hospital records, most likely as they gave birth outside Landspitali University Hospital. The additional 26 women who had multiple births and another 19 who had missing dietary data were excluded, resulting in 1651 women being eligible for analyses. No major differences were found in the baseline characteristics or dietary measures among those who were included in the full analysis and those who were excluded because of missing data [18].

2.1.1. The Outcome Variable

The information regarding GDM cases was retrieved from maternal hospital records (ICD-10 codes O24.4 and O24.9, but O24.9 is used at Landspitali GDM treated with medications). The criteria for GDM diagnoses was according to the 2010 International Association of Diabetes and Pregnancy Study Groups (IADPSG) Consensus Panel [6].

2.1.2. The Dietary Assessment and the Dietary Risk Score

The details about the dietary assessment and construction of the dietary risk score have been described in detail elsewhere [18]. In short, the dietary screening questionnaire consisted of a 40-item list of common foods and food groups for which the frequency of consumption was recorded (see Supplemental File S1). The list was designed to give a rough overview of the participant's general diet in comparison to current food-based dietary guidelines. The dietary data collected was converted to frequency per week for all food groups, which was then transformed into 13 predefined dietary risk factors for inadequate diet (Figure 1). The 13 factors used to construct the risk score are based on the Nordic [19] and Icelandic dietary recommendations [20] and supported by evidence from studies conducted in pregnant women [21–25].

Risk factors for inadequate diet	
1. Not eating a varied diet	8. Sugar and artificially sweetened beverages ≥5 times/week
2. Vegetables and fruits<5 times/day	9. Sweets, ice cream, cakes, cookies ≥2.5 times/week
3. Fish intake <2 times/week	10. French fries and fried potatoes ≥1 time/week
4. Dairy intake <2 times/day	11. High dairy intake ≥5 times/day
5. Wholegrain products <2 times/day	12. Processed meat products ≥1 time/week
6. Beans, nuts, seeds <3.5 times/week	13. Quality of fat - using butter (or other unsaturated fat sources) rather than oil (≥50%)
7. Vitamin-D <5 times/week	

Figure 1. The predefined dietary risk factors for inadequate diet. The risk factors were mainly based on the Nordic Nutrition Recommendations [19] and the Icelandic Food-Based Dietary Recommendations [20]. If the women excluded/avoided any of the main food groups (cereal, vegetables/fruits, fish, meat, eggs, high-fat foods or dairy), they were categorized to the group of not eating a varied diet.

Using these 13 predefined dietary risk factors as inputs, a stepwise backward elimination was used to identify a reduced set of variables with the highest maximum likelihood that best predicted GDM. The model performance was assessed by Nagelkerke's R^2. The following set of seven dietary risk factors (predictors) were included in the final model: Non-varied diet; sugar/artificially sweetened beverages ≥5 times/week; sweets, ice cream, cakes, cookies ≥2.5 times/week; processed meat products ≥1 time/week; whole grain products <2 times/day; dairy <2 times/day and vitamin D intake <5 times/week. The set of seven variables was then used to calculate a combined dietary risk score. Each participant got 1 score for fulfilling the risk criteria, and 0 for not fulfilling the risk criteria. The scores of the dietary risk factors were then summed up, ranging from 0 to 7.

To verify the the stability of our findings in terms of variable selection, comparable risk scores were created based on either a fewer or a larger number of dietary factors being retained in the model. The associations between these different scores in relation to GDM risk are shown in Table A1 (Appendix A).

2.2. The Pilot Intervention Study

For the pilot intervention study, 100 women with pre-pregnancy body mass ≥25 kg/m^2, attending prenatal care at the Health Care Institution of North Iceland were recruited. At recruitment, i.e., at the first antenatal care visit, the women answered the same dietary questionnaire as described above for the cohort study. The participants were then randomized into a control group receiving the habitual care of brochures on the recommended diet during pregnancy according to clinical guidelines ($n = 50$; 9 dropouts), and an intervention group ($n = 50$; 3 dropouts), receiving personalized feedback on their diet quality through an interactive website [26]. This website was designed to give each woman simple personalized feedback, aimed at improving diet quality, in accordance with the answers provided by the dietary questionnaire. At baseline, a nutritionist showed the participants in the intervention group the website and went through the personalized feedback with them. Dietary intake in gestation weeks 24–26 and 35–38 was assessed by two 24-h recalls. These recalls were performed by another nutritionist who was blinded to the intervention assignment.

2.3. Statistical Analyses

The students t-tests were used to compare the normally distributed continuous variables, whereas, for skewed and categorical variables, the Mann-Whitney U test and Chi-square tests were used, respectively.

For the cohort study, the associations between the diet reported at baseline and GDM was assessed using multivariable Poisson log-linear regression. The covariates included in the adjusted models were selected, a priori, based on their potential influence on dietary habits and GDM [27–31]. The covariates included in the regression analyses were: Maternal pre-pregnancy BMI (<25, 25–29.99, ≥30 kg/m^2); maternal age (quartiles); parity (nulliparous versus primi/multiparous); education (elementary schooling, high school and/or technical school, university education, and higher academic education); maternal smoking during pregnancy (yes/no) and family history of type 2 diabetes. The information on these covariates was recorded at recruitment with the exception of maternal age and family history of type 2 diabetes, which was retrieved from hospital records. The missing values for covariates (maternal pre-pregnancy BMI (0.7%), parity (1.2%), educational level (0.9%), and maternal smoking during pregnancy (1.5%) were assumed to be missing at random and were imputed using multiple imputations as implemented in *proc MI* in SAS v9.2 8. Statistical significance was accepted at $p < 0.05$.

2.4. Ethics

The ethics committee of Landspitali University Hospital approved the study protocol (21/2015) for the cohort study. For the intervention study, ethical approval was received from The National Bioethics committee (VSN-15-111-S1). Written consent was obtained from all participants in both studies.

3. Results

The characteristics of the PREWICE cohort are presented in Table 1. The mean age was 30 years, and most (94%) participants were non-smokers, 39% were nulliparous and 58% of the women had a university education or higher academic degree. In total, 16% ($n = 265$) were diagnosed with GDM during pregnancy. Stratified by pre-pregnancy weight, the prevalence of GDM among women of normal weight (BMI < 25 kg/m^2), overweight (BMI 25–29.99 kg/m^2) or obesity (BMI ≥ 30 kg/m^2) was 5%, 15% and 49%, respectively. The mothers who developed GDM were also more likely to be older, Primi/multiparous and have a lower educational level (Table 1).

Table 1. Birth outcomes and characteristics of mothers at baseline in relation to gestational diabetes mellitus diagnoses.

	All [a] (n = 1651)	GDM [a,b] (16%)	No GDM [a] (84%)	p Value [c]
Maternal age (year)	30.3 ± 5.2	31.8 ± 5.4	30.0 ± 5.1	<0.01 [d]
Height (cm)	167.5 ± 6.1	166.5 ± 6.3	167.7 ± 6.1	<0.01 [d]
Birth weight (g)	3670 ± 552	3686 ± 587	3667± 545	0.64 [d]
Gestational age (weeks)	40.0 (1.0)	39.0 ± 2.0	40.0 ± 2.0	<0.01 [e]
Pre-pregnancy weight (kg)	68.0 (20.0)	85.0 (19.5)	66.0 (16.0)	<0.01 [e]
Pre-pregnancy BMI (kg/m^2)	24.2 (6.7)	30.5 (7.6)	23.5 (5.3)	<0.01 [e]
Pre-pregnancy BMI (groups)				<0.01 [f]
<18.5 kg/m^2 (%)	3	1	4	
18.5–24.99 kg/m^2 (%)	54	17	61	
25–29.99 kg/m^2 (%)	24	24	23	
≥30 kg/m^2 (%)	19	59	11	
Exc. GWG (%)	36	33	36	0.38 [f]
Parity (%)				<0.01 [f]
Nulliparous	39	31	41	
Primi/multiparous	61	69	59	
Single (%)	6	7	5	0.34 [f]
Smoking during pregnancy (%)	6	7	6	0.74 [f]
Family history of type 2 diabetes (%)	18	15	39	<0.01 [f]
Education (%)				<0.01 [f]
Elementary schooling	13	18	12	
High sch. and technical sch.	30	32	29	
University education	34	37	34	
Higher academic	24	14	26	

Abbreviations: BMI, body mass index; GDM, gestational diabetes mellitus; GWG, gestational weight gain. [a] Values are mean ± standard deviation or median (IQR) for continuous variables and percentages for categorical variables; [b] The criteria that was used [6] [c] Differences between GDM and no GDM. [d] F-test (Type III) of differences among groups. [e] Mann-Whitney U test of differences among groups. [f] Chi-square test of differences among groups.

The number of women who fulfilled the risk criteria for each of the identified dietary risk factors is shown in Table 2. In total, 21% reported that they had a nonvaried diet, i.e., that they avoided or excluded some food groups. In total, 28% frequently consumed sugar and artificially sweetened beverages (≥5 times/week), 59% had a frequent intake of sweets, ice creams, cakes and cookies (≥2.5 times/week), and 31% ate processed meat products weekly (≥1 time/week). Most women did neither meet the public recommendations for whole grain intake of at least two portions per day (91%) nor the two recommended dairy portions per day (78%), and 30% of the women reported intake of vitamin D supplements less than <5 times per week. A higher proportion of women with GDM fulfilled the risk criteria for the consumption of sugar and artificially sweetened beverages ($p \leq 0.01$) and processed meat products ($p = 0.04$) compared with women with no GDM. The other dietary risk factors did not differ significantly (Table 2).

Table 2. Percent of women fulfilling the predefined risk criteria.

Risk factors	All (n = 1651)	GDM [a] (16%)	No GDM (84%)	p [b]
Not eating a varied diet	21%	23%	21%	0.43
Sugar and artificially sweetened beverages ≥5 times/week	28%	37%	27%	<0.01
Sweet, ice cream, cakes, cookies ≥2.5 times/week	59%	63%	58%	0.14
Processed meat products ≥1 time/week	31%	37%	30%	0.04
Whole grain products <2 times/day	91%	93%	91%	0.26
Dairy <2 times/day	78%	81%	77%	0.18
Vitamin D intake <5 times/week	30%	34%	29%	0.12

[a] The criteria that was used [6]. [b] Chi-square test of differences among groups (GDM vs. no GDM).

In Table 3, the results for the multivariable association between the dietary risk score and GDM are presented. When dichotomizing the exposure, women with a high (≥5, $n = 302$) versus low (≤2, $n = 407$) dietary risk scores had 38% higher relative risk (RR) (95%CI: 3, 85%) of being diagnosed with GDM. The effect modification by pre-pregnancy BMI was formally tested. This was done by including the dietary risk score (continuous variable), BMI (continuous variable) and an interaction term between the two in the logistic regression model, along with the remaining covariates. An interaction was not observed ($p = 0.81$). In accordance to these results, similar results were found when comparing those with a high versus low dietary risk score among women with BMI < 25 (RR = 1.11 95%CI: 0.90, 1.36) vs. BMI ≥ 25 (RR = 1.09 95%CI: 1.002, 1.19).

Table 3. The association between the dietary risk score and gestational diabetes [a].

	Cases (%)/*n*	RR (95% CI) [b]	
		Crude	Adjusted [c]
Dichotomized score			
≤2 scores	49 (12%)/407	ref	ref
3 scores	76 (15%)/503	1.26 (0.90, 1.75)	0.96 (0.72, 1.30)
4 scores	69 (16%)/439	1.31 (0.93, 1.83)	1.00 (0.74, 1.37)
≥5 scores	71 (24%)/302	1.95 (1.40, 2.72)	1.38 (1.03, 1.85)
p for trend		<0.01	0.02
Stratified analyses, continuous score			
All women	265 (16%)/1651	1.20 (1.10, 1.32)	1.10 (1.02, 1.20)
BMI < 25 kg/m^2 [d]	51 (5%)/947	1.20 (0.96, 1.52)	1.11 (0.90, 1.36)
BMI ≥ 25 kg/m^2 [d]	214 (30%)/704	1.12 (1.02, 1.23)	1.09 (1.002, 1.19)

Abbreviations: BMI, body mass index; [a] The criteria that was used [6]. [b] Logistic regression model reflecting the odds of GDM. [c] Adjusted for maternal pre-pregnancy BMI, age, parity, smoking during pregnancy, educational level and family history of type 2 diabetes. [d] Pre-pregnancy BMI not included as a covariate.

Table 4. Baseline characteristics and dietary habits at the endpoint among pregnant women participating in the pilot intervention.

	Control ($n = 41$) [a]	Intervention ($n = 47$) [a]	*p*-Value [b]
Baseline Characteristics			
Pre-pregnancy BMI (kg/m^2)	28.7 (27.1–31.5)	29.4 (27.5–35.2)	0.40
Gestational length at baseline (weeks)	15.0 ± 2.5	14.8 ± 2.7	0.83
Age			0.27
18–24, *n* (%)	10 (24)	10 (21)	
25–34, *n* (%)	28 (68)	28 (60)	
≥35, *n* (%)	3 (7)	9 (19)	
Parity			0.27
Nulliparous, *n* (%)	13 (32)	10 (21)	
Primi/multiparous, *n* (%)	28 (68)	37 (79)	
Smoking during pregnancy, *n* (%)	5 (12)	5 (11)	0.82
Dietary habits at endpoint [c]			
Milk and cultured milk products (g/d)	217 (138–396)	247 (102–376)	0.91
Vegetables (g/d)	91 (23–148)	101 (57–135)	0.18
Fruits and berries (g/d)	105 (73–220)	150 (70–215)	0.67
Fish ≥300g/week (%)	22%	32%	0.30
Processed meat (g/d)	14 (0–42)	10 (0–25)	0.69
Soft drinks (g/d)	125 (25–365)	75 (0–200)	0.03
French fries or chips ≥100g/week (%)	27%	19%	0.38
Cakes, biscuits, and/or sweets (g/d)	62 (19–114)	37 (18–88)	0.25

[a] Values are mean ± standard deviation or median (25th–75th centiles) for continuous variables and percentages for categorical variables. [b] F test (Type III) or Mann-Whitney U test was used to assess differences among groups for continuous variables and Chi-square test for categorical variables. [c] Mean of two 24 h recalls in gestational weeks 24–26. and 35–38.

In the pilot study, neither differences in the background variables (Table 4) nor dietary intake at baseline (Table A2) were observed. In total, 88 women completed both 24 h recalls (47 in the intervention group and 41 in the control group). Table 4 shows the median intake of selected food groups based on the two 24 h recalls. At the endpoint, soft drink consumption was significantly lower in the intervention group compared with the control group, corresponding to approximately one liter less consumption per week. Other differences in dietary intake between the groups were not statistically significant.

4. Discussion

This study found that a dietary risk score, partly characterized by frequent consumption of sugar/artificially sweetened beverages, sweets, cookies, ice creams and processed meat products, was associated with GDM diagnoses. The most pronounced differences in dietary habits of GDM versus non-GDM cases, as recorded at baseline, was excessive (≥5 times/week) consumption of soft drinks. The pilot intervention study, conducted in parallel, showed that internet-based personalized feedback on diet, reported early in pregnancy, could substantially reduce soft drink consumption. Whether such reduction can reduce GDM risks needs to be explored further in an intervention setting.

The results of this study are in line with previous studies using more detailed dietary assessment methods. For example, a recent Icelandic study showed that women who were overweight or obese but had a healthy diet were not at higher risk of gestational diabetes in comparison to women with normal weight [9]. Moreover, unhealthy dietary patterns, soft drinks and the intake of foods high in added sugar have previously been linked to a higher risk of GDM [10–12,32,33]. The regular intake of processed meat products has also commonly been associated with a higher risk of Type 2 diabetes [34,35] and GDM [8,12] and there are some indications that poor vitamin D status, commonly observed at Northern latitudes, may also be important for glucose homeostasis [36].

The Finnish Gestational Diabetes Prevention Study (RADIEL) [37] succeeded in reducing the overall incidence of GDM. However, here the focus was on obese women (and women with previous history of gestational diabetes) without taking into account the baseline dietary habits. Although high pre-pregnancy BMI status is a strong risk factor for GDM, not all overweight or obese women develop GDM [28] and as a substantial proportion of the general population is overweight and obese [38] more precise cost-effective risk assessment is needed.

Apart from GDM, a healthy diet in pregnancy has also been associated with a decreased risk for several other pregnancy and birth outcomes [23,24,39–45]. However, the translation and implementation of these results into clinical practice is still a challenge. One reason for this is that dietary assessment tools used in research settings are very time-consuming and not suitable for use in maternal care. The motivation for the studies reported here was to develop and test a diet screening questionnaire to be used in combination with a web-based platform that automatically gives users feedback on their diet during pregnancy [26]. This application is currently being tested for integration into the National Citizen Health Portal in Iceland. The portal is a centralized web-application where all citizens have secure, digital access to their own health information (e.g., maternal records) and official eHealth services currently available in the country. The inclusion of dietary screening into the portal may increase the feasibility of implementing dietary screening in early pregnancy on a national level and for use in clinical practice. To the authors' best knowledge, information on dietary intake (other than supplement use) is not recorded anywhere in national prenatal health registries, but valid information about diet quality in early pregnancy might change the way women in need for dietary support during pregnancy are defined.

The main strengths of our cohort study include prospective data collection, high participation rates (77%), and information on GDM retrieved from medical records. However, as with all observational studies, the role of confounding cannot be excluded. It is important to note that the methodology used in our cohort study is based on both predefined and data-driven methods, tested in Iceland. The observed association with GDM might therefore not apply directly to other populations. However, this approach, i.e., to use a short FFQ (that takes into consideration population's dietary habits) and to identify the potential risk factors based on existing recommendations, can be used in other settings to generate comparable (but perhaps not identical) results valuable for use in clinical practice. Using the same methodology as used in the present study, the authors have previously identified a dietary risk score that predicts the risk of excessive gestational weight gain and giving birth to a child weighing >4500 g (defined as macrosomia) independent of other known risk factors [18]. These findings need to be tested further in well-powered intervention settings. The short dietary screening questionnaire has been validated against 4-day weighed food records in a pilot study among 25 pregnant women (Spearman's correlation >+0.3). The validation against biochemical analysis is part of an ongoing project (PREWICE II). Its ability to rank subjects according to consumption will be assessed, as well as its ability to detect the risk of predefined nutrient deficiency.

The pilot study had several limitations including a few participants. Moreover, the intervention consisted only of one contact with the participants at baseline. More frequent conversations about the results of the diet screening might have resulted in a greater difference between the groups [43,44]. However, the strength of this approach was its simplicity. This study showed that a simple intervention can result in dietary changes, i.e., lower soft drink consumption, in a population where excessive soft drink intake (≥5 times/week) was relatively common (~28%). While there was a trend towards improvement for other factors, no significant differences were observed. However, in the context of the result from the cohort study, these results are important as the most pronounced difference in the diet between GDM and non GDM cases was excessive consumption of soft drink (see Table 2). Previous intervention studies aimed at encouraging lifestyle changes to reduce the risk of GDM have often selected participants and tested interventions [46] regardless of the participants baseline diet and other lifestyle habits. The results from our studies here and recent work [47] suggest that a sensible way forward would be to select participants based on their baseline diet or other lifestyle factors that can be improved. Prioritizing and identifying a few factors to focus on might also be more attainable for women and more practicable in the clinical setting.

In summary, our results showed that a simple dietary screening tool administered in the 1st trimester could be used to identify dietary habits associated with GMD. This approach could be used to identify women in more need of support and diet counselling. Moreover, the results from the pilot intervention indicate that improvements in dietary quality can be achieved using low intensity and cost-effective measures. This procedure might strengthen preventative measures and enable targeted intervention among individuals most likely to benefit.

Author Contributions: Conceptualization, I.G., L.H. and T.I.H.; data curation, L.H., I.G. and T.I.H. formal analysis, L.H. and T.I.H.; funding acquisition, I.G., T.I.H. and L.H.; investigation, L.H., I.G., B.E.B., I.T.H., A.K.S., H.H. and T.I.H.; methodology, I.G., L.H. and T.I.H.; project administration, I.G.; resources, I.G., H.H., I.T.H. and T.I.H.; supervision, I.G. and L.H.; visualization, I.G., L.H. and T.I.H.; writing—original draft, L.H. and T.I.H.; writing—review and editing, L.H., I.G., B.E.B., I.T.H., A.K.S., H.H. and T.I.H.

Acknowledgments: We are particularly grateful to the women who participated in the studies. We would also like to acknowledge the work of the PREWICE staff and the great staff at the Ultrasound Department at Landspitali National University Hospital and the Health Care Institution of North Iceland who made the study possible.

Appendix A

As the use of backward elimination for selecting factors that predict gestational diabetes involves some arbitrary decisions in terms of where to stop the elimination process, we examined the stability of our findings by creating standardized risk scores based on fewer and more dietary factors being retained in the model (Table A1).

SCORE-1 included two dietary risk factors, i.e., the factors most strongly associated with GDM in the multivariable model: sugar and artificially sweetened beverages ≥5 times/week and processed meat products ≥1 time/week.

SCORE-2 included seven dietary risk factors, i.e., a non-varied diet, sugar and artificially sweetened beverages ≥5 times/week, sweet, ice cream, cakes, cookies ≥2.5 times/week, processed meat products ≥1 time/week, whole grain products <2 times/day, dairy <2 times/day and vitamin D intake <5 times/week.

SCORE-3 included all 13 dietary risk factors, i.e., not eating a varied diet, vegetables and fruits <5 times/day, fish intake <2 times/day, dairy intake <2 times/day, whole grain products <2 times /day, beans, nuts, seeds <3.5 times/week, vitamin D <5 times/week, quality of fat—using butter rather than oil (≥50%), french fries and fried potatoes ≥1 time/week, sweets, ice cream, cakes, cookies ≥2.5 times/week, sugar and artificially sweetened beverages ≥5 times/week, dairy intake ≥5 times/day, processed meat products ≥1 time/week.

As can be seen in Table A1, The combination of the seven dietary risk factors resulted in the most significant association.

Table A1. Different combinations of the dietary risk score and the risk of gestational diabetes mellitus (GDM) [a].

	Crude [b] RR (95%CI)	**Adjusted [b,c] RR (95%CI)**
SCORE-1	1.23 (1.10, 1.36)	1.11 (1.00, 1.22)
SCORE-2	1.26 (1.13, 1.40)	1.13 (1.02, 1.25)
SCORE-3	1.22 (1.09, 1.36)	1.10 (0.99, 1.22)

[a] The criteria that was used [6]. [b] Standardized coefficient reflecting the risk of GDM per standard deviation increase in the dietary risk score. [c] Adjusted for maternal pre-pregnancy BMI, age, parity, smoking during pregnancy, educational level and family history of type 2 diabetes.

Table A2. Baseline dietary intake (frequency per week) of subjects in the pilot study.

5	**Control (n = 41) [a]**	**Intervention (n = 47) [a]**	**p Value [b]**
Milk	5.3 (2.2–7.6)	5.4 (2.1–14.4)	0.289
Cultured milk	5.0 (1.0–5.0)	2.5 (1.0–5.0)	0.876
Beans, nuts and/or seeds	0.5 (0.1–1.0)	0.5 (0.1–2.5)	0.244
Vegetables	7.0 (3.8–7.0)	7.0 (2.5–14)	0.202
Fruits and berries	14.0 (7.0–14)	7.0 (5.0–14)	0.655
Fish	1.1 (1.0–2.8)	1.5 (0.8–2.8)	0.803
Processed meat	0.5 (0.3–0.8)	0.5 (0.3–1.0)	0.158
Soft drinks	2.0 (0.6–5.0)	2.0 (0.6–3.5)	0.556
French fries or chips	0.5 (0.5–1.0)	0.5 (0.5–1.0)	0.554
Cakes, biscuits, ice and sweets	3.5 (1.5–6.0)	2.7 (1.5–5.0)	0.058

[a] Values are median (25th–75th centiles). [b] Mann-Whitney U test was used to assess differences among groups.

References

1. Zhu, Y.; Zhang, C. Prevalence of Gestational Diabetes and Risk of Progression to Type 2 Diabetes: A Global Perspective. *Curr. Diabetes Rep.* **2016**, *16*, 7. [CrossRef] [PubMed]
2. Wendland, E.M.; Torloni, M.R.; Falavigna, M.; Trujillo, J.; Dode, M.A.; Campos, M.A.; Duncan, B.B.; Schmidt, M.I. Gestational diabetes and pregnancy outcomes—A systematic review of the World Health Organization (WHO) and the International Association of Diabetes in Pregnancy Study Groups (IADPSG) diagnostic criteria. *BMC Pregnancy Childbirth* **2012**, *12*, 23. [CrossRef] [PubMed]
3. Alberico, S.; Montico, M.; Barresi, V.; Monasta, L.; Businelli, C.; Soini, V.; Erenbourg, A.; Ronfani, L.; Maso, G. The role of gestational diabetes, pre-pregnancy body mass index and gestational weight gain on the risk of newborn macrosomia: Results from a prospective multicentre study. *BMC Pregnancy Childbirth* **2014**, *14*, 23. [CrossRef] [PubMed]

4. Bellamy, L.; Casas, J.P.; Hingorani, A.D.; Williams, D. Type 2 diabetes mellitus after gestational diabetes: A systematic review and meta-analysis. *Lancet* **2009**, *373*, 1773–1779. [CrossRef]
5. Vohr, B.R.; Boney, C.M. Gestational diabetes: The forerunner for the development of maternal and childhood obesity and metabolic syndrome? *J. Matern. Fetal Neonatal Med.* **2008**, *21*, 149–157. [CrossRef] [PubMed]
6. Metzger, B.E.; Gabbe, S.G.; Persson, B.; Buchanan, T.A.; Catalano, P.A.; Damm, P.; Dyer, A.R.; Leiva, A.; Hod, M.; Kitzmiler, J.L.; et al. International association of diabetes and pregnancy study groups recommendations on the diagnosis and classification of hyperglycemia in pregnancy. *Diabetes Care* **2010**, *33*, 676–682. [CrossRef] [PubMed]
7. Donazar-Ezcurra, M.; Lopez-Del Burgo, C.; Martinez-Gonzalez, M.A.; Basterra-Gortari, F.J.; de Irala, J.; Bes-Rastrollo, M. Pre-pregnancy adherences to empirically derived dietary patterns and gestational diabetes risk in a Mediterranean cohort: The Seguimiento Universidad de Navarra (SUN) project. *Br. J. Nutr.* **2017**, *118*, 715–721. [CrossRef] [PubMed]
8. Zhang, C.; Schulze, M.B.; Solomon, C.G.; Hu, F.B. A prospective study of dietary patterns, meat intake and the risk of gestational diabetes mellitus. *Diabetologia* **2006**, *49*, 2604–2613. [CrossRef] [PubMed]
9. Tryggvadottir, E.A.; Medek, H.; Birgisdottir, B.E.; Geirsson, R.T.; Gunnarsdottir, I. Association between healthy maternal dietary pattern and risk for gestational diabetes mellitus. *Eur. J. Clin. Nutr.* **2016**, *70*, 237–242. [CrossRef] [PubMed]
10. He, J.R.; Yuan, M.Y.; Chen, N.N.; Lu, J.H.; Hu, C.Y.; Mai, W.B.; Zhang, R.F.; Pan, Y.H.; Qiu, L.; Wu, Y.F.; et al. Maternal dietary patterns and gestational diabetes mellitus: A large prospective cohort study in China. *Br. J. Nutr.* **2015**, *113*, 1292–1300. [CrossRef] [PubMed]
11. Shin, D.; Lee, K.W.; Song, W.O. Dietary Patterns during Pregnancy Are Associated with Risk of Gestational Diabetes Mellitus. *Nutrients* **2015**, *7*, 9369–9382. [CrossRef] [PubMed]
12. Schoenaker, D.A.; Mishra, G.D.; Callaway, L.K.; Soedamah-Muthu, S.S. The Role of Energy, Nutrients, Foods, and Dietary Patterns in the Development of Gestational Diabetes Mellitus: A Systematic Review of Observational Studies. *Diabetes Care* **2016**, *39*, 16–23. [CrossRef] [PubMed]
13. Hu, F.B.; Manson, J.E.; Stampfer, M.J.; Colditz, G.; Liu, S.; Solomon, C.G.; Willett, W.C. Diet, lifestyle, and the risk of type 2 diabetes mellitus in women. *N. Engl. J. Med.* **2001**, *345*, 790–797. [CrossRef] [PubMed]
14. Shim, J.S.; Oh, K.; Kim, H.C. Dietary assessment methods in epidemiologic studies. *Epidemiol. Health* **2014**, *36*, e2014009. [CrossRef] [PubMed]
15. Walsh, J.M.; McGowan, C.A.; Mahony, R.; Foley, M.E.; McAuliffe, F.M. Low glycaemic index diet in pregnancy to prevent macrosomia (ROLO study): Randomised control trial. *BMJ* **2012**, *345*, e5605. [CrossRef]
16. Khoury, J.; Henriksen, T.; Christophersen, B.; Tonstad, S. Effect of a cholesterol-lowering diet on maternal, cord, and neonatal lipids, and pregnancy outcome: A randomized clinical trial. *Am. J. Obstet. Gynecol.* **2005**, *193*, 1292–1301. [CrossRef] [PubMed]
17. Briley, A.L.; Barr, S.; Badger, S.; Bell, R.; Croker, H.; Godfrey, K.M.; Holmes, B.; Kinnunen, T.I.; Nelson, S.M.; Oteng-Ntim, E.; et al. A complex intervention to improve pregnancy outcome in obese women; the UPBEAT randomised controlled trial. *BMC Pregnancy Childbirth* **2014**, *14*, 74. [CrossRef]
18. Hrolfsdottir, L.; Halldorsson, T.I.; Birgisdottir, B.E.; Hreidarsdottir, I.T.; Hardardottir, H.; Gunnarsdottir, I. Development of a dietary screening questionnaire to predict excessive weight gain in pregnancy. *Matern. Child Nutr.* **2018**, e12639. [CrossRef]
19. Nordic Nutrition Recommendations. *Integrating Nutrition and Physical Activity*; Nordic Council of Ministers: Copenhagen, Denmark, 2014.
20. Embætti Landlæknis. *Grundvöllur Ráðlegginga um Mataræði og Ráðlagðir Dagskammtar Næringarefna*; Embætti Landlæknis: Reykjavík, Iceland, 2016.
21. Gunnarsdottir, I.; Tryggvadottir, E.A.; Birgisdottir, B.E.; Halldorsson, T.I.; Medek, H.; Geirsson, R.T. Diet and nutrient intake of pregnant women in the capital area in Iceland. *Laeknabladid* **2016**, *102*, 378–384.
22. Olsen, S.F.; Halldorsson, T.I.; Willett, W.C.; Knudsen, V.K.; Gillman, M.W.; Mikkelsen, T.B.; Olsen, J. Milk consumption during pregnancy is associated with increased infant size at birth: Prospective cohort study. *Am. J. Clin. Nutr.* **2007**, *86*, 1104–1110. [CrossRef]
23. Renault, K.M.; Carlsen, E.M.; Norgaard, K.; Nilas, L.; Pryds, O.; Secher, N.J.; Olsen, S.F.; Halldorsson, T.I. Intake of Sweets, Snacks and Soft Drinks Predicts Weight Gain in Obese Pregnant Women: Detailed Analysis of the Results of a Randomised Controlled Trial. *PLoS ONE* **2015**, *10*, e0133041. [CrossRef]

24. Englund-Ogge, L.; Brantsaeter, A.L.; Haugen, M.; Sengpiel, V.; Khatibi, A.; Myhre, R.; Myking, S.; Meltzer, H.M.; Kacerovsky, M.; Nilsen, R.M.; et al. Association between intake of artificially sweetened and sugar-sweetened beverages and preterm delivery: A large prospective cohort study. *Am. J. Clin. Nutr.* **2012**, *96*, 552–559. [CrossRef]
25. Zhu, Y.; Olsen, S.F.; Mendola, P.; Halldorsson, T.I.; Rawal, S.; Hinkle, S.N.; Yeung, E.H.; Chavarro, J.E.; Grunnet, L.G.; Granstrom, C.; et al. Maternal consumption of artificially sweetened beverages during pregnancy, and offspring growth through 7 years of age: A prospective cohort study. *Int. J. Epidemiol.* **2017**, *46*, 1499–1508. [CrossRef]
26. Nutrition Mother and Baby; In Icelandic Næring Móðir og Barn. Available online: https://nmb.is/ (accessed on 1 April 2019).
27. White, S.L.; Lawlor, D.A.; Briley, A.L.; Godfrey, K.M.; Nelson, S.M.; Oteng-Ntim, E.; Robson, S.C.; Sattar, N.; Seed, P.T.; Vieira, M.C.; et al. Early Antenatal Prediction of Gestational Diabetes in Obese Women: Development of Prediction Tools for Targeted Intervention. *PLoS ONE* **2016**, *11*, e0167846. [CrossRef]
28. Torloni, M.R.; Betran, A.P.; Horta, B.L.; Nakamura, M.U.; Atallah, A.N.; Moron, A.F.; Valente, O. Prepregnancy BMI and the risk of gestational diabetes: A systematic review of the literature with meta-analysis. *Obes. Rev.* **2009**, *10*, 194–203. [CrossRef]
29. Bouthoorn, S.H.; Silva, L.M.; Murray, S.E.; Steegers, E.A.; Jaddoe, V.W.; Moll, H.; Hofman, A.; Mackenbach, J.P.; Raat, H. Low-educated women have an increased risk of gestational diabetes mellitus: The Generation R Study. *Acta Diabetol.* **2015**, *52*, 445–452. [CrossRef]
30. England, L.J.; Levine, R.J.; Qian, C.; Soule, L.M.; Schisterman, E.F.; Yu, K.F.; Catalano, P.M. Glucose tolerance and risk of gestational diabetes mellitus in nulliparous women who smoke during pregnancy. *Am. J. Epidemiol.* **2004**, *160*, 1205–1213. [CrossRef]
31. Lawlor, D.A.; Emberson, J.R.; Ebrahim, S.; Whincup, P.H.; Wannamethee, S.G.; Walker, M.; Smith, G.D. Is the association between parity and coronary heart disease due to biological effects of pregnancy or adverse lifestyle risk factors associated with child-rearing? Findings from the British Women's Heart and Health Study and the British Regional Heart Study. *Circulation* **2003**, *107*, 1260–1264.
32. Donazar-Ezcurra, M.; Lopez-Del Burgo, C.; Martinez-Gonzalez, M.A.; Basterra-Gortari, F.J.; de Irala, J.; Bes-Rastrollo, M. Soft drink consumption and gestational diabetes risk in the SUN project. *Clin. Nutr.* **2018**, *37*, 638–645. [CrossRef]
33. Ruiz-Gracia, T.; Duran, A.; Fuentes, M.; Rubio, M.A.; Runkle, I.; Carrera, E.F.; Torrejon, M.J.; Bordiu, E.; Valle, L.D.; Garcia de la Torre, N.; et al. Lifestyle patterns in early pregnancy linked to gestational diabetes mellitus diagnoses when using IADPSG criteria. The St Carlos gestational study. *Clin. Nutr.* **2016**, *35*, 699–705. [CrossRef]
34. Battaglia Richi, E.; Baumer, B.; Conrad, B.; Darioli, R.; Schmid, A.; Keller, U. Health Risks Associated with Meat Consumption: A Review of Epidemiological Studies. *Int. J. Vitam. Nutr. Res.* **2015**, *85*, 70–78. [CrossRef]
35. Boada, L.D.; Henriquez-Hernandez, L.A.; Luzardo, O.P. The impact of red and processed meat consumption on cancer and other health outcomes: Epidemiological evidences. *Food Chem. Toxicol.* **2016**, *92*, 236–244. [CrossRef]
36. Zhang, Y.; Gong, Y.; Xue, H.; Xiong, J.; Cheng, G. Vitamin D and gestational diabetes mellitus: A systematic review based on data free of Hawthorne effect. *BJOG* **2018**, *125*, 784–793. [CrossRef]
37. Koivusalo, S.B.; Rono, K.; Klemetti, M.M.; Roine, R.P.; Lindstrom, J.; Erkkola, M.; Kaaja, R.J.; Poyhonen Alho, M.; Tiitinen, A.; Huvinen, E.; et al. Gestational Diabetes Mellitus Can Be Prevented by Lifestyle Intervention: The Finnish Gestational Diabetes Prevention Study (RADIEL): A Randomized Controlled Trial. *Diabetes Care* **2016**, *39*, 24–30. [CrossRef]
38. NCD Risk Factor Collaboration (NCD-RisC). Trends in adult body-mass index in 200 countries from 1975 to 2014: A pooled analysis of 1698 population-based measurement studies with 19.2 million participants. *Lancet* **2016**, *387*, 1377–1396.
39. Assaf-Balut, C.; Garcia de la Torre, N.; Duran, A.; Fuentes, M.; Bordiu, E.; Del Valle, L.; Familiar, C.; Valerio, J.; Jimenez, I.; Herraiz, M.A.; et al. A Mediterranean Diet with an Enhanced Consumption of Extra Virgin Olive Oil and Pistachios Improves Pregnancy Outcomes in Women Without Gestational Diabetes Mellitus: A Sub-Analysis of the St. Carlos Gestational Diabetes Mellitus Prevention Study. *Ann. Nutr. Metab.* **2019**, *74*, 69–79. [CrossRef]

40. Chen, L.W.; Aris, I.M.; Bernard, J.Y.; Tint, M.T.; Chia, A.; Colega, M.; Gluckman, P.D.; Shek, L.P.; Saw, S.M.; Chong, Y.S.; et al. Associations of Maternal Dietary Patterns during Pregnancy with Offspring Adiposity from Birth Until 54 Months of Age. *Nutrients* **2016**, *9*, 2. [CrossRef]
41. Brantsaeter, A.L.; Haugen, M.; Samuelsen, S.O.; Torjusen, H.; Trogstad, L.; Alexander, J.; Magnus, P.; Meltzer, H.M. A dietary pattern characterized by high intake of vegetables, fruits, and vegetable oils is associated with reduced risk of preeclampsia in nulliparous pregnant Norwegian women. *J. Nutr.* **2009**, *139*, 1162–1168. [CrossRef]
42. Hillesund, E.R.; Bere, E.; Haugen, M.; Overby, N.C. Development of a New Nordic Diet score and its association with gestational weight gain and fetal growth—A study performed in the Norwegian Mother and Child Cohort Study (MoBa). *Public Health Nutr.* **2014**, *17*, 1909–1918. [CrossRef]
43. Martin, C.L.; Sotres-Alvarez, D.; Siega-Riz, A.M. Maternal Dietary Patterns during the Second Trimester Are Associated with Preterm Birth. *J. Nutr.* **2015**, *145*, 1857–1864. [CrossRef]
44. Wolff, S.; Legarth, J.; Vangsgaard, K.; Toubro, S.; Astrup, A. A randomized trial of the effects of dietary counseling on gestational weight gain and glucose metabolism in obese pregnant women. *Int. J. Obes. (Lond.)* **2008**, *32*, 495–501. [CrossRef]
45. Haby, K.; Glantz, A.; Hanas, R.; Premberg, A. Mighty Mums—An antenatal health care intervention can reduce gestational weight gain in women with obesity. *Midwifery* **2015**, *31*, 685–692. [CrossRef]
46. Rogozinska, E.; Marlin, N.; Jackson, L.; Rayanagoudar, G.; Ruifrok, A.E.; Dodds, J.; Molyneaux, E.; van Poppel, M.N.; Poston, L.; Vinter, C.A.; et al. Effects of antenatal diet and physical activity on maternal and fetal outcomes: Individual patient data meta-analysis and health economic evaluation. *Health Technol. Assess. (Winch. Engl.)* **2017**, *21*, 1–158. [CrossRef]
47. Guo, X.Y.; Shu, J.; Fu, X.H.; Chen, X.P.; Zhang, L.; Ji, M.X.; Liu, X.M.; Yu, T.T.; Sheng, J.Z.; Huang, H.F. Improving the effectiveness of lifestyle interventions for gestational diabetes prevention: A meta-analysis and meta-regression. *BJOG* **2019**, *126*, 311–320. [CrossRef]

7

Prenatal Intervention with Partial Meal Replacement Improves Micronutrient Intake of Pregnant Women with Obesity

Suzanne Phelan [1,*], Barbara Abrams [2] and Rena R. Wing [3]

1 Department of Kinesiology & Public Health, California Polytechnic State University, 1 Grand Ave, San Luis Obispo, CA 93407, USA

2 Division of Epidemiology, University of California at Berkeley School of Public Health, 2121 Berkeley Way #5302, Berkeley, CA 94720-7360, USA; babrams@berkeley.edu

3 Warren Alpert Medical School at Brown University Department of Psychiatry and Human Behavior, 197 Richmond Street, Providence, RI 02906, USA; rwing@lifespan.org

* Correspondence: sphelan@calpoly.edu

Abstract: A behavioral lifestyle intervention with partial meal replacement reduced excess gestational weight gain in ethnically diverse women with overweight/obesity, but the effects on micronutrient intake remained unknown. A secondary analysis of a randomized, controlled trial tested whether the intervention improved micronutrient intake relative to usual care. Pregnant women (n = 211; 30.5 years of age, body mass index, BMI, of 32.0 kg/m^2) were enrolled and randomized within site and ethnicity (40% were Hispanic) into intervention (n = 102) or usual care (n = 109) groups. Two 24 h dietary recalls were conducted on random days at study entry and late pregnancy (35–36 weeks gestation). Nutrient adequacy was defined using the Estimated Average Requirement cut-point method. At study entry and including prenatal vitamins, ≥90% of participants reported inadequate intake of vitamins D and E and iron; 40–50% reported inadequate intake of calcium, protein, vitamins A, C, B_6, folate, magnesium, and zinc. From study entry to late pregnancy, the behavioral intervention with partial meal replacement increased the overall intake of vitamins A, E, and D and copper and reduced the odds of inadequate intake of calcium (odds ratio (OR) = 0.37 (0.18, 0.76)), vitamins A (OR = 0.39 (0.21, 0.72)) and E (OR = 0.17 (0.06, 0.48)), and magnesium (OR = 0.36 (0.20, 0.65)). A behavioral intervention with partial meal replacement during pregnancy improved the intake of several micronutrients in Hispanic and non-Hispanic women with overweight/obesity.

Keywords: prenatal intervention; meal replacements; randomized clinical trial; lifestyle intervention; obesity; RDA; micronutrients

1. Introduction

Maternal pre-pregnancy obesity and excess gestational weight gain are well established risk factors for several adverse short- and long-term maternal and child health outcomes, including pregnancy complications, diabetes, obesity, and cardio-metabolic comorbidities [1]. Compounding risks, pregnant women with obesity are more likely than those with normal weight to have micronutrient insufficiency [2–4], conferring additional potential risks of pregnancy complications and chronic conditions in later life [5,6].

The Academy of Nutrition and Dietetics recommends that the optimal prenatal diet should limit overconsumption yet prevent micronutrient insufficiency [5]. A varied and balanced diet, rich in fruits, vegetables, and whole grains is recommended. Several studies have shown that comprehensive lifestyle interventions that target reduced calorie intake and balanced nutrition can effectively reduce excess gestational weight gain in women with obesity [7], but less is known about intervention effects on micronutrient intake. Micronutrient needs increase during pregnancy, particularly for folic acid, iron, zinc, calcium, vitamin C, and vitamin D [8]. While supplementation can reduce micronutrient deficiencies and some associated maternal and fetal complications [9–12], adherence to prenatal multivitamins may be limited by gastrointestinal distress or nausea [13]. The provision of micronutrient-rich foods [14,15] and nutrition educational interventions [16] can also improve dietary quality and pregnancy outcomes, but few randomized clinical trials have been done, particularly in pregnant women with obesity who are at risk of micronutrient insufficiency [15].

Healthy Beginnings/Cominezos Saludables was a randomized clinical trial designed to test the efficacy of a partial meal replacement program versus usual care to reduce excessive gestational weight gain in 257 pregnant women with overweight or obesity. The intervention significantly reduced excess gestational weight gain, which was related to increased use of meal replacements during pregnancy [17]. No significant treatment effect was seen on energy or macronutrient composition [17]. Since the provided meal replacements were fortified with vitamins and minerals, it is possible that they could address underlying micronutrient inadequacies in pregnant women with overweight or obesity. The purpose of this study was to determine if the behavioral intervention with partial meal replacement compared with usual care improved micronutrient intake of pregnant women with overweight and obesity.

2. Materials and Methods

2.1. Design

Healthy Beginnings/Comienzo Saludables was a randomized controlled trial conducted at California Polytechnic State University, San Luis Obispo, California, and at the Miriam Hospital with Women & Infants Hospital in Providence, Rhode Island, and was part of the Lifestyle Interventions for Expectant Moms (LIFE-Moms) consortium [18]. Clinical Trial Registry Number: ClinicalTrials.gov, www.clinicaltrials.gov, NCT01545934.

2.2. Participants

The study was conducted in accordance with the ethical principles of research; the protocol was approved by the Institutional Review Boards of California Polytechnic State University (2018-264) and the Miriam Hospital (2144-11), and all participants provided written informed consent. As previously described [17,19], recruitment occurred November 2012 and October 2015 in California and Rhode Island. Eligibility criteria included gestational age between 9 and 16 weeks, body mass index (BMI) ≥25, being English or Spanish-speaking, age ≥18 years, and singleton pregnancy. Participants were excluded if they had glycosylated hemoglobin (Hb A1c) ≥ 6.5 or self-reported major health diseases (e.g., heart disease, cancer, renal disease, and diabetes), and other (Figure 1). Of the 5381 screened women, 24% were excluded due to BMI < 25, and 24% were excluded due to gestational age >16 weeks. Other prevalent reasons for exclusions are shown in Figure 1.

Figure 1.

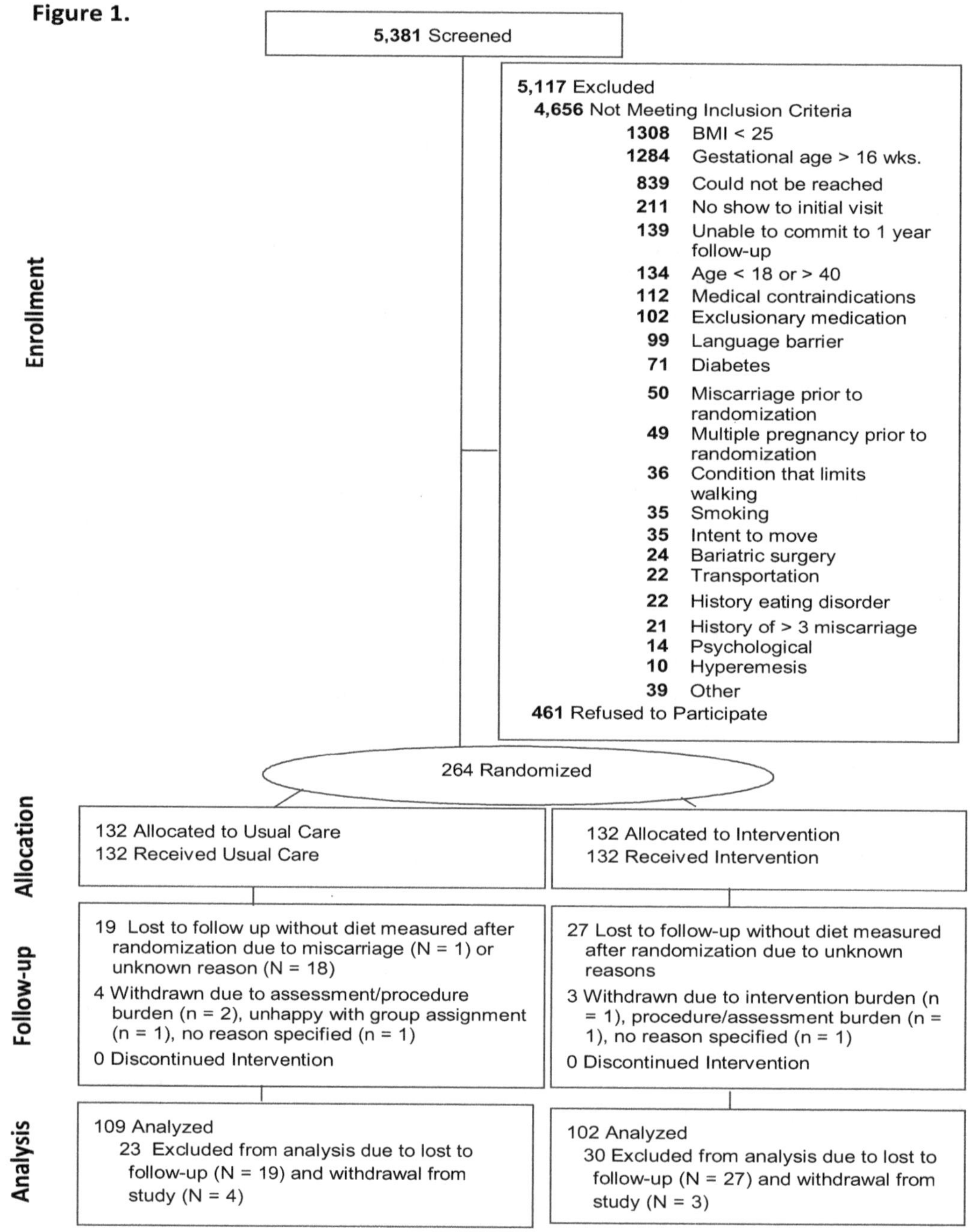

Figure 1. Participant flow and Retention in Healthy Beginnings/Comienzos Saludables. BMI = body mass index.

2.3. *Interventions*

In this two-site trial, randomization was computer-generated by the study statistician, and women were randomly assigned within site and ethnicity (Hispanic versus non-Hispanic) to one of the two treatment conditions: (1) usual care or (2) behavioral lifestyle intervention with partial meal replacement.

2.4. *Usual Care*

Participants in the usual care group received all aspects of usual care offered by their prenatal care providers [20]. Usual prenatal care visits typically occur monthly until 28 weeks of gestation, bi-weekly between 28 and 36 weeks of gestation, and weekly until delivery. Also, in this group at the time of study randomization, participants attended a ~20 min welcome visit with a study interventionist, providing general information about healthy eating, physical activity, and the Institte of Medicine (IOM)recommendations for total gestational weight gain [21]. Study interventionists were bilingual registered dietitians or counselors with degrees in nutrition, community health, psychology, kinesiology, or a related field. Participants received study newsletters with general information about pregnancy-related health, including consuming prenatal vitamins, quitting smoking, planning to breastfeed, and fetal growth.

2.5. *Behavioral Lifestyle Intervention with Partial Meal Replacement during Pregnancy*

Participants in the intervention group received all aspects of usual care plus a behavioral lifestyle intervention designed to prevent excessive weight gain during pregnancy. As described previously [17], the intervention targeted healthy eating, activity, and behavioral strategies. Each woman received ~20 min, individual, face-to-face counseling sessions with a study interventionist every two weeks until 20 weeks of gestation and then monthly visits until delivery. Women were encouraged to gain approximately one-half pound (0.23 kg) per week, on the basis of the 2009 IOM guidelines [21]. To promote adherence to weight gain guidelines, women were provided with a structured meal plan [22] that was individually tailored to meet each participant's self-reported dietary needs, including food aversions, cravings, lactose intolerance, and specialized diets, such as vegetarianism. The plan provided a caloric prescription of ~18 kcal/kg of body weight at study entry [23] and consisted of 30% of calories from fat, 15–20% from protein, and 50–55% from carbohydrates [24]. Women were instructed to replace two meals with a provided meal replacement shake or bar and to consume at least one meal of regular foods and two to four healthy snacks each day. The meal replacement products were provided free of charge at every intervention visit and in the quantities needed until the next scheduled intervention visit. The study's meal replacement options were selected at study onset by the investigators after an analysis of various meal plan scenarios that considered the micronutrient and macronutrient composition of specific meal replacement products, the participant's use of prenatal vitamins, the intervention's calorie and nutritional goals, and the current micronutrient and macronutrient recommendations for pregnant women [24]. Options included organic and lactose-free drinks and bars in a variety of flavors and brands (Supplemental Table S1).

2.6. *Outcome Assessments*

Assessments were conducted early in pregnancy (between 9 and 16 weeks) and at 35–36 weeks of gestation. The participants received $25 for completing each assessment. The assessment staff was masked to randomization to minimize potential bias. Dietary intake was assessed at study entry and 35–36 weeks of gestation using interview-administered 24 h recalls on two random days over a week and completed using the National Cancer Institute Automated Self-Administered 24 h recall (ASA-24; http://riskfactor.cancer.gov/tools/instruments/asa24.html) [25]. The ASA-24 provided values (combined from food, beverages, and supplements) for thiamin, riboflavin, niacin, vitamin B6, folate, vitamin B12, vitamin C, vitamin A, vitamin E, iron, zinc, calcium, magnesium, phosphorous, copper, selenium, water, energy, carbohydrate, total fat, and protein and included intake of supplements [26]. Dietary intake was categorized as meeting or not meeting the Recommended Daily Allowance (RDA) based on the Estimated Average Requirement (EAR) of the Institute of Medicine (IOM) for pregnant women [27–32]. The RDA represents an estimate of the average daily intake level sufficient to meet the nutrient requirements for 97–98% of healthy individuals. To assess the prevalence of inadequacy, the cut-point method was used [29,33] to classify individuals with intakes below versus at or above the median EAR considered needed for half of the individuals in the population (Table 1) [27–32,34,35]. For micronutrients in which an RDA and EAR had not been established (i.e., vitamin K, choline, potassium, sodium), cutoffs based on Adequate Intakes (AI) were used, albeit interpreted with less confidence [27–32]. The ASA-24 was also used to measure meal replacement intake, quantified as the total number of meal replacement products including shakes and bars that were consumed each day, on average, during the assessment period.

Table 1. Estimated average requirements (EAR) [1] for pregnancy.

Nutrient	Recommended Amount
Total Water (L/d) **	3.0 **
Calcium (mg/d)	800
CHO (g/d)	135
Fiber (g/d) **	28 **
Added sugars	≤25% of TE
Protein (g/kg/d)	0.88
Vit A μg, RAE/d	550
Vit C (mg/d)	70
Vit D (μg/d)	10
Vit E (mg/d)	12
Vit K μg/d **	90 **
Thiamin (mg/d)	1.2
Riboflavin (mg/d)	1.2
Niacin (mg/d)	14
Vit B6 (mg/d)	1.6
Folate (μg/d)	520
Vit B12 (μg/d)	2.2
Choline mg/d **	450 **
Copper (μg/d)	800
Iron (mg/d)	22
Magnesium (mg/d)	290
Phosphorus (mg/d)	580
Selenium (μg/d)	49
Zinc (mg/d)	9.5
Potassium mg/d **	4.7 **
Sodium g/d **	1.5 **

Abbreviations: Vit: vitamin; TE: total energy; d: day; RAE: retinol activity equivalents; CHO: carbohydrates: [1] EAR is the average daily nutrient intake level estimated to meet the requirements of half of the healthy individuals who are pregnant and aged 19–30 years [27–32]. Vitamin A based on RAEs; vitamin E based on α-tocopherol; niacin expressed as niacin equivalents; folate expressed as folate equivalents. Food and Nutrition Board, Institute of Medicine, National Academies reports may be accessed via www.nap.edu [27–32], ** Adequate Intakes (AI) because EARs have not been established; this cutoff is made with less confidence [27–32].

Weight and height were assessed in duplicate to the nearest 0.1 kg or 0.1 cm using a calibrated standard digital scale and stadiometer with the participant in lightweight clothing without shoes. Heritage and ethnicity were assessed by self-report using questionnaires with fixed categories. Marital status, income, education, employment status, and childbearing history were also assessed by self-report questionnaires. Gestational age in weeks at study entry was measured via clinical ultrasound.

2.7. Statistical Methods

Analysis Plan

To compare participants in the two groups and completers versus non-completers, Independent *t*-test for continuous variables and Pearson $\chi 2$ test or exact tests for categorical variables were used. To test if the intervention versus usual care affected micronutrient values, a repeated measures analysis of variance was used. The models included the terms treatment group and group × time interactions (fixed effect) and a priori defined covariates that included weeks of gestation at randomization, age, ethnicity (Hispanic versus non-Hispanic), parity (multiparity versus primiparity), study entry BMI category (overweight versus obese), household family income (≥50,000/year versus <50,000/year), and baseline value of variable of interest [36]; site (California versus Rhode Island) was also included as a fixed effect. (A sensitivity analysis that divided the income into four categories and also included education did not alter the results). To test whether the intervention versus usual care improved micronutrient adequacy (meeting versus not meeting RDA's EAR cutpoint), logistic regression was used that included the treatment group and the same covariates. Within the intervention group alone, number of meal replacement products/day and changes in micronutrients status were also analyzed via Pearson's partial correlations, adjusting for the same covariates. Statistical significance was set to $p < 0.05$. The SPSS (23.0.0; IBM Corporation; Armonk, NY, USA) statistical package was used for all analyses.

3. Results

Figure 1 summarizes the participant flow and retention into Healthy Beginnings/Comienzos Saludables. Participant characteristics were well balanced by randomized group (Table 2). At the 35–36 weeks of gestation visit, 82.1% (211/257) of participants completed the dietary assessment, including 85.2% (109/128) of usual care and 79.1% (102/129) of intervention participants, with no statistically significant ($p = 0.55$) differences in retention by group. The demographic characteristics (site, group, BMI, age, education, parity, weeks of gestation at randomization) did not significantly differ between participants who completed and those who did not complete the 35–36 weeks gestation visit. Completers were more likely than non-completers to have adequate intake of phosphorus (38/43 versus 209/211; chi square test $p = 0.002$), niacin (32/46 versus 187/211; $p = 0.002$), riboflavin (33/46 versus 185/211; $p = 0.011$), and thiamin (23/46 versus 144/211; $p = 0.03$); no other significant differences were observed.

Table 2. Baseline characteristics of the participants by condition.

Characteristic	Total $n = 211$	Usual Care $n = 109$	Intervention $n = 102$
Age, years, Mean (SD)	30.5 (5.3)	30.0 (5.6)	31.0 (4.9)
Hispanic/Latino, No. (%)			
Yes	85 (40.3)	43 (39.4)	42 (41.2)
No	126 (59.7)	66 (60.6)	60 (58.8)
Heritage, No. (%) (participants could select multiple)			
American Indian or Alaskan Native	7 (3.3)	3 (2.8)	4 (3.9)
Asian	2 (0.9)	0 (0)	2 (2.0)
Black or African American	15 (7.1)	7 (6.4)	8 (7.8)
Native Hawaiian or Pacific Islander	4 (1.9)	3 (2.8)	1 (1.0)
White	131 (62.1)	67 (61.5)	64 (62.7)
Other	60 (28.4)	30 (27.5)	30 (29.4)
Marital Status, No. (%)			
Married or living with significant other	148 (70.1)	97 (89.0)	51 (50.0)
Never married/divorced/widowed	63 (29.9)	12 (11.0)	51 (50.0)
Annual household Income $, No. (%)			
<$24,999	49 (23.2)	28 (25.7)	21 (20.6)
$25,000–49,999	62 (29.4)	30 (27.5)	32 (31.4)
$50,000–99,999	60 (28.4)	30 (27.5)	30 (29.4)
≥$100,000	40 (19.0)	21 (19.3)	19 (18.6)
Education, No. (%)			
High school or less	48 (22.7)	29 (26.6)	19 (18.6)
Some college/College	130 (61.6)	62 (56.9)	68 (66.7)
Post-graduate work	33 (15.6)	18 (16.5)	15 (14.7)
Employment, No. (%)			
Employed Full Time (at least 35 hours/week)	121 (57.3)	62 (56.9)	59 (57.8)
Employed Part-Time (less than 35 hours/week)	38 (18.0)	22 (20.2)	16 (15.7)
Unemployed	52 (24.6)	25 (22.9)	27 (26.5)
Childbearing history, No. (%)			
Primiparous	53 (25.1)	25 (22.9)	28 (27.5)
Multiparous	154 (73.0)	82 (75.2)	72 (70.6)
Weeks of gestation at study entry, Mean (SD)	13.6 (1.7)	13.5 (1.9)	13.8 (1.5)
Weight, kg, at study entry, Mean (SD)	84.9 (16.5)	86.1 (17.9)	83.6 (14.8)
BMI, kg/m^2, at study entry, Mean (SD)	32. (5.3)	32.5 (5.4)	32.1 (5.3)

Table 2. *Cont.*

Characteristic	Total n = 211	Usual Care n = 109	Intervention n = 102
Weight status			
Overweight, No. (%)	86 (40.8)	42 (38.5)	44 (43.1)
Obese, No. (%)	125 (59.2)	67 (61.5)	58 (56.9)
Preconception weight, Mean (SD)	83.0 (16.5)	81.9 (14.8)	84.1 (17.9)
Preconception weight status			
Overweight, No. (%)	94 (44.5)	44 (40.4)	50 (49.0)
Obese, No. (%)	114 (54.0)	63 (57.8)	51 (50.0)
Weight gain from preconception to study entry, kg, Mean (SD)	1.9 (4.4)	1.8 (3.3)	19 (5.0)
Daily prenatal vitamin intake, No. (%)	105 (96.7%)	105 (96.3)	99 (97.0)

Abbreviations: SD: standard deviation; BMI is calculated as weight in kilograms divided by the square of height in meters. Y: years. No.: number.

3.1. Intervention Effects on Micronutrient Intake

When examining the average changes in micronutrients from study entry to 35–36 weeks gestation (Table 3), significant group × time interactions indicated that the intervention relative to usual care increased the average intake of vitamins A (178.3 versus 34.6, μg/day, respectively; p = 0.0001), E (1.9 versus −0.3 mg/day; p = 0.0001), and K (23.4 versus −11.7 μg/day; p = 0.04). In addition, the intervention significantly increased (relative to usual care) the intakes of vitamin D (1.5 versus 0.5 μg/day; p = 0.045) and copper (259.2 versus −34.5, μg/day; p = 0.001) and significantly decreased the intake of selenium (−11.0 versus −7.2 μg/day; p = 0.002).

Table 3. Micronutrient intake from early pregnancy (baseline) to 35 weeks of gestation by treatment group.

	EAR	Usual Care; n = 109 Mean (SD)		Intervention; n = 102 Mean (SD)		Statistical Results [1]	
		Baseline	35 Weeks	Baseline	35 Weeks	T	G × T
Total Water, L/d	3.0 **	2.6 (0.9)	2.8 (1.1)	2.5 (0.8)	2.8 (0.9)	0.20	0.72
Calcium, mg/d	800	973.5 (355.8)	1026.0 (387.8)	928.9 (352.1)	1097.2 (378.0)	0.06	0.14
CHO, g/d	135	219.6 (68.3)	225.1 (71.9)	219.7 (75.6)	217.7 (63.3)	0.001	0.783
Fiber, g/d	28 **	16.5 (6.3)	15.6 (6.6)	16.7 (6.9)	14.2 (6.4)	0.02	0.07
Added sugars, % TE	<25% of TE	9.6 (4.6)	10.3 (7.0)	10.5 (6.1)	12.3 (10.3)	0.28	0.35
Protein, g/kg/d,	0.88	0.9 (0.3)	0.8 (0.3)	0.9 (.31665)	0.8 (0.3)	0.92	0.76
Vit A μg, RAE/d·	**550**	**631.2 (336.6)**	**667.6 (372.3)**	**720.0 (378.9)**	**898.0 (402.9)**	**0.10**	**0.0001**
Vit C, mg/d	70	90.1 (62.4)	78.0 (57.3)	103.3 (70.5)	94.6 (64.8)	0.03	0.09
Vit D, μg/d	**10**	**4.1 (2.6)**	**4.6 (2.9)**	**4.0 (2.5)**	**5.5 (3.3)**	**0.55**	**0.045**
Vit E, mg/d	**12**	**7.2 (4.4)**	**6.9 (3.1)**	**7.3 (3.7)**	**9.2 (5.0)**	**0.03**	**0.0001**
Vit K, μg/d	**90 ***	**111.8 (108.6)**	**100.0 (105.0)**	**116.1 (114.3)**	**140.0 (175.3)**	**0.07**	**0.04**
Thiamin, mg/d	1.2	1.5 (0.5)	1.6 (0.6)	1.5 (0.6)	1.5 (0.62)	0.04	0.91
Riboflavin, mg/d	1.2	1.9 (0.6)	2.1 (0.7)	1.9 (0.8)	2.0 (0.8)	0.63	0.77
Niacin, mg/d	14	22.2 (7.6)	22.3 (8.6)	22.2 (7.8)	22.4 (7.4)	0.01	0.95
Vit B6, mg/d	1.6	1.9 (0.9)	2.0 (0.9)	1.9 (0.8)	2.0 (2.0)	0.02	0.72
Folate, μg/d	520	519.4 (218.2)	554.1 (248.7)	557.9 (267.5)	550.3 (287.3)	0.01	0.71
Vit B12, μg/d	2.2	4.8 (3.1)	5.3 (2.8)	5.4 (4.2)	5.2 (2.9)	0.9	0.70
**Choline, mg/d ** **	**450 ****	**285.1 (160.4)**	**294.0 (150.3)**	**291.5 (208.6)**	**230.4 (138.5)**	**0.11**	**0.005**
Copper, μg/d	**800**	**1270 (471)**	**1236 (390)**	**1208 (363)**	**1467 (473)**	**0.14**	**0.0001**
Iron, mg/d	22	14.0 (5.3)	15.1 (5.5)	15.1 (6.0)	15.7 (6.2)	0.003	0.70
Magnesium, mg/d	290	280.7 (90.5)	282.4 (93.7)	269.6 (79.4)	326.5 (99.3)	**0.09**	**0.001**
Phosphorus, mg/d	580	1246.6 (391.9)	1262.9 (407.4)	1172.6 (360.1)	1255.3 (353.4)	0.035	0.91
Selenium, μg/d	**49**	**108.9 (37.9)**	**101.6 (28.3)**	**100.4 (38.4)**	**88.1 (28.9)**	**0.012**	**0.002**
Zinc, mg/d	9.5	11.2 (4.6)	11.0 (4.0)	10.6 (4.0)	12.2 (4.8)	0.635	0.06
Potassium mg/d	4.7**	2.4 (0.7)	2.4 (0.8)	2.4 (0.8)	2.4 (0.7)	0.003	0.63
Sodium g/d	**1.5 ****	**3.2 (1.0)**	**3.1 (0.9)**	**3.1 (1.0)**	**2.8 (1.1)**	**0.118**	**0.04**

Bold font used to highlight nutrients that statistically differed by randomized group. Abbreviations: TE: total energy; T: time; G × T: group by time, Vitamin A based on RAEs; [1] Repeated measures ANOVA adjusted for weeks gestation at randomization, age, ethnicity (Hispanic versus non-Hispanic), parity (multiparity versus primiparity), study entry BMI category (overweight verssu obese), household family income (>50,000/year versus <50,000/year), and baseline value of the variable of interest. However, the mean (SD) values in table are shown unadjusted. ** AI because EARs have not been established; this cutoff is made with less confidence [27–32].

3.2. Intervention Effects on Micronutrient Adequacy Based on the RDAs

Study Entry. Despite the prevalent intake of prenatal vitamins (97%, Table 2), significant proportions of participants reported inadequate intakes of nearly every micronutrient on the basis of the EARs for pregnant women (Table 4). The vast majority (≥90%) reported inadequate intakes of fiber, vitamin D, Vitamin E, iron. Nearly half (between 40 and 50%) of the participants also reported inadequate intakes of calcium, protein, vitamin A, vitamin C, vitamin B_6, folate, magnesium, and zinc. On the basis of AI cutoffs, inadequate intakes of choline and vitamin K were also quite prevalent (Table 4). Few participants reported intakes that were at or above the recommended tolerable limit for the micronutrients. Exceptions were that a majority of participants had higher than recommended as tolerable levels of sodium (170/211; 81.0%), and a minority had excess magnesium (39/211; 18.5%), folate (12/211; 5.7%), and niacin (19/211; 9.0%) at study entry (Table 5).

Table 4. Proportions with micronutrient inadequacy at 35 weeks of gestation by treatment group.

	EAR	Usual Care; *n* = 109 No. (%)		Intervention; *n* = 102 No. (%)					
		Baseline	35 Weeks	Baseline	35 Weeks	Sig [1]	OR [1]	95% CI [1] Lower	Upper
Total Water, L/d; No. (%)	3.0 **	74 (67.9)	72 (66.1)	85 (83.3)	64 (62.8)	0.27	0.70	0.37	1.33
Calcium, mg/d; No. (%)	**800**	**43 (39.5)**	**34 (31.2)**	**41 (40.2)**	**18 (17.7)**	**0.007**	**0.37**	**0.18**	**0.76**
CHO, g/d; No. (%)	135	9 (8.3)	9 (8.3)	11 (10.8)	5 (4.9)	0.34	0.55	0.16	1.88
Fiber, g/d; No. (%)	28 **	102 (93.6)	104 (95.4)	98 (96.1)	100 (98.0)	0.32	2.54	0.41	15.91
Added sugars, % TE; No. (%)	<25% of TE	0 (0.00)	5 (4.6)	2 (2.0)	6 (5.9)	0.53	0.52	0.07	4.10
Protein, g/kg/d; No. (%)	0.88	53 (48.6)	71 (65.2)	52 (51.0)	71 (69.6)	0.42	1.30	0.69	2.45
Vit A, μg_RAE/d; No. (%)	**550**	**53 (48.6)**	**50 (45.9)**	**44 (43.1)**	**26 (25.5)**	**0.003**	**0.39**	**0.21**	**0.72**
Vit C, mg/d; No. (%)	70	45 (41.3)	56 (51.4)	39 (38.2)	41 (40.2)	0.17	0.66	0.37	1.18
Vit D, μg/d; No. (%)	10	106 (97.3)	103 (94.5)	99 (97.1)	95 (93.1)	0.53	0.68	0.20	2.27
Vit E, mg/d; No. (%)	**12**	**98 (89.9)**	**104 (95.4)**	**91 (89.2)**	**79 (77.5)**	**0.001**	**0.17**	**0.06**	**0.48**
Vit K, μg/d; No. (%)	**90 ****	**65 (59.6)**	**70 (64.2)**	**57 (55.9)**	**49 (48.0)**	**0.023**	**0.49**	**0.26**	**0.91**
Thiamin, mg/d; No. (%)	1.2	29 (26.6)	24 (22.0)	38 (37.3)	31 (30.4)	0.08	1.61	0.95	2.73
Riboflavin (mg/d; No. (%)	1.2	10 (9.2)	9 (8.3)	16 (15.7)	10 (9.8)	0.25	1.43	0.77	2.66
Niacin (mg/d; No. (%)	14	12 (11.0)	15 (13.8)	12 (11.8)	11 (10.8)	0.58	1.18	0.66	2.11
Vit B6 (mg/d; No. (%)	1.6	46 (42.2)	44 (40.4)	36 (35.3)	27 (26.5)	0.06	0.56	0.31	1.03
Folate (μg/d; No. (%)	520	63 (57.8)	59 (54.1)	52 (51.0)	55 (53.9)	0.85	1.06	0.59	1.89
Vit B12 (μg/d; No. (%)	2.2	13 (11.9)	8 (7.3)	11 (10.8)	10 (9.8)	0.37	1.62	0.57	4.60
Choline mg/d; No. (%)	**450 ****	**98 (89.9)**	**99 (90.8)**	**91 (89.2)**	**100 (98.0)**	**0.048**	**5.00**	**1.02**	**24.60**
Copper (μg/d; No. (%)	800	13 (11.9)	10 (9.2)	8 (7.8)	7 (6.7)	0.85	1.11	0.37	3.32
Iron (mg/d; No. (%)	22	102 (93.6)	102 (93.6)	90 (88.2)	90 (88.2)	0.55	0.72	0.25	2.08
Magnesium (mg/d; No. (%))	290	69 (63.3)	64 (58.7)	70 (68.6)	38 (37.3)	**0.001**	**0.36**	**0.20**	**0.65**
Phosphorus (mg/d; No. (%)	580	1 (0.9)	3 (2.8)	1 (1.0)	3 (2.9)	0.99	1.01	0.18	5.74
Selenium (μg/d; No. (%)	49	2 (1.8)	3 (2.8)	8 (7.8)	9 (8.8)	0.08	3.67	0.88	15.30
Zinc (mg/d; No. (%)	9.5	42 (38.5)	47 (43.1)	44 (43.1)	36 (35.3)	0.25	0.71	0.39	1.27
Potassium mg/d; No. (%)	4.7 **	0 (0)	0 (0)	0 (0)	0 (0)	–	–	–	–
Sodium, g/d; No. (%)	1.5 **	2 (1.8)	2 (1.8)	5 (4.9)	7 (6.9)	0.68	0.91	0.57	1.45

Bold font used to highlight nutrients that statistically differed by randomized group. Abbreviations: [1] Logistic regression analysis adjusted for weeks of gestation at randomization, age, ethnicity (Hispanic versus non-Hispanic), parity (multiparity versus primiparity), study entry BMI category (overweight versus obese), household family income (>50,000/year versus <50,000/year), and baseline value of the variable of interest. ** AI because EARs have not been established; this cutoff is made with less confidence [27–32].

Study Entry to 35–36 Weeks of Gestation. Significant group x time interactions were observed that indicated that the intervention significantly reduced the odds at 35–36 weeks of gestation of inadequate intake based on the EARs for calcium (odds ratio (OR) = 0.34 (0.18, 0.76) p = 0.007), vitamin A (OR = 0.39 (0.21, 0.72) p = 0.003;), vitamin E (OR = 0.17 (0.06, 0.48) p = 0.001), and magnesium (OR = 0.36 (0.20, 0.65) p = 0.001), as shown in Table 4. Based on AIs, the intervention also decreased the odds of inadequate intake of vitamin K (OR = 0.49 (0.26, 0.91)) and increased the odds of inadequate intake of choline (OR = 5.0 (1.0, 24.6) p = 0.04).

From study entry to 35–36 weeks of gestation, the intervention reduced the odds of intake above tolerable limits for sodium (OR = 0.47 (0.24, 0.91) p = 0.026) and increased the odds of intake above tolerable limits for magnesium (OR = 2.0 (1.0, 3.7); p = 0.038) (Table 5).

Table 5. Proportions with micronutrient levels above recommended tolerable limits.

	Upper Limit [1]	Usual Care $n = 109$		Intervention $n = 102$		Sig [2]	OR [2]	95% CI	
								Lower	Upper
		Baseline	35 Weeks	Baseline	35 Weeks				
Calcium no., %	2500 (mg/d)	0	0	0	0	–	–	–	–
Vit A no., %	3000 (μg/d)	0	0	0	0	–	–	–	–
Vit C no., %	2000 (mg/d)	0	0	0	0	–	–	–	–
Vit E no., %	1000 (mg/d)	0	0	0	0	–	–	–	–
Niacin no., %	35 (mg/d)	9 (8.2)	5 (4.6)	10 (9.8)	5 (4.9)	0.89	0.91	0.23	3.52
Vit B6 no., %	1000 (mg/d)	0	0	0	0	–	–	–	–
Folate no., %	100 (μg/d)	4 (3.7)	7 (6.4)	8	4 (3.9)	0.10	0.27	0.05	1.30
Choline no., %	3500 mg/d	0	0	0	0	–	–	–	–
Copper no., %	10,000 (μg/d)	0	0	0	0	–	–	–	–
Magnesium no., %	350 (mg/d)	23 (21.1)	24 (22.0)	16 (15.7)	36 (35.3)	0.038	1.97	1.04	3.74
Phosphorus no., %	3500(mg/d)	0	0	0	0	–	–	–	–
Selenium no., %	400 (μg/d)	0	0	0	0	–	–	–	–
Zinc no., %	40 (mg/d)	0	0	0	0	–	–	–	–
Sodium no., %	2.3 g/d	90 (82.6)	85 (78.0)	80 (78.4)	64 (62.7)	0.026	0.47	0.24	0.91

Abbreviations: [1] Upper limit (UL) is the highest level of daily nutrient intake that is likely to pose no risk of adverse health effects to almost all pregnant women aged 19–30 years. As intake increases above the UL, the risk for adverse effects increases. ULs are not intended to be a recommended level of intake, rather a level of intake that most individuals can likely tolerate. [2] Logistic regression analysis adjusted for weeks of gestation at randomization, age, ethnicity (Hispanic versus non-Hispanic), parity (multiparity versus primiparity), study entry BMI category (overweight versus obese), household family income (>50,000/year versus <50,000/year), baseline value of the variable of interest.

3.3. *Intervention Adherence*

From baseline to weeks 35–36, the intervention increased the average number of meal replacement products reported each day by an additional 0.63 (SD 0.83) products/day. Increased reported intake of meal replacement products/day was significantly related to increased intake of micronutrients (Figure 2), including vitamin A ($r = 0.33$; $p = 0.002$), vitamin E ($r = 0.30$; $p = 0.004$), niacin ($r = 0.21$; $p = 0.043$), thiamin ($r = 0.31$; $p = 0.003$), copper ($r = 0.50$; $p = 0.0001$), iron ($r = 0.28$; $p = 0.008$), magnesium ($r = 0.47$; $p = 0.0001$), phosphorus ($r = 0.22$; $p = 0.04$), and zinc ($r = 0.241$ $p = 0.02$). Trend positive partial correlations were observed for calcium ($r = 0.21$; $p = 0.05$), riboflavin ($r = 0.20$; $p = 0.058$), vitamin B_6 ($r = 0.20$; $p = 0.06$), and choline ($r = 0.20$; $p = 0.06$), and a trend inverse correlation was observed for vitamin K ($r = -0.18$; $p = 0.08$) (Figure 2). No significant correlations were observed for changes in meal replacements and vitamin C, K, folic acid, B_{12}, selenium, potassium, or sodium.

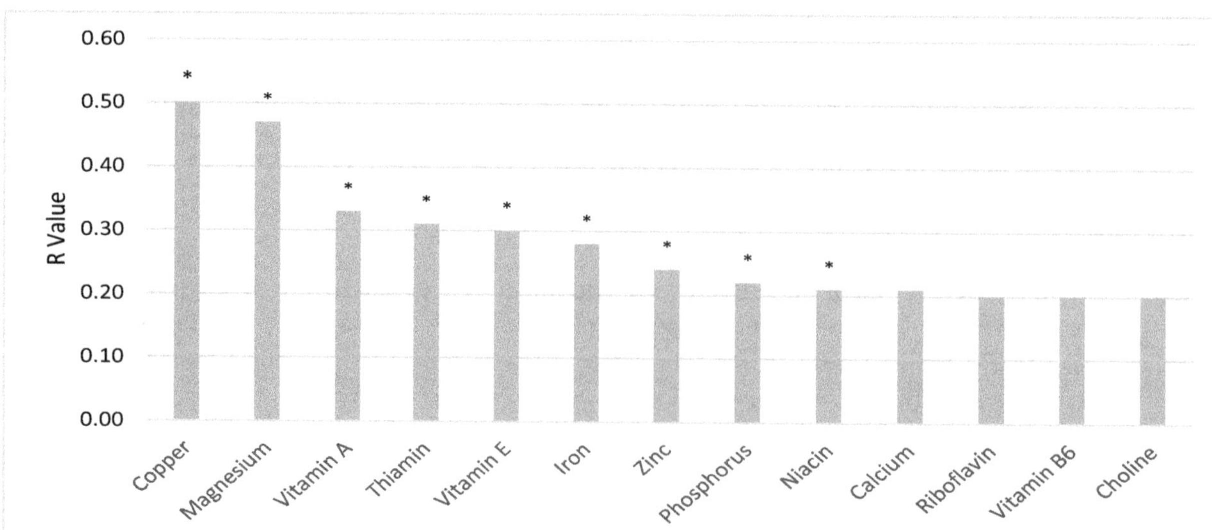

Figure 2. R values for changes in daily meal replacement servings/day and micronutrients from study entry to 35 weeks gestation among the intervention participants. * $p < 0.05$.

4. Discussion

A prenatal meal replacement intervention that reduced excess gestational weight gain also improved the micronutrient intake of pregnant women with overweight and obesity. At study entry, despite the intake of prenatal vitamins, more than 90% of participants reported inadequate intakes of vitamin E, and about 50% reported inadequate intakes of calcium, vitamins A and K, and magnesium. By 35 weeks of gestation, the prenatal lifestyle intervention with partial meal replacement had cut by more than half the odds of these micronutrient insufficiencies. Given the association between inadequate levels of nutrients during pregnancy and later adverse maternal and child health conditions [5], these findings highlight an additional potential benefit of the lifestyle intervention that reduced excess gestational weight gain [17].

At study entry, the vast majority of participants (81%) had higher than recommended intakes for sodium. By 35 weeks gestation, the intervention reduced by nearly 90% the odds of excess sodium intake based on AI cutoffs. The effects of excess sodium intake during pregnancy remain unclear [37]. Animal and some human studies have suggested that excess sodium may negatively affect the immune system [38] and placental functioning [37,39,40] and contribute to the development of high blood pressure and pre-eclampsia [41]. However, mixed findings and lack of evidence that restricting sodium during pregnancy has any long-term health benefits to mothers or children have led the current guidelines not to recommend sodium restriction during pregnancy, unless a woman has high blood pressure [42,43]. In the current trial, the intervention did not have a significant effect on lowering blood pressure [17], despite the reductions in sodium intake reported here.

The intervention-related increases in micronutrient intake generally occurred without promoting an excess in micronutrients—with the exception of magnesium. The intervention increased the odds of exceeding the recommended tolerable limit for intake of magnesium (i.e., 350 mg/day). The upper limits are not intended to be a recommended "cap" but rather a level of intake that most individuals could likely tolerate [29,30,34,35]. Nevertheless, high amounts of magnesium could result in diarrhea, nausea, and abdominal cramping [29,30,34,35], which were not measured in the current study.

Also of note, the intervention increased the odds of inadequate intake of choline. Choline does not yet have an established EAR, so cutoffs were based on AI, which should be interpreted with less confidence [27–32]. Nevertheless, the reasons for an intervention-related decline in choline remain unclear. The meal replacements likely did not contain adequate amounts of choline and might have displaced typical consumption of choline-containing foods, such as eggs and milk. However, group differences in milk intake were not observed (data not shown). Adequate intake of dietary choline may be important for optimal fetal outcome (birth defects, brain development) and for maternal liver and placental function [44]. Future research of the intervention approach should consider the promotion of both egg and milk consumption or other choline-rich foods or a diet supplement that might assist women in the intervention in meeting the daily choline intake recommendations.

This study is the first to examine whether a prenatal lifestyle intervention with partial meal replacement that reduced excess gestational weight gain had positive effects on micronutrient intake of pregnant women with overweight and obesity. The study's strengths include its randomized design, diverse population, blinded assessors, and two repeated, random, and interview-administered 24 h recalls to measure the dietary intake. Limitations of this study include the fact that the assessment of micronutrients was solely based on self-report, which could have overestimated the proportions with inadequate intake [45]. Also, data were lacking for some micronutrients, including molybdenum and iodine. Also, for micronutrients in which an RDA and EAR had not been established (i.e., vitamin K, choline, potassium, sodium), cutoffs were based on AIs, which should be interpreted with less confidence, since the amount and quality of data currently available may not be sufficient to make reliable estimates [46]. The study design tested a treatment "package" and did not allow for isolation of the independent contribution of meal replacements from other intervention components. Future randomized clinical trials are needed to tease apart the intervention "package" and identify the independent contribution of meal replacements and other intervention components on improving micronutrient adequacy. Only 82% of the original sample completed the dietary assessment, although the characteristics of completers versus non-completers were similar. Also, the study's sample size was not powered to examine the effect of changes in micronutrients on maternal and fetal complications.

5. Conclusions

A comprehensive prenatal lifestyle intervention that reduced excess gestational weight gain [17] also improved micronutrient intake and reduced the odds of inadequate intake of several micronutrients. A low nutritional quality of the diet and inadequate intakes of micronutrients can have significant consequences for both the mother and the developing fetus. Future research is now needed to examine the generalizability and effectiveness of this prenatal lifestyle modification program in other populations and settings.

Author Contributions: S.P., B.A., R.R.W. designed the research; S.P., R.R.W. conducted the research; S.P. analyzed the data; S.P., R.R.W., B.A. wrote the paper; S.P. had primary responsibility for the final content. All authors read and approved the final manuscript.

Acknowledgments: We thank the participants in the study. We thank our unpaid recruitment sites, including in California, Pacific Central Coast Health Centers, including Santa Maria Women's Health Center, Bishop's Peak Women's Health Center, and Templeton Women's Health Center and the Community Health Centers (CHC) in Templeton, San Luis Obispo, Santa Maria, and Nipomo, and Creating Harmony Women's Healthcare, French Hospital Medical Center, and Marian Regional Medical Center, and San Luis Obispo and Santa Barbara WIC clinics, and, in Rhode Island, the Women's Primary Care Center at Women and Infants Hospital, Center for OB-GYN, Women's Care, Inc. in Providence, Pawtucket and East Greenwich, Beitle, Bayside OB-GYN, Broadway OB/GYN, RI WIC Clinics. We thank the paid research team members in CA, including Adilene Quintana-Diaz, Noemi Alarcon, Martha La Spina, Maria Legato, Samantha Lalush, Adrian Mercado, Nick Katsantones, Megan Ershov, Natali Valdez, Ana Stewart, Vanessa Rodriguez, Jill Jacoby, Hannah Feldman, and in RI, including Juliana Duszlak (Luciani), Erica Ferguson-Robichaud, Denise Fernandes-Pierre, Kristen DeLayo, Kathryn Story, Stephanie Guerra, Patricia Sandoval, Zeely Sylvia-Denmat, Isabella Cassell, Julie Krol, Sarah Morris, Briana Borgolini, Molly La Rue, Kaitlyn Dahlborg, Genevieve Ramos, Whitney Howie, and Leah Sabatino. We thank the LIFE-Moms consortium members for their paid contributions to the development and oversight of the common measures and procedures shared across the trials. We thank Orgain and Pure Fit bar for providing product purchase discounts in support of this study.

References

1. Koletzko, B.; Godfrey, K.M.; Poston, L.; Szajewska, H.; van Goudoever, J.B.; de Waard, M.; Brands, B.; Grivell, R.M.; Deussen, A.R.; Dodd, J.M.; et al. Nutrition during pregnancy, lactation and early childhood and its implications for maternal and long-term child health: The early nutrition project recommendations. *Ann. Nutr. Metab.* **2019**, *74*, 93–106. [CrossRef] [PubMed]
2. Nesby-O'Dell, S.; Scanlon, K.S.; Cogswell, M.E.; Gillespie, C.; Hollis, B.W.; Looker, A.C.; Allen, C.; Doughertly, C.; Gunter, E.W.; Bowman, B.A. Hypovitaminosis D prevalence and determinants among African American and white women of reproductive age: Third National Health and Nutrition Examination Survey, 1988–1994. *Am. J. Clin. Nutr.* **2002**, *76*, 187–192. [CrossRef]
3. Agarwal, S.; Reider, C.; Brooks, J.R.; Fulgoni, V.L. Comparison of prevalence of inadequate nutrient intake based on body weight status of adults in the United States: An analysis of NHANES 2001–2008. *J. Am. Coll. Nutr.* **2015**, *34*, 126–134. [CrossRef]
4. Astrup, A.; Bugel, S. Overfed but undernourished: recognizing nutritional inadequacies/deficiencies in patients with overweight or obesity. *Int. J. Obes.* **2018**. [CrossRef] [PubMed]
5. Procter, S.B.; Campbell, C.G. Position of the Academy of Nutrition and Dietetics: Nutrition and lifestyle for a healthy pregnancy outcome. *J. Acad. Nutr. Diet.* **2014**, *114*, 1099–1103. [CrossRef] [PubMed]
6. Shapira, N. Prenatal nutrition: A critical window of opportunity for mother and child. *Womens Health* **2008**, *4*, 639–656. [CrossRef]
7. Peaceman, A.M.; Clifton, R.G.; Phelan, S.; Gallagher, D.; Evans, M.; Redman, L.M.; Knowler, W.C.; Joshipura, K.; Haire-Joshu, D.; Yanovski, S.Z.; et al. Lifestyle Interventions Limit Gestational Weight Gain in

Women with Overweight or Obesity: LIFE-Moms Prospective Meta-Analysis. *Obesity (Silver Spring)* **2018**, *26*, 1396–1404. [CrossRef]
8. Marangoni, F.; Cetin, I.; Verduci, E.; Canzone, G.; Giovannini, M.; Scollo, P.; Corsello, G.; Poli, A. Maternal diet and nutrient requirements in pregnancy and breastfeeding. An italian consensus document. *Nutrients* **2016**, *8*, 629. [CrossRef]
9. Milman, N.; Bergholt, T.; Byg, K.E.; Eriksen, L.; Graudal, N. Iron status and iron balance during pregnancy. A critical reappraisal of iron supplementation. *Acta. Obstet. Gynecol. Scand.* **1999**, *78*, 749–757. [CrossRef]
10. Czeizel, A.E. Periconceptional folic acid containing multivitamin supplementation. *Eur. J. Obstet. Gynecol. Reprod. Biol.* **1998**, *78*, 151–161. [CrossRef]
11. Murphy, M.M.; Scott, J.M.; McPartlin, J.M.; Fernandez-Ballart, J.D. The pregnancy-related decrease in fasting plasma homocysteine is not explained by folic acid supplementation, hemodilution, or a decrease in albumin in a longitudinal study. *Am. J. Clin. Nutr.* **2002**, *76*, 614–619. [CrossRef] [PubMed]
12. Zeghoud, F.; Vervel, C.; Guillozo, H.; Walrant-Debray, O.; Boutignon, H.; Garabedian, M. Subclinical vitamin D deficiency in neonates: Definition and response to vitamin D supplements. *Am. J. Clin. Nutr.* **1997**, *65*, 771–778. [CrossRef] [PubMed]
13. Koren, G.; Pairaideau, N. Compliance with prenatal vitamins. Patients with morning sickness sometimes find it difficult. *Can. Fam. Phys.* **2006**, *52*, 1392–1393. [PubMed]
14. Dobbing, J.; Rybar Laboratories. *Prevention of Spina Bifida and Other Neural Tube Defects*; Academic Press: London, UK; New York, NY, USA, 1983; p. xiv. 251p.
15. Fall, C.H.; Yajnik, C.S.; Rao, S.; Davies, A.A.; Brown, N.; Farrant, H.J. Micronutrients and fetal growth. *J. Nutr.* **2003**, *133*, S1747–S1756. [CrossRef]
16. Long, V.A.; Martin, T.; Janson-Sand, C. The great beginnings program: Impact of a nutrition curriculum on nutrition knowledge, diet quality, and birth outcomes in pregnant and parenting teens. *J. Am. Diet. Assoc.* **2002**, *102*, S86–S89. [CrossRef]
17. Phelan, S.; Wing, R.R.; Brannen, A.; McHugh, A.; Hagobian, T.A.; Schaffner, A.; Jelalian, E.; Hart, C.N.; Scholl, T.O.; Munoz-Christian, K.; et al. Randomized controlled clinical trial of behavioral lifestyle intervention with partial meal replacement to reduce excessive gestational weight gain. *Am. J. Clin. Nutr.* **2018**, *107*, 183–194. [CrossRef]
18. Clifton, R.G.; Evans, M.; Cahill, A.G.; Franks, P.W.; Gallagher, D.; Phelan, S.; Pomeroy, J.; Redman, L.M.; Van Horn, L.; Group, L.I.-M.R. Design of lifestyle intervention trials to prevent excessive gestational weight gain in women with overweight or obesity. *Obesity (Silver Spring)* **2016**, *24*, 305–313. [CrossRef]
19. Phelan, S.; Wing, R.R.; Brannen, A.; McHugh, A.; Hagobian, T.; Schaffner, A.; Jelalian, E.; Hart, C.N.; Scholl, T.O.; Munoz-Christian, K.; et al. Does Partial Meal Replacement During Pregnancy Reduce 12-Month Postpartum Weight Retention? *Obesity (Silver Spring)* **2019**, *27*, 226–236. [CrossRef]
20. Conner, P.; Bartlett, S.; Mendelson, M.; Condon, K.; Sutcliffe, C. (Eds.) *WIC Participant and Program Characteristics 2008, WIC-08-PC*; U.S. Department of Agriculture, Food and Nutrition Service, Office of Research and Analysis: Alexandria, VA, USA, 2010.
21. Phelan, S.; Phipps, M.G.; Abrams, B.; Darroch, F.; Schaffner, A.; Wing, R.R. Randomized trial of a behavioral intervention to prevent excessive gestational weight gain: The Fit for Delivery Study. *Am. J. Clin. Nutr.* **2011**, *93*, 772–779. [CrossRef]
22. Wing, R.R.; Jeffery, R.W.; Burton, L.R.; Thorson, C.; Nissinoff, K.S.; Baxter, J.E. Food provision vs structured meal plans in the behavioral treatment of obesity. *Int. J. Obes. Relat. Metab. Disord.* **1996**, *20*, 56–62.
23. Artal, R.; Catanzaro, R.B.; Gavard, J.A.; Mostello, D.J.; Friganza, J.C. A lifestyle intervention of weight-gain restriction: Diet and exercise in obese women with gestational diabetes mellitus. *Appl. Physiol. Nutr. Metab.* **2007**, *32*, 596–601. [CrossRef]
24. Otten, J.J.; Hellwig, J.P.; Meyers, L.D. *DRI, Dietary Reference Intakes: The Essential Guide to Nutrient Requirements*; National Academies Press: Washington, DC, USA, 2006; p. xiii. 543p.
25. Kirkpatrick, S.I.; Subar, A.F.; Douglass, D.; Zimmerman, T.P.; Thompson, F.E.; Kahle, L.L.; George, S.M.; Dodd, K.W.; Potischman, N. Performance of the Automated Self-Administered 24-h Recall relative to a measure of true intakes and to an interviewer-administered 24-h recall. *Am. J. Clin. Nutr.* **2014**, *100*, 233–240. [CrossRef]
26. Subar, A.F.; Kirkpatrick, S.I.; Mittl, B.; Zimmerman, T.P.; Thompson, F.E.; Bingley, C.; Willis, G.; Islam, N.G.; Baranowski, T.; McNutt, S.; et al. The Automated Self-Administered 24-h dietary recall (ASA24): A resource

for researchers, clinicians, and educators from the National Cancer Institute. *J. Acad. Nutr. Diet.* **2012**, *112*, 1134–1137. [CrossRef] [PubMed]

27. Institute of Medicine (U.S.). Standing Committee on the Scientific Evaluation of Dietary Reference Intakes. *Dietary Reference Intakes: For Calcium, Phosphorus, Magnesium, Vitamin D, and Fluoride*; National Academy Press: Washington, DC, USA, 1997; p. xv. 432p.
28. Institute of Medicine (U.S.). Standing Committee on the Scientific Evaluation of Dietary Reference Intakes; Institute of Medicine (U.S.). Panel on Folate Other B Vitamins and Choline; Institute of Medicine (U.S.). Subcommittee on Upper Reference Levels of Nutrients. *Dietary Reference Intakes for Thiamin, Riboflavin, Niacin, Vitamin B_6, Folate, Vitamin B_{12}, Pantothenic Acid, Biotin, and Choline*; National Academy Press: Washington, DC, USA, 1998; p. xxii. 564p.
29. Institute of Medicine (U.S.). Panel on Dietary Antioxidants and Related Compounds. *Dietary Reference Intakes for Vitamin C, Vitamin E, Selenium, and Carotenoids: A Report of the Panel on Dietary Antioxidants and Related Compounds, Subcommittees on Upper Reference Levels of Nutrients and of Interpretation and Use of Dietary Reference Intakes, and the Standing Committee on the Scientific Evaluation of Dietary Reference Intakes, Food and Nutrition Board, Institute of Medicine*; National Academy Press: Washington, DC, USA, 2000; p. xx, 506p.
30. Institute of Medicine (U.S.). Panel on Micronutrients. *DRI: Dietary Reference Intakes for Vitamin A, Vitamin K, Arsenic, Boron, Chromium, Copper, Iodine, Iron, Manganese, Molybdenum, Nickel, Silicon, Vanadium, and Zinc: A Report of the Panel on Micronutrients and the Standing Committee on the Scientific Evaluation of Dietary Reference Intakes, Food and Nutrition Board, Institute of Medicine*; National Academy Press: Washington, DC, USA, 2001; p. xxii, 773p.
31. Institute of Medicine (U.S.). Panel on Macronutrients; Institute of Medicine (U.S.). Standing Committee on the Scientific Evaluation of Dietary Reference Intakes. *Dietary Reference Intakes for Energy, Carbohydrate, Fiber, Fat, Fatty Acids, Cholesterol, Protein, and Amino Acids*; National Academies Press: Washington, DC, USA, 2005; p. xxv, 1331p.
32. Ross, A.C. Dietary Reference Intakes for Adequacy: Calcium and Vitamin D. In *Dietary Reference Intakes for Calcium and Vitamin D*; National Academies Press: Washington, DC, USA, 2011; pp. 345–402.
33. Beaton, G.H. Approaches to analysis of dietary data: relationship between planned analyses and choice of methodology. *Am. J. Clin. Nutr.* **1994**, *59*, 253S–261S. [CrossRef]
34. Institute of Medicine (U.S.). Food and Nutrition Board; Suitor, C.W.; Meyers, L.D. *Dietary Reference Intakes Research Synthesis Workshop Summary*; National Academies Press: Washington, DC, USA, 2007; p. xii, 297p.
35. Institute of Medicine (U.S.). Panel on Dietary Reference Intakes for Electrolytes and Water. *DRI, Dietary Reference Intakes for Water, Potassium, Sodium, Chloride, and Sulfate*; National Academies Press: Washington, DC, USA, 2005; p. xviii, 617p.
36. Rasmussen, K.M.; Yaktine, A.L.; Institute of Medicine (U.S.). Committee to Reexamine IOM Pregnancy Weight Guidelines. *Weight Gain during Pregnancy: Reexamining the Guidelines*; National Academies Press: Washington, DC, USA, 2009.
37. Asayama, K.; Imai, Y. The impact of salt intake during and after pregnancy. *Hypertens. Res.* **2018**, *41*, 1–5. [CrossRef]
38. Luo, T.; Ji, W.J.; Yuan, F.; Guo, Z.Z.; Li, Y.X.; Dong, Y.; Ma, Y.Q.; Zhou, X.; Li, Y.M. Th17/Treg Imbalance Induced by Dietary Salt Variation Indicates Inflammation of Target Organs in Humans. *Sci. Rep.* **2016**, *6*, 26767. [CrossRef]
39. Lenda, D.M.; Boegehold, M.A. Effect of a high salt diet on microvascular antioxidant enzymes. *J. Vasc. Res.* **2002**, *39*, 41–50. [CrossRef]
40. Lenda, D.M.; Boegehold, M.A. Effect of a high-salt diet on oxidant enzyme activity in skeletal muscle microcirculation. *Am. J. Physiol. Heart. Circ. Physiol.* **2002**, *282*, H395–H402. [CrossRef] [PubMed]
41. Dishy, V.; Sofowora, G.G.; Imamura, H.; Nishimi, Y.; Xie, H.G.; Wood, A.J.; Stein, C.M. Nitric oxide production decreases after salt loading but is not related to blood pressure changes or nitric oxide-mediated vascular responses. *J. Hypertens.* **2003**, *21*, 153–157. [CrossRef] [PubMed]
42. Visintin, C.; Mugglestone, M.A.; Almerie, M.Q.; Nherera, L.M.; James, D.; Walkinshaw, S.; Guideline Development Group. Hypertension in Pregnancy: The Management of Hypertensive Disorders During Pregnancy. *BMJ* **2010**. [CrossRef] [PubMed]

43. Hypertension in pregnancy. Report of the American College of Obstetricians and Gynecologists' Task Force on Hypertension in Pregnancy. Hypertension in pregnancy. Report of the American College of Obstetricians and Gynecologists' Task Force on Hypertension in Pregnancy. *Obstet. Gynecol.* **2013**, *122*, 1122–1131.
44. Zeisel, S.H. Nutrition in pregnancy: The argument for including a source of choline. *Int. J. Womens Health* **2013**, *5*, 193–199. [CrossRef] [PubMed]
45. Garriguet, D. Impact of identifying plausible respondents on the under-reporting of energy intake in the Canadian Community Health Survey. *Health Rep.* **2008**, *19*, 47–55. [PubMed]
46. Institute of Medicine (U.S.). *DRI Dietary Reference Intakes: Applications in Dietary Assessment*; National Academies Press: Washington, DC, USA, 2000. [CrossRef]

8

Preterm Birth: A Narrative Review of the Current Evidence on Nutritional and Bioactive Solutions for Risk Reduction

Tinu M. Samuel [1], Olga Sakwinska [1], Kimmo Makinen [1], Graham C. Burdge [2], Keith M. Godfrey [3] and Irma Silva-Zolezzi [4,*]

1 Nestlé Research, 1000 Lausanne, Switzerland
2 School of Human Development and Health, Faculty of Medicine, University of Southampton, Southampton SO16 6YD, UK
3 MRC Lifecourse Epidemiology Unit and NIHR Southampton Biomedical Research Centre, University of Southampton & University Hospital Southampton NHS Foundation Trust, Southampton SO16 6YD, UK
4 Nestlé Research, Singapore 618802, Singapore
* Correspondence: irma.silvazolezzi@rdsg.nestle.com

Abstract: Preterm birth (PTB) (<37 weeks of gestation) is the leading cause of newborn death and a risk factor for short and long-term adverse health outcomes. Most cases are of unknown cause. Although the mechanisms triggering PTB remain unclear, an inappropriate increase in net inflammatory load seems to be key. To date, interventions that reduce the risk of PTB are effective only in specific groups of women, probably due to the heterogeneity of its etiopathogenesis. Use of progesterone is the most effective, but only in singleton pregnancies with history of PTB. Thus, primary prevention is greatly needed and nutritional and bioactive solutions are a promising alternative. Among these, docosahexaenoic acid (DHA) is the most promising to reduce the risk for early PTB. Other potential nutrient interventions include the administration of zinc (possibly limited to populations with low nutritional status or poor zinc status) and vitamin D; additional preliminary evidence exists for vitamin A, calcium, iron, folic acid, combined iron-folate, magnesium, multiple micronutrients, and probiotics. Considering the public health relevance of PTB, promising interventions should be studied in large and well-designed clinical trials. The objective of this review is to describe, summarize, and discuss the existing evidence on nutritional and bioactive solutions for reducing the risk of PTB.

Keywords: preterm birth; preterm labor; etiology; nutrition; DHA; probiotics

---

1. Introduction

Preterm birth (PTB) is defined as birth at <37 weeks of gestation or at <259 days since the first day of a woman's last menstruation, and it is broadly classified into extremely preterm (PT) (<28 weeks), very PT (28 to <32 weeks), and moderate PT (32 to <37 completed weeks of gestation). Moderate PTB is further categorized as early PTB (EPTB) and late PTB (LPTB) depending on whether the infant was born <34 weeks or between 34 and <37 weeks of gestation, respectively [1]. PTB is a risk factor for adverse short and long-term health outcomes. Short term, it is the leading cause of neonatal death and the second cause of all under-5 mortality [2]. Long term, it is associated with increased risks of hypertension, cardiovascular and cerebrovascular diseases, type 2 diabetes, chronic kidney disease, asthma and abnormalities in pulmonary function, and neurocognitive disorders [3,4]. In addition, PTB is associated with increased health care costs [5] and socioeconomic disadvantages in adulthood [6].

Estimates based on most recent data from 107 countries suggest that in 2014 an estimated 10.6% of livebirths worldwide (14.84 million) were preterm, with 81.1% occurring in Asia and sub-Saharan

Africa. There are also significant disparities in PTB rates between countries (8.7% in Europe vs. 13.55% in North Africa) [7]. PTB rates have been increasing in most countries with reliable data, attributed to factors including but not limited to, better detection, older maternal age, multiple pregnancies from assisted reproductive technologies, and higher rates of underlying conditions such as diabetes and hypertensive disorders [8]. The reported prevalence may be an underestimate due to lack of routine collection, and within and between country comparisons are challenging due to inconsistencies in reporting pregnancy outcomes and utilizing standard definitions of PTB.

A series of maternal factors have been identified that impact the risk of PTB. Of these, some are non-modifiable, such as history of PTB, extremes in maternal age (<19 and >35 years) [9–11], multiple pregnancies [12], short cervical length (CL) [13], uterine abnormalities, prior cervical excision [14], dilation/curettage [15], ethnicity and family history [16], and genetic factors [17–20]. In addition, some are modifiable, such as nutrition, low socioeconomic status, low body mass index (BMI), obesity, poor pregnancy weight gain, smoking, substance abuse, short inter-pregnancy interval, periodontal disease, bacterial vaginosis, late or no prenatal care, untreated antenatal depression, and the use of assisted reproductive technologies [21].

The clinical presentation of PTB is either "spontaneous" (70%) or "indicated". Spontaneous PTB is characterized by preterm labor (PTL) with cervical dilation or preterm premature rupture of membranes (PPROM), while indicated PTB is initiated by obstetricians due to complications in absence of labor or PPROM [22,23]. Recent evidence indicates that etiologist of spontaneous and indicated LPTB overlap and are often characterized by placental vascular mal-perfusion lesions. However, the etiologies of EPTB differ, with indicated PTB typically characterized by placental vascular mal-perfusion lesions and spontaneous PTB by placental infectious inflammatory lesions [24]. This suggests that the underlying molecular mechanisms associated with EPTB differ to those of LPTB and thus potentially efficacy of preventive interventions may differ between EPTB and LPTB.

Differential mechanisms underlying PTB are also inherent to a series of clinical conditions that trigger labor and have been associated with PTB (see Figure 1): (1) decidual hemorrhage caused by placental abruption [25], possibly triggered by infection, inflammation, hypoxia, or oxidative stress [26]; (2) uterine factors such as cervical insufficiency [27] and uterine distension or stretch [21]; (3) maternal mood and distress involving activation of the hypothalamic–pituitary–adrenal axis [28–30] and increased production of prostaglandins (e.g., prostaglandin E2) [31,32]; (4) extra and intra-uterine infections [33], as well as intra-amniotic infection (IAI) [34,35], including intrauterine and systemic viral infections [36]; (5) inflammation in the absence of infection (e.g., via production of parturition-triggering cytokines) [37]; and (6) PPROM [38] representing a common final pathway to PTB associated with other of these clinical conditions [39].

Although the molecular mechanisms underlying labor onset remain puzzling, it is generally accepted that a "parturition cascade" triggers spontaneous PTL by premature stimulation of pro-inflammatory pathways within the uterus triggered by different clinical conditions (see Figure 1) [33,40,41]. At a molecular level, this cascade is mediated by progesterone and involves the coordinated activation of progesterone receptor-B (PR-B) and its truncated and much less active nuclear PR isoform progesterone receptor-A (PR-A) (see Figure 1) [41]. The balance between inflammation and progesterone activity seems key for timing of delivery.

Novel approaches to reduce the risk of PTB are needed due to the very limited success of different medical strategies to achieve this goal. For example, for women experiencing PTL, tocolytics (cyclooxygenase inhibitors, calcium channel blockers, or betamimetics) are used to stop contractions and delay delivery; unfortunately, these do not remove the underlying stimulus that initiated parturition or reverse parturition [42]. Thus, early identification of risk factors, as well as effective preventive interventions, are needed. Currently, screening, while imperfect, is done based on measuring CL (the strongest clinical predictor of PTB in asymptomatic women), as well as fetal fibronectin levels and CL assessment, the latter in singleton pregnancies with acute PTL symptoms. These approaches remain to be proven in multiple pregnancies [43]. Stopping smoking early in pregnancy has also been shown to reduce the risk of PTB, and other more specific strategies exist for scenarios of low- and high-risk pregnancies [9,44].

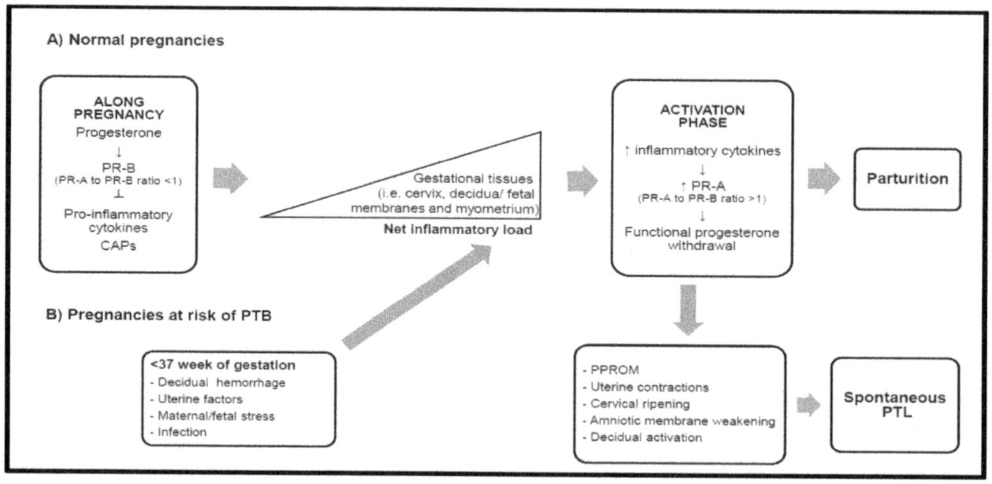

Figure 1. Parturition cascade in normal term and preterm pregnancies. PR-A and PR-B: progesterone receptors A and B, respectively; CAPs: contraction-associated proteins, PTL: preterm labor; PTB: preterm birth; PPROM: preterm premature rupture of membranes.

In asymptomatic pregnancies with a shortened cervix (CL ≤25 mm) identified at mid-trimester, vaginal progesterone is efficacious for preventing PTB, particularly in multiple pregnancies [45,46]. In singleton at-risk pregnancies and those with history of PTB, vaginal progesterone administered from 16 to 36 weeks of gestation is efficacious [47]. Also, serial CL screening is indicated between 16 and 24 weeks of gestation. In pregnancies with a shortened cervix (CL ≤25 mm) or with history of PTB, vaginal progesterone is the preferred option, with tightening the cervix with a stitch (cerclage) and closing the cervix with a silicone ring (cervical pessary) being alternatives [47,48].

Although promising, no approach is uniformly effective as primary-prevention to lower PTB rates because most cases are of unknown cause [49]. Inadequate nutrition preconception and during pregnancy has been associated with the risk of PTB and intervention studies suggest roles for specific nutrients in reducing PTB risk and/or increasing the duration of gestation [50]. The aim of this review is to summarize the evidence on nutritional and bioactive solutions for reducing the risk of PTB.

2. Materials and Methods

Literature search and selection criteria: We conducted a narrative literature review and search using SCOPUS and PubMed databases limited to English language original research, literature reviews and conference abstracts/papers/presentations published before May 2019. For omega-3 fatty acids (with the largest body of evidence today), we reviewed intervention studies of either docosahexaenoic acid (DHA) or eicosapentaenoic acid (EPA) alone or using varying combinations of both, food-based intervention studies, and systematic reviews/meta-analyses. We only reviewed those studies in which long-chain polyunsaturated fatty acid (LC-PUFA) administration was started no later than 12–32 weeks of gestation. The key words used were LC-PUFA, omega 3, eicosapentaenoic acid (EPA) and docosahexaenoic acid (DHA), intervention studies, clinical trials, pregnancy, gestational age at birth, preterm birth, and early preterm birth. For all other macro and micronutrients, we summarized the evidence based on the latest systematic reviews and meta-analyses. The key words used were nutrients, systematic review, meta-analyses, pregnancy, gestational age at birth, preterm birth, and early preterm birth. For probiotics, we included studies that reported PTB as either the primary or secondary outcome, and those that reported outcomes relevant to PTB such as the gestational age at birth or vaginal health during pregnancy; we only included studies where probiotic administration was started no later than 12–32 weeks gestation.

3. Results

3.1. *The Role of Nutrition in Reducing the Risk of PTB*

In the preceding sections, while a broad overview of the pathophysiology of PTB has been presented, there is increasing evidence that infection and/or inflammation are the pathological process for which the molecular pathophysiology has been best defined and a causal link with PTB has been fairly well established [51]. It is therefore of significant relevance to evaluate whether specific diet patterns and nutritional/bioactive interventions targeted to modulate inflammation/infection can be efficacious in reducing the risk of PTB. In the following sections of this review we document the evidence of maternal diet patterns, nutrients, and bioactives on PTB risk reduction and/or increasing gestational age at birth, probably via an anti-inflammatory and/or an immunomodulatory effect.

3.1.1. Evidence from Dietary Pattern Analyses

Observational studies indicate that poor maternal nutrition preconception and during early pregnancy may influence PTB risk [12]. In observational studies, consumption of specific foods such as >1 serving/day of artificially sweetened and sugar-sweetened beverages have been associated with increased PTB risk (adjusted odds ratios: 1.11 and 1.24, respectively), [52], but other studies have found no association [53]. Assessment of dietary patterns found that high scores on a "prudent" dietary pattern (higher intakes of vegetables, salad, onion/leek/garlic, fruit and berries, nuts, vegetable oils, water as beverage, whole grain cereals, poultry, and fiber rich bread, as well as low intake of processed meat products, white bread, and pizza/tacos) was associated with significant reductions in the risk of PTB (by 12%) and spontaneous PTB (by 15%), comparing the highest and lowest thirds of the population. Several mechanisms are postulated through which a prudent diet may reduce PTB risk, including an anti-stressor effect of a low fat diet on the hypothalamic–pituitary–adrenal axis or an anti-inflammatory effect due to an increased antioxidant intake or attributable to a diet low in saturated fat [54]. Adherence to a Mediterranean diet has been linked with a reduced PTB risk. Among Danish women, intake of a Mediterranean diet (fish bi-weekly or more, using olive or rape seed oil, >5 portions of fruit and vegetables/day, meat other than poultry and fish at most twice a week, and at most 2 cups of coffee/day) lowered the risk of EPTB by 72%, although PTB risk was not significantly reduced [55]. Adherence to a dietary pattern similar to Mediterranean diet was associated with a 30% decreased risk of PTD specifically in overweight and obese pregnant women in a French Caribbean island where the population is largely of African descent [56]. Similarly, in a randomized controlled trial (RCT) in healthy Norwegian pregnant women, those adhering to a dietary pattern resembling the Mediterranean diet had a 90% reduction in PTB risk [57]. However, Norwegian women who met the Mediterranean Diet criteria (fish ≥2 times a week, fruit and vegetables ≥5 times/day, use of olive/canola oil, red meat intake ≤2 times/week, and ≤2 cups of coffee/day) did not have reduced risk of PTB [58]. In addition, a vegetarian diet or pre-dominantly plant-based diet, both low in vitamin B12, vitamin D, zinc [59], EPA and DHA [60], as well as marginal intakes or low status of these nutrients have been associated with increased PTB risk [61]. These observational studies are reinforced by three recent systematic reviews showing that a "healthy" dietary pattern during pregnancy higher in fruits, vegetables, legumes and whole grains is associated with a lower risk of PTB (21% to 25% reduced risk) [62–64].

3.1.2. Nutrient-Based Interventions

Omega 3 Fatty Acids

Omega-3 fatty acids are long-chain, polyunsaturated fatty acids (PUFAs) of plant and marine origin. Alpha linolenic acid (ALA) and linoleic acid (LA) cannot be synthesized by the human body and must be derived from dietary sources. ALA is the parent omega-3 fatty acid that can be converted into longer chain n-3 PUFA including EPA and DHA [65]. The conversion of ALA to EPA and DHA is inefficient in humans and varies markedly between individuals; only 8–12% ALA is converted to EPA and less than 0.05% to DHA [66]. The efficiency of the conversion is dependent on epigenetic and genetic processes influencing the transcription of the fatty acid desaturase (*FADS*) genes [67]. Dietary factors can reduce conversion efficiency. In particular, greater conversion is observed among women compared to men, probably due to the influence of estrogen or other hormones [65,66]. It is recommended to obtain EPA and DHA preformed from additional dietary sources including fish/seafood and oils from marine animals, such as fish oil and cod liver oil. DHA intake across the world is variable [68,69].

The following sections briefly describe the evidence relating to EPA and DHA and PTB risk reduction. The first evidence that omega 3 fatty acids may play a role in reducing the risk of PTB was observed in women from Faeroe Islands who consumed a diet high in fish and showed an increased duration of gestation (4 days) and birth weight (194 g) compared to Danish women [70]. Additional supportive observational evidence included a prospective study in pregnant women reporting that non-consumers of fish had a shorter gestational length and higher odds of PTB, compared to fish eaters [71], another showing that any intake of seafood was associated with a lower prevalence of PTB [72], and a dose–response relationship observed for the association between seafood intake and risk of PTB [73]. However, other large cohort studies in the United States [74] and the United Kingdom [75] did not support the association of n-3 PUFA intake and/or seafood intake with length of gestation or PTB risk.

Ten clinical trials have investigated the role of omega 3 fatty acids on the duration of gestation and/or the incidence of PTB and/or EPTB [76–85] (Table 1). Eight of these 10 trials were interventions constituting of either DHA or EPA alone or used varying combinations of both, and two were predominantly food based [84,85]. Only two trials were carried out among pregnant women from low or middle-income countries (Mexico and Chile) [78,84]. Three trials were conducted in women with high-risk pregnancies (history of PTB, history or high risk of developing intra-uterine growth restriction (IUGR), or pregnancy-induced hypertension (PIH), women diagnosed with pre-eclampsia in current pregnancy or twin pregnancies) [80–82]. While most of the trials started the intervention around mid-pregnancy and followed through to delivery, one trial recruited women as early as 12–14 weeks gestation [82], and another at approximately 30 weeks of gestation [83].

The Kansas DHA Outcome Study (KUDOS trial), demonstrated that a daily administration of 600 mg DHA/day in pregnant women improved gestation duration (2.9 days) [76], and while an overall reduction in PTB was not observed, there was a reduction in EPTB (<34 weeks gestation). The results of this study are in accordance with those of another very large Australian trial (DHA to Optimize Mother Infant Outcome, DOMInO) in which positive findings in secondary outcomes such as an increase in the duration of gestation (1 day) and a 51% reduced risk of EPTB were also observed [77]. A trial among Danish pregnant women also demonstrated an improvement in the duration of gestation (4 days) with fish oil supplementation (2.7 g n-3 fatty acids) compared to olive oil. In this study, the effect of supplementation on the length of gestation seemed to depend on the habitual intake of fish. Among women who had the highest intake of fish at randomization, no difference could be detected between the groups, while in the women with the lowest intake for fish; a significant difference of 7.4 day was observed [83]. In contrast, a large trial among predominantly middle-class Mexican women from urban areas with access to health care indicated no benefit of supplementation of 400 mg DHA/day on gestational age, incidence of PTB, birth weight, length, or head circumference [78]. The results from the Norway [79], United Kingdom [81] and the Netherlands [82] trials concurred with the Mexican trial and did not find that omega 3 fatty acids lengthened the duration of gestation or reduced the incidence of PTB or early PTB. Two food-based interventions have assessed the effect of a dairy product fortified with multiple micronutrients, ALA and LA [84] or DHA-enriched eggs [85], on the length of gestation and birth weight. Both these trials reported a lower incidence of EPTB and an increase in the length of gestation. The latter trial [85] demonstrated an increase of 6 days of gestation with as little as 133 mg DHA/day.

Table 1. Characteristics and efficacy of clinical trials investigating the role of omega-3 fatty acids in reducing risk of early and any PTB.

Ref.	Study				Ingredient, Daily Dosage	Main Results	Comments
	Objective	Design	Population/Sample Size	Duration			
Carlson et al. 2013 [76]	To assess if DHA supplementation can increase maternal and newborn DHA status, gestation duration, birth weight, and length	RCT, DB, PC.	Healthy pregnant women between 8 and 20 weeks of gestation from the USA, $n = 350$	<20 weeks of gestation until delivery	Intervention: 3 capsules/day of a marine algae-oil source of DHA (600 mg DHA/day) Placebo: 3 capsules containing half soybean and half corn oil	Compared to placebo, DHA supplementation resulted in: (1) Longer gestation duration (2.9 day; $p = 0.041$). (2) Fewer infants born <34 weeks of gestation ($p = 0.025$). EPTB reduced by 87.5%. (3) Shorter hospital stays for PT infants (40.8 compared with 8.9 day; $p = 0.026$). (4) Similar PTB incidence between groups, with more EPTB in the placebo group (4.8% vs. 0.6%, $p = 0.025$). (5) Greater birth weight (172 g; $p = 0.004$), length (0.7 cm; $p = 0.022$), and head circumference (0.5 cm; $p = 0.012$). (6) Higher maternal and cord Red Blood Cell-phospholipid-DHA (2.6%; $p < 0.001$).	Women taking supplements <300 mg DHA/day were not excluded. Dietary n−3 LC-PUFA intakes were not assessed Many secondary variables were studied but without adjustment for multiple comparisons. Incidence of PTB and EPTB were secondary outcomes.
Makrides et al. 2010 [77]	To assess if DHA supplementation during the last half of pregnancy has a beneficial effect on maternal depressive symptoms and child neurodevelopment	RCT, DB, PC.	Healthy pregnant women <21 weeks gestation from Australia $n = 2399$	<21 weeks of gestation until delivery	Intervention: 3 capsules/day of DHA-rich fish oil concentrate (800 mg DHA/day A + 100 mg EPA/day) Placebo: 3 capsules/day of vegetable oil containing a blend of rapeseed, Sunflower, and palm oil	Compared to placebo, DHA+EPA supplementation resulted in (1) No differences in the rate of women with depressive symptoms, as well as the cognitive and language composite scores of their children. (2) A small to modest increase in the duration of gestation (precise estimate of effect size could not be determined due to obstetric interventions). (3) Fewer infants born <34 weeks gestation (1.09 % vs. 2.25% adjusted Relative Risk (RR), 0.49; $p = 0.03$), and association with fewer low birth weight infants and fewer admissions to neonatal intensive care. EPTB was reduced by 51.6%.	Dietary intake of n-3 LC-PUFAs was not assessed. The study failed to demonstrate an improvement in primary outcomes such as reduction in depressive symptoms among women and improvement in cognitive and language scores of their children.
Ramakrishnan et al. 2010 [78]	To assess if prenatal DHA supplementation increases gestational age and birth size	RCT, DB, PC.	Healthy pregnant women from 18 to 22 weeks of gestation from Mexico $n = 1094$	From 18 to 22 weeks of gestation until delivery	Intervention: 2 capsules/day of 200 mg of DHA derived from an algal source (400 mg DHA/day) Placebo: 2 capsules/day containing olive oil	Compared to placebo, DHA supplementation resulted in (1) No differences in mean gestational age, PTB, weight, length and head circumference at birth.	

Table 1. *Cont.*

Ref.	Study				Ingredient, Daily Dosage	Main Results	Comments
	Objective	Design	Population/Sample Size	Duration			
Helland et al. 2001 [79]	To evaluate the effect of n-3 or n-6 long-chain PUFAs on birth weight, gestational length, and infant development	RCT, DB, PC.	Healthy, nulli- or primiparous women in weeks 17 to 19 of pregnancy from Norway $n = 590$	17 to 19 weeks of gestation until 3 months after delivery	Intervention: 10 mL/day of cod liver oil, providing around 2 g daily of the long chain omega-3 fatty acids. Placebo: 10 mL/day of corn oil, providing around 5 g daily of omega-6 fatty acid linoleic acid.	In comparison with placebo, cod liver oil supplementation resulted in (1) No differences in gestational length or birth weight, length or head circumference. (2) Higher concentrations of n-3 fatty acids EPA, DHA, and DHA in umbilical plasma phospholipids. (3) Neonates with high concentration of DHA in umbilical plasma phospholipids (upper quartile) had longer gestational length than those with low concentration (lower quartile; 282.5 (8.5) vs. 275.4 (9.3) days).	Substantial numbers of women excluded from the two groups post randomization due to withdrawals. It does not mention gestational lengths to facilitate undertaking of an ITT analyses. In this population, baseline intake of long-chain n-3 fatty acids was estimated to be relatively high (0.5 g/day) and less than one 1% had a PTB.
Olsen et al. 2000 [80]	To test the preventive effects of dietary n-3 fatty acids on Pre-term delivery, Intrauterine growth retardation, and pregnancy-induced hypertension	Multicenter RCT, PC (4 prophylactic + 2 therapeutic trials)	High risk pregnancies from 19 hospitals in 7 different countries in Europe Four prophylactic trials: previous pre-term ($n = 232$), IUGR ($n = 280$), PIH ($n = 386$) and twin pregnancies ($n = 579$) Two therapeutic trials: threatening pre-eclampsia ($n = 79$) and suspected IUGR ($n = 63$)	From ~20 weeks (prophylactic trials) or 33 weeks (therapeutic trials) until delivery.	Intervention: prophylactic trials (4 capsules/day of fish oil, 1.3 g EPA and 0.9 g DHA) and therapeutic trials (9 capsules/day of fish oil, 2.9 g EPA and 2.1g DHA) (32% EPA, 23% DHA, 2 mg tocopherol/mL) Placebo: identical looking capsules of olive oil (72% oleic acid, 12% linoleic acid)	Compared to placebo, fish oil supplementation resulted in the following among women with a previous Pre-term delivery in the prophylactic trial: (1) Reduced recurrence risk of PTB from 33% to 21% (Odds Ratio (OR) 0.54 (95% Confidence Interval (CI) 0.30–0.98)) (2) Reduced recurrence risk of EPTB from 13.3% to 4.6% (OR 0.32 (95% CI 0.11–0.89)). (3) Longer mean gestational length by 8.5 day (95% CI 1.9–15.2. (4) No effect on PTB in twin pregnancies.	
Onwude et al. 1995 [81]	To determine whether n-3 fatty acid (EPA/DHA) prophylaxis is beneficial in high-risk pregnancies	RCT, DB, PC.	Pregnant women at high risk of developing PIH and asymmetrical IUGR from an antenatal clinic from UK $n = 233$	From around 25 weeks of gestation until 38 weeks of gestation	Intervention: 9 capsules/day of fish oil providing 2.7 g omega-3 fatty acids/day (1.62 g of EPA and 1.08 g of DHA) Placebo: matching air-filled capsules	Compared to placebo, fish oil supplementation resulted in (1) No difference in the duration of gestation or other outcomes such as proteinuric PIH, non-proteinuric PIH, or birth weight within the lowest 3% on the growth charts.	This study failed to support the hypothesis that fish oil supplementation improved pregnancy outcome in an at risk population for impaired fetal growth or PIH.
Bulstra Ramakers et al. 1995 [82]	To study the effects of adding 3 g/day of EPA to the diet, on recurrence rate of IUGR and PIH in a high-risk population	RCT, DB, PC.	Pregnant women with a history of IUGR with or without PIH in the previous pregnancy from the Netherlands $n = 63$	From 12 to 14 weeks of gestation until delivery	Intervention: 4 capsules 3 times daily, which corresponded to a daily dose of 3 g of EPA Placebo: Identical capsules with coconut oil	Compared to placebo, EPA supplementation resulted in (1) No difference in the rates of PTB	No information was provided about content of DHA No estimate of mean gestational length was provided

Table 1. *Cont.*

Ref.	Study				Ingredient, Daily Dosage	Main Results	Comments
	Objective	Design	Population/Sample Size	Duration			
Olsen et al. 1992 [83]	To study the effect of a fish-oil supplement, a control olive-oil supplement, and no supplementation on pregnancy duration, birthweight, and birth length	RCT	Healthy pregnant women from Denmark $n = 533$	From gestation week 30 until delivery	Intervention: Four 1 g fish oil capsules/day containing 2.7 g n-3 fatty acids- 32% EPA, 23% DHA, 2 mg tocopherol Placebo: Four 1 g olive oil capsules/day No supplement group	Compared to placebo fish oil supplementation resulted in: (1) The highest mean length of gestation when all 3 groups were compared in a single analysis (fish oil, olive oil and no supplement: 283, 279.4 and 281.7 days respectively, $p = 0.006$). (2) On an average 4 days longer pregnancies in the fish-oil group compared to the olive oil group (95% CI: 1.5–6.4, $p = 0.005$). (3) The effect seemed to depend on the baseline intake of fish. -Among those 20% of the women who had the highest intake of fish at randomization, no difference could be detected between the oil groups. -In those 20% who had the lowest intake for fish, a difference of 7.4 days was observed (95% CI 2.2–12.6 days, $p = 0.01$). -In the middle 60%, the groups differed by 4.8 days (95 CI 1.8–7.8, $p = 0.005$).	Maternal baseline dietary intake could explain differences in the duration of gestation and higher intakes may have a saturating effect
Mardones et al. 2008 [84]	To study the effect of maternal food fortification with omega-3 fatty acids and multiple micronutrients on birth weight and gestation duration	Non-blinded, RCT, PC.	Healthy pregnant women up to 20 weeks Gestation from Chile $n = 972$	From up to 20 weeks of gestation until delivery	Intervention: 2 kg/month of powdered milk fortified with multiple micronutrients and both a-linolenic acid and linoleic acid; iron was supplied in an amino-chelated form Placebo: 2 kg/month powdered milk fortified with small amounts of iron sulphate, copper, zinc, and vitamin C.	Based on ITT analyses and in comparison with placebo, the intervention resulted in (1) Lower incidence of EPTB (0.4% vs. 2.1%; crude OR (95% CI): 5.26 (1.08–34.90), $p = 0.02$). (2) Increase in gestation duration (1.40 days difference, 95% CI: -0.02–2.82 d, $p = 0.05$). (3) Higher mean birth weight (65.4 g difference, 95% CI: 5–126 g; $p = 0.03$). (4) Higher infant length (0.37 cm difference, 95% CI: 0.06–0.68 cm, $p = 0.019$).	Impossibility to perform a blinded design and have strict control of compliance with the prescribed amounts of the products taken to the homes of the study subjects Slight difference in gestational age at recruitment Associations with gestation duration would need a larger sample size for confirmation (the statistical power reached only 0.61 in ITT analyses)
Smuts et al. 2003 [85]	To assess whether higher intake of DHA would increase duration of gestation and birth weight in US women	RCT, DB, PC.	Healthy pregnant women between the 24th and 28th week of pregnancy from the US (predominant black population) $n = 291$	From 24–28 weeks of gestation until delivery	Intervention: 1 DHA enriched egg/day (133 mg DHA) Placebo: 1 ordinary egg/day (33 mg DHA)	Compared to the placebo group, the supplementation with DHA-enriched egg resulted in (1) Increased duration of gestation (6.0 ± 2.3 days, $p = 0.009$) (based on analyses adjusted for maternal BMI at enrollment and number of prior pregnancies).	The unadjusted analysis showed a difference of 2.6 days (not statistically significant), while adjustment for maternal BMI at enrollment and number of prior pregnancies resulted in an increased duration of gestation by 6 days. The adjustments may have introduced a post hoc element into the interpretation of the result.

BMI: body mass index, DHA: docosahexaenoic acid, EPA: eicosapentanoic acid, EPTB: early PTB, PTB: preterm birth, IUGR: intrauterine growth retardation, LC-PUFA: long-chain polyunsaturated fatty acids, PIH: pregnancy-induced hypertension, RCT: randomized controlled trial, DB: double blind, PC: placebo controlled.

Many factors may influence the response to supplementation and variability in outcomes observed in these trials, including variability in the dose of n−3 LC-PUFA, differences in the source of DHA, population differences in gestation duration, PTB rates and birth weight within the control arm, differences in habitual intakes of DHA from food, differences in baseline n-3 fatty acid status, and high-risk pregnancies with a history of PTB. The role of *FADS* gene variants as determinants of PUFA levels should also be considered as depending on genetic variants, requirements of dietary PUFA or LC-PUFA intakes to achieve comparable biological effects may differ [86] In the Child, parent and health: lifestyle and genetic constitution (KOALA—acronym of the Dutch title) birth cohort, both maternal DHA intake and the maternal FADS rs174556 Single Nucleotide Polymorphism (SNP) genotype were associated with pregnancy duration, and women who were homozygous for the minor allele (indicating their lower n–3 LC-PUFA interconversion and hence higher dependence on dietary supply) had significantly shorter pregnancies (2 days) [87]. In all of the trials with DHA supplementation, PTB or EPTB was never a primary outcome, but rather a secondary or safety-related outcome. Two ongoing RCTs (Assessment of DHA On Reducing Early preterm birth, ADORE and Omega-3 fats to Reduce the Incidence of Prematurity, ORIP) will examine the efficacy and safety of high dose DHA supplementation to reduce early PTB as a primary outcome (1000 mg/day and 800 mg/day DHA, respectively) [88,89].

Six meta-analyses/systematic reviews/Cochrane reviews have evaluated the effect of EPA + DHA (n-3 LC-PUFA) supplementation during pregnancy on gestation duration and risk of PTB and found that supplementing pregnant women with n−3 LC-PUFA appears to be beneficial in reducing the risk of EPTB (magnitude of the effect ranging from 26% to 61%) [90–94]. However, the clinical relevance of a minor increment in gestation duration is questionable. The most recent Cochrane systematic review of RCTs comparing omega-3 fatty acids during pregnancy with placebo or no omega-3 showed a risk reduction of 42% for EPTB (nine RCTs, 5204 participants; high-quality evidence) and 11% for PTB (26 RCTs, 10,304 participants; high-quality evidence). The mean gestational length was also greater in women who received omega-3 LC-PUFA (mean difference (MD) 1.67 days, 41 trials, 12,517 participants; moderate-quality evidence) [95]. Another recent meta-analysis (nine RCTs) demonstrated that n-3 LC-PUFA are effective at reducing the risk of EPTB by 58%, any PTB by 17%, increasing the length of gestation by 1.95 weeks and increasing birth weight by 122.1 g, and that these effects did not differ according to the risk status of women or dose or timing of the intervention [93]. Evidence from recent trials that have used DHA alone (600 mg DHA/day) [76] or DHA as the main n-3 fatty acid in terms of dose (800 mg DHA/day + 100 mg EPA/day) [77] also showed reduction of the risk of EPTB (magnitude of the effect from 51.6% to 87.5%). It also appears that higher doses of DHA (≥600 mg DHA/day) may be needed to have a protective effect, as trials providing <600 mg DHA/day have not found a reduction in EPTB, and ongoing studies will test the efficacy of doses up to 1000 mg DHA/day.

It could be hypothesized that DHA supplementation reduces the inflammation responsible for both cervical ripening and spontaneous EPTB [87] or that it increases circulating EPA through enhanced biosynthesis via retro conversion from supplemented DHA [96]. Other mechanisms may explain a lengthened duration of gestation. EPA competes with arachidonic acid (ARA), which is the source of pro-constriction mediators such as the 2-series prostaglandins E2 and F2α that can cause contraction of myometrium and cervical ripening and result in an increase the production of prostacyclins (PGI2 and PGI3), with a relaxant effect on the myometrium [70]. Omega 3 fatty acids are also thought to have an "antiarrhythmic" effect on the myometrium that may delay the initiation of labor [97]. Increased intake of marine PUFA is hypothesized to attenuate inflammation by modifying the membrane phospholipid fatty acid composition, altering the physical properties of the cell membrane such as membrane fluidity, through its effects on cell signaling pathways or by altering the pattern of the lipid mediators produced [98].

Other Macro and Micronutrients

Zinc is key for protein synthesis, cellular division, and nucleic acid metabolism [99]. Inadequate intakes (diets lacking in animal food sources rich in zinc) coupled with the limited zinc absorption (high consumption of phytate from cereals) and chronic infections result in reduced maternal plasma concentrations, resulting in reduced supply of zinc to the fetus [100,101]. Zinc deficiency alters the circulating levels of a number of hormones associated with the onset of labor such as progesterone and prolactin [100]. Zinc supplementation has been proposed to reduce the incidence or the severity of maternal infections, and thereby lower the risk of PTB [102]. A Cochrane review (16 RCTs, 7637 women) demonstrated moderate quality evidence of a small but significant 14% reduction in PTB with antenatal supplementation of zinc alone or in combination with other micronutrients compared to placebo. However, this was not accompanied by a similar reduction in the proportion of low birth weight infants or a difference in the gestational age at birth. Most of the studies included women from low- and middle-income settings who had, or were likely to have, low zinc concentrations and overall low nutritional status, making these findings particularly relevant in low-income countries with high perinatal mortality [103]. To the contrary, a more recent systematic review found no association between maternal zinc status and spontaneous PTB, however the authors expressed uncertainty on the evidence due to the heterogeneity in the studies included and the need for further studies populations at increased risk of zinc deficiency [104].

The hormonal form of vitamin D3 (1α,25-dihydroxyvitamin D3) plays a role in the mineralization of the skeleton and regulation of parathyroid hormone, and affects physiological pathways involved in PTB, including inflammation, immunomodulation, and transcription of genes involved in placental function [105]. Vitamin D deficiency in reproductive-age women is widespread and low maternal vitamin D status during pregnancy is a risk factor for various adverse birth outcomes including PTB [106]. Vitamin D is suggested to have an effect on PTB due to its immunomodulatory role and anti-inflammatory effects [107,108]. Two recent meta-analyses of observational studies have shown that vitamin D deficiency as indicated by serum 25 hydroxyvitamin D (25-OHD) levels <50 nmol/L is associated with an increased risk of PTB (by an odds of 1.25 to 1.29 times) [109,110]. Another meta-analysis of observational studies found that 25(OH) D levels >50 nmol/L was associated with longer gestation duration (difference of 0.2 week) [111]. A Cochrane review showed that supplementation with vitamin D alone versus no intervention/placebo reduced the risk of PTB by 64% (three trials and 477 women, moderate quality evidence), while supplementation with vitamin D and calcium versus no treatment/placebo significantly increased the risk of PTB (3 trials and 798 women); however, most trials included were of low methodological quality [112] Recent high quality trials such as The Maternal Vitamin D Osteoporosis Study (MAVIDOS) [113] were not included in the review; in the MAVIDOS trial PTB was reported only as a safety-related outcome but there was no effect of vitamin D supplementation on PTB.

Magnesium is key in the regulation of body temperature, synthesis of nucleic acids and proteins, and maintenance of electrical potentials in nerves and muscle membranes. Ionized and total magnesium levels are shown to decrease with increasing gestational age [114]. Insufficient magnesium intake is common in women [115] and magnesium deficiency during pregnancy is associated with a higher risk of chronic hypertension, preeclampsia, placental dysfunction and premature labor [116]. Reduced placental vascular flow is considered responsible for placental insufficiency and fetal intra-uterus growth restriction and magnesium is believed to have an immediate effect on placental vascular flow [117]. A 2001 Cochrane review (seven trials, 2689 women) reported that oral magnesium supplementation starting before 25 weeks of gestation compared to placebo was associated with a 27% reduction in risk of PTB, without any effect on gestational age at birth. However, when one of the studies that had a cluster design was excluded, there was no effect of magnesium supplementation on any of the outcomes [118]. A recent update of this review reported no significant differences in outcomes such as gestational age at birth (five trials, 5564 women) and PTB (seven trials, 5981 women) between the magnesium supplemented group and the control group [119]. Overall, both reviews reported a lack of high quality evidence. Magnesium sulphate has been used as a tocolytic agent to inhibit uterine activity in women in the setting of preterm labor with the aim of preventing PTB. However, a Cochrane review (37 trials, 3571 women), concluded that magnesium sulphate is ineffective at delaying birth or preventing PTB, has no clear benefits on neonatal and maternal outcomes and may be associated with an increased risk of fetal, neonatal, or infant mortality [120]. A multicenter double-blind, placebo-controlled randomized clinical trial of oral magnesium citrate supplementation (the BRAzil MAGnesium (BRAMAG) trial) among high-risk pregnant women starting at 12 to 20 weeks of gestation through to delivery is currently ongoing [121], with the primary perinatal outcome being a composite of PTB < 37 weeks gestation, stillbirth >20 weeks gestation, neonatal death < 28 days, or Small for Gestational Age (SGA) birthweight <3rd percentile.

Calcium plays a role in nerve cell function, muscle contraction, enzyme and hormone actions, and bone mineralization. A recent Cochrane review suggested that there are no benefits of calcium supplementation during pregnancy in reducing the risk for either PTB or EPTB. The significant heterogeneity among studies (13 trials), led the investigators to perform sub-group analyses stratified by the total dose of calcium per day (<1000 mg/day or ≥1000 mg/day), starting time of calcium supplementation (before or after 20 weeks), and type of calcium (calcium carbonate, lactate and gluconate). There were no statistically significant differences between sub-groups for either the starting time of supplementation or the type of calcium [122]. The effects of baseline calcium intake ($n = 5$ trials) and risk for hypertensive disorders of pregnancy ($n = 4$ trials) have also been studied, however, no protective effect of calcium supplementation on PTB risk reduction was observed [123]. Iron is key for oxygen transport from lungs to tissues, in energy transfer and facilitating oxygen use and storage in muscles. Iron deficiency is the most common nutrient deficiency among pregnant women and results from an increased requirement for iron during pregnancy, a diet poor in absorbable iron, and parasitic infections [124]. Folate is essential for the synthesis of nucleic acid, amino acids, phospholipids and, consequently, lipoproteins, cell division, tissue growth, and DNA methylation. Supplementation with folic acid in the immediate period before and early in pregnancy reduces the risk of neural tube defects [125]. Observational studies show that both anemia [126] and iron deficiency [127] are associated with increased risk of PTB. Recent Cochrane reviews have analyzed the efficacy of a range of interventions containing iron alone, folic acid alone or iron and folic acid together on reduction of PTB. There were no reported differences in the number of women experiencing PTB receiving supplements with iron alone versus no treatment/placebo (six trials, 1713 women) [124], folic acid alone (three trials, 2959 women) [128], daily iron and folic acid supplements versus no treatment or placebo (three trials, 1497 women), or any supplements containing iron and folic acid versus same supplements without iron nor folic acid or placebo (three trials, 1497 women) [124,128]. The studies were of low quality and used a heterogeneous definition of PTB ranging from anywhere between 36 to 38 weeks.

Vitamin A plays a role in visual function and modulation of the expression of genes involved in immune function, reproduction, tissue growth and embryonic development. Vitamin A deficiency (low serum and breast milk vitamin A concentrations) is highly prevalent among pregnant women from Asia, South Asia, and Africa [129]. Vitamin A or beta carotene supplementation during pregnancy has been shown to improve hematologic status of women by improving hemoglobin levels and reducing the risk of anemia [130]. A large trial in Nepal demonstrated that vitamin A supplementation during pregnancy was associated with a 40% reduced risk for pregnancy-related maternal mortality [131]. However, a meta-analysis reported no significant effect of vitamin A supplementation either on PTB (five studies) or EPTB (two studies) risk reduction, and only one trial among South African women reported a significant 33% reduction in the prevalence of PTB and a 66% reduction in EPTB, but this effect disappeared after excluding multiple pregnancies [130].

Sub-optimal micronutrient intakes and micronutrient deficiencies during pregnancy are a global problem and have been associated with placental oxidative stress and complications of pregnancy such as PTB and preeclampsia [100,132]. Although mechanisms linking the use of multivitamins with PTB are not fully understood, they are thought to be involved in the process of normal placentation, and deficiencies in vitamin B12 and folate have been implicated in the development of defects within the placental vascular bed [133]. Impaired placentation has been associated with recurrent PTB [134]. Results from the Danish National Birth Cohort show that peri-conceptional multivitamin use was associated with a 16% reduced risk of PTBs, with a 20% risk reduction of preterm labor in non-overweight women [135]. However, a recent Cochrane review showed no significant differences in PTB between women who were supplemented with Multiple Micronutrient (MMN) containing iron and folic acid versus those receiving iron, with or without folic acid (15 trials, 90892 women, high quality evidence). A sub-group analysis, however, showed that MMN supplementation led to significantly fewer PTB in women with a BMI <20 kg/m^2 (RR 0.85, 95% CI 0.80–0.90, $n = 4$) [136].

Balanced protein-energy supplementation (protein <25% of the total energy content) was found to reduce the risk of intrauterine growth retardation (IUGR) (23% risk reduction) [137] and was associated with modest increases in maternal weight gain (on average 21 g/week), birth weight (on average 38 g) and a substantial 32% reduction in risk of small-for-gestational-age (SGA) [137]. However, evidence from five trials with 2436 pregnant women reported a non-significant reduction in PTB with balanced protein energy supplementation (without any effect on mean gestational age), possibly related to lack of data on gestational age or problems in gestational age measurement, highlighting the need for confirmatory trials in this area [138].

3.2. *Role of Probiotics in Reducing the Risk for PTB*

The main rationale for intervention with probiotics stems from observational data suggesting a link between vaginal infections, dysbiosis, and PTB [139]. It is universally accepted that a certain proportion of PTB is caused by ascending infections from vagina underlying the importance of vaginal health. Moreover, it has been suggested that vaginal dysbiosis (bacterial vaginosis, BV) could trigger an inflammatory cascade leading to PTB even in the absence of ascending infection. Antibiotics such as metronidazole are the standard of care treatment for BV, but there is conflicting evidence whether such treatment results in the risk reduction of PTB [140]. The modest, at best, efficacy of antibiotics is not be surprising, because bacterial vaginosis is characterized by the absence of lactobacilli in addition to the presence of specific pathogenic organisms, and antibiotics cannot restore the depleted lactobacilli. *Lactobacillus* probiotics could fulfill this role through the production of lactic acid, lowering vaginal pH and helping to prevent the growth of potentially pathogenic microorganisms through production of hydrogen peroxide, bacteriocins, and surface-binding proteins that inhibit adhesion of pathogens. Indeed, oral or vaginal administration of probiotics have improved vaginal microbiota composition or alleviated BV in several studies [141]. In addition, and independently of maintenance of vaginal health, oral probiotics may act directly in the gut, down-modulating local and systemic inflammation [142].

3.2.1. Probiotic Intervention studies

We identified 71 publications derived from 21 individual clinical studies that described health outcomes following the administration of probiotics during pregnancy. One reported PTB as the primary outcome and four as a secondary outcome. The rest reported other outcomes informative of PTB such as the gestational age at birth or vaginal health during pregnancy. Of the 21 studies, only eight, where probiotic administration was started no later than at 12–32 weeks of gestation, were considered here (Table 2).

3.2.2. The effect of Oral Probiotics on PTB Rates

Two studies (NCT00217308 and NCT00303082), were designed to test the effect of oral administration of *Lactobacillus rhamnosus* GR-1 and *Lactobacillus reuteri* RC-14 or placebo on the incidence of BV and PTB (co-primary outcomes [143]). Both were discontinued due to difficulties with recruitment, but the partial results were published [144]. The PTB rate was 1.6% in the treatment and 3.3% in the placebo group (RR:0.495; 95% CI: 0.17,1.43; $p = 0.14$). The overall PTB rate (2.5%) was lower than the national average for Brazil (9%) [8].

The same combination of probiotics was tested in a German study [145] with BV as the primary outcome, and PTB rate reported as a secondary outcome. The investigators expected BV rates of 28–42%, but only 6% at baseline was observed, decreasing to 2.5% by the end of the study. There were no differences in BV incidence between the probiotic and placebo groups. PTB rate (4%) was lower than the national average of 9.2% [8].

PTB rates were reported as a secondary outcome in two studies testing different combinations of probiotics. *Lactobacillus rhamnosus* GG and *Bifidobacterium lactis* Bb12 were tested in Finland [146], and *Lactobacillus rhamnosus* LPR and *Bifidobacterium lactis* NCC 2818 in the Philippines [147]. Both studies found PTB rates much lower than national averages reported by WHO, 1.7% vs. 5.5% in Finland and 2.4% vs. 15% in the Philippines [8].

In all the above studies, no firm conclusions could be drawn regarding the effect of probiotics on PTB due to its lower than expected rates, but also raised questions about causes of the observed low PTB rates. The enrollment biases resulting in inadvertent exclusion of women at highest risk is the likely explanation.

Four studies in which probiotic administration was started at 24–32 weeks of pregnancy reported that the gestational age and its range did not differ between the probiotic and the placebo groups [148]. However, because direct data on PTB rates were not reported and the statistical power of the studies with regards to PTB is unknown, no conclusions on the potential effect of probiotics on PTB can be drawn from them.

A prospective cohort study conducted based on Norwegian Mother and Child Cohort Study (MoBa) examined the consumption of probiotic milk during pregnancy and concluded that the intake in early pregnancy (around 17 weeks of gestation) was associated with reduced risk of preterm birth, while late intake (around 30 weeks of gestation) was not [149,150]. The main probiotic milks available in Norway at that time contained *Lactobacillus acidophilus* LA-5, *B. lactis* Bb12, and *L. rhamnosus* GG. Regarding systematic reviews and meta-analyses, a 2007 Cochrane review on the efficacy of probiotics for preventing preterm labor [151] concluded that there were insufficient data as only one study with PTB as an outcome (not primary) was found [146]. The review was updated in 2010 with unchanged conclusions. A recent systematic review and meta-analysis which included unpublished data from previous studies concluded that there was no evidence that taking probiotics or prebiotics in pregnancy decreases the risk of preterm birth [152]. However, even though thirteen studies with 2484 participants were included, the overall PTB rate was only 3.6%. Moreover, the probiotic administration was started in early pregnancy (before 18 weeks of gestation) in only two studies. A recent Cochrane review examined the impact of probiotics on prevention of morbidity and mortality in preterm infants, and the rate of PTB [153]. The overall conclusion was that there is insufficient evidence and more research is needed. Therefore, it appears that the question about potential benefits of probiotic administration in early pregnancy remains open.

3.2.3. The Effect of Vaginal Probiotics on Outcomes Related to PTB

Stojanovic et al. 2012 [154] reported a study testing the effect of a vaginal tablet containing *Lactobacillus rhamnosus* BMX 54 on vaginal health. However, the probiotic had a favorable impact on parameters considered indicative of increased risk of PTB or miscarriage, such as the length, consistency and dilatation of the cervix, the level of the presenting part of the fetus as well as the prevalence of pathogenic microorganisms in vaginal and/or cervical swabs, lower vaginal pH, and lower vaginal discharge "whiff test" positivity. Since the study did not follow the women until delivery, and no data on PTB or other birth outcomes are available but the improvement in parameters associated with PTB was observed. Two ongoing studies in US (NCT00635622, NCT02766023), conducted in non-pregnant women, are testing the benefits of vaginal application of *Lactobacillus crispatus* CTV-05 on BV, as recent data indicate that absence of *L. crispatus*, as opposed to any lactobacilli, is most strongly correlated with adverse vaginal health outcomes [155,156].

Table 2. Characteristics, efficacy and safety of clinical trials investigating the role of probiotics in reducing risk of any preterm delivery.

Ref.	Study				Ingredient, Daily Dose	Main Results	Comments
	Objective	Design	Population/ Sample Size	Duration			
Gille et al. 2016 [145]	To assess whether probiotic supplementation with *Lactobacillus rhamnosus* GR-1 and *Lactobacillus reuteri* RC-14 can improve maternal vaginal microbiota	RCT, DB, PC	Healthy pregnant women (first trimester) from Germany, $n = 320$, 2010–2012	8 weeks to assess Nugent scores; entire pregnancy for PTB (secondary outcome)	Capsules with 10^9 CFU, once daily	Compared to placebo, DHA supplementation resulted in No effect on vaginal microbiota (improvement in Nugent scores). No effect on PTB rates.	Low rate of preterm of 4% Very low rate of bacterial vaginosis 3%. Trend increase on miscarriages in treated (7.7% vs. 3.1%, $p = 0.08$).
Luoto et al. 2010 [146]	To assess whether dietary counselling and probiotic supplementation with (*Lactobacillus rhamnosus* GG and *Bifidobacterium lactis* Bb12) can improve pregnancy outcomes	RCT, PC 3 groups: (1) Probiotics and dietary counselling vs. (2) Placebo and dietary counselling (DB); (3) Placebo without dietary counselling (SB)	Healthy pregnant women in the first trimester from Finland, $n = 256$, late 1990s	From the first antenatal visit to the end of pregnancy	Capsules with 10^{10} CFU, once daily	Compared to placebo, probiotic supplementation resulted in 1. No effect on PTB rate.2. No effect on duration of gestation.	Very low rate of PTB: 1.7%.
Kraus Silva 2011 et al. [143]	To assess whether probiotic supplementation with (*L. rhamnosus* GR-1 and *L. reuteri* RC-14) can reduce BV and PTB	RCT, DB, PC	Pregnant women (8 to 20 weeks gestation), With asymptomatic BV: Vaginal pH >4.5, Nugent >4 from Brazil $n = 644$ randomized, late 1990s	<20 weeks gestation to 24 or 26 weeks	Capsules with 10^6 colony-forming units each, twice daily	Compared to placebo, probiotics supplementation resulted in no effect on PTB rate. However, the PTB rates were lower with treatment (ITT: 1.6%, 5 in 304; vs. 3.3% 10 in 301)	Low rate of PTB 2.5% Low probiotics dose Exclusion criteria were very broad: previous history of PTB, hypertension, diabetes, asthma, cervical incompetence, atypical vaginal bleeding, atypical vaginal secretion, HPV, gonorrhea, syphilis, dysuria, pruritus, burning, corticotherapy, recent antibiotic therapy (within 8 weeks prior to screening)
Rautava et al. 2012 [148]	The effect of maternal administration of probiotics on atopic disease in infants.	RCT, DB, PC.	Pregnant women with atopic sensitization and either a history of or active allergic disease from Finland $n = 241$	Probiotics given to the mother 8 weeks before and 8 weeks after delivery.	(1) Dietary food supplement with *Lactobacillus rhamnosus* LPR + *Bifidobacterium longum* NCC 3001 (10^9 CFU/day) (2) Dietary food supplement with *Lactobacillus paracasei* ST11 + NCC 3001 (1^9 CFU/day) (3) Placebo	No information on preterm birth rates. Gestational age in all groups was 39 weeks with a similar range (34–41 weeks).	Not possible to draw firm conclusions about effects on preterm delivery. However, papers seems to suggest lack of effect because gestational ages were similar between groups.
Kim et al. 2010 [157]	The effect of maternal and infant administration of probiotics on atopic disease in infants	RCT, DB, PC.	Pregnant women with a family history of allergic diseases day $n = 112$, and their infants. from Korea	Probiotic was given to mothers from 8 weeks before delivery until 3 months post-delivery, then to infants from 4 months until 6 months	(1) Bifido Inc mix (*Bifidobacterium bifidum* BGN4, *Bifidobacterium lactis* AD011, *Lactobacillus acidophilus* AD030), 1.6×10^9 CFU/day each, in powder (2) Placebo powder (maltodextrin and alpha-corn)	Infants delivered before 36 weeks were excluded. No difference observed in the number of infants removed between the two groups, suggesting no difference in PTB rates. In both groups the gestational ages were around 40 weeks, and birth weights were similar.	Not possible to draw conclusions about effects on PTB. However, papers seems to suggest lack of effect.

Table 2. *Cont.*

Ref.	Study				Ingredient, Daily Dose	Main Results	Comments
	Objective	Design	Population/ Sample Size	Duration			
Ou et al. 2012 [158]	The effect of maternal administration of probiotics on atopic disease in infants	RCT, DB, PC	Pregnant women with atopic diseases history and Total IgE >100 kU/L from Taiwan $n = 191$	From 24 weeks gestation until delivery. After delivery, administration was exclusively to breastfeeding mothers	(1) *L. rhamnosus* GG (Valio, ATCC 53103) 10^{10} CFU/ day (2) Placebo (microcrystalline cellulose)	PTB rates were not reported. However, gestational age was 39 weeks in both groups (range 31–41 weeks in the *L. rhamnosus* GG group and 35–41 weeks in placebo group), which suggests lack of efficacy on PTB rates.	The study suggests that *L. rhamnosus* GG probably has no impact on PTB rates.
Vitali et al. 2012 [159]	The effect of probiotic supplementation during late pregnancy on vaginal microbiota and cytokine secretion	Non-randomized, controlled, pilot	Healthy pregnant women with no symptoms of vaginal or urinary tract infection from Italy $n = 27$	Probiotic was given during weeks 32–37 of gestation.	(1) Probiotic group: one sachet of VSL #3 (*Lactobacillus acidophilus, Lactobacillus plantarum, Lactobacillus casei, Lactobacillus delbrueckii ssp. bulgaricus, Bifidobacterium breve, Bifidobacterium longum, Bifidobacterium infantis, S. salivaris ssp. thermophilus*) ($n = 12$) 9×10^{11} total CFU/day (2) Control group: no supplementation ($n = 12$)	PTB rates were not reported, but the gestational ages were not different between the two groups. This suggests that the probiotic did had no effect on PTB rates. No significant changes were found in the amounts of the principal vaginal bacterial populations in women administered with VSL#3, but qPCR results suggested a potential role of the probiotic product in counteracting the decrease of *Bifidobacterium* and the increase of *Atopobium*, that occurred in control women during late pregnancy. Incidence of vaginal infections was not reported.	The study is too small to draw conclusions, but it did not show any effect of VSL3 on gestational age.
Stojanovic et al. 2012 [154]	The effect of probiotics on vaginal microflora, cervical length, cervical consistency, and fetal positioning.	Observational, randomized, prospective	Pregnant women	Probiotic was administered for 12 weeks during pregnancy	(1) untreated arm of the study ($n = 30$) (2) vaginal application of one tablet containing *L. rhamnosus* BMX 54 (Normogin™-($n = 30$) once a week	No data on PTB rates as women were not followed until delivery. Increase in pathogenic microorganisms in the vaginal and/or cervical swabs of untreated women ($p < 0.05$), also in average pH values ($p < 0.05$), amount ($p < 0.05$) and "whiff test" positivity ($p < 0.05$) of vaginal discharge. Significant trend was also found for decrease in length ($p < 0.0001$) and increase in dilatation ($p < 0.05$) of cervix, as well as for lower position of the fetus ($p < 0.0001$). In the group treated with *L. rhamnosus* BMX 54, none of these values significantly changed throughout the observation period, with the exception of cervical length that was significantly decreased at T3 ($p < 0.01$).	Cannot conclude on PTB rates. However, it suggests that vaginally administered probiotic had a positive impact on parameters associated with PTB.

CFU: colony forming unit, RCT: randomized controlled trial, DB: double blind, PC: placebo controlled.

3.2.4. Ongoing Probiotic Studies

In an ongoing study (NCT02693041), *L. rhamnosus* GG or placebo is administered orally in pregnancy starting at 17 weeks gestation, to test the hypothesis that the probiotic decreases the rate of PTB and the incidence of pre-eclampsia (PE) by affecting the inflammatory state. In addition, several registered trials (NCT02430246, NCT02692820, NCT02150655) target the treatment of bacterial vaginosis in pregnancy, all with the combination of *L rhamnosus* GR-1 and *L. reuteri* RC-14. Even though PTB prevention is not a primary outcome in these trials, one of them will report it as a secondary outcome. All trials also refer, in their scientific rationale, to PTB prevention, which could be targeted in subsequent trials once the efficacy of probiotics to decrease BV during pregnancy is proven.

4. Conclusions

Worldwide about 15 million preterm babies are born annually, and despite intensive research the specific mechanisms triggering the PTB remain unclear. An increase in the net pro-inflammatory load has been proposed as main driver of progesterone withdrawal, leading to the onset of parturition. Progesterone has been shown to be the most effective pharmacological intervention to reduce the risk of PTB in singleton pregnancies among at-risk women with a previous PTB, but most approaches tested, mainly directed at at-risk pregnancies, have not proven effective at lowering the rate of PTB, probably because the majority of cases are of unknown cause. Though great effort has been placed on early diagnosis, only a small proportion of PTB are successfully predicted using CL measurements, alone and in combination with fetal fibronectin quantification. In the absence of predictive tests that are sensitive, specific, and feasible to implement, more general approaches for primary prevention are needed. In this respect, nutritional and bioactive interventions seem a promising alternative. This review provides a comprehensive overview of the existing literature on the role of nutritional approaches to reducing the risk of PTB. The beneficial effect of n−3 LC-PUFAs (combinations of EPA and DHA) in reducing the risk of EPTB has been demonstrated in large intervention studies and several meta-analyses. Also, the role of only DHA is supported by two large RCTs. Higher doses of DHA (doses ≥600 mg DHA/day) may be needed to have a protective effect, although the optimal dosage is yet to be determined. The evidence of n−3 LC PUFA and in particular DHA appears to be quite substantial, and the two large ongoing studies should provide further clarity and confirmation as to whether DHA could be brought into clinical practice and recommended for all pregnant women or specific populations at risk. Other nutrients that may help reduce the risk of PTB include zinc (effects might be limited to populations with low overall nutritional status or poor zinc status) and vitamin D (Table 3). The emerging evidence is promising; however, larger and well-designed studies with EPTB and/or PTB as primary outcome are needed before conclusions can be drawn or recommendations made. Current data do not permit any conclusions to be drawn for the efficacy of vitamin A, calcium, iron, folic acid, iron folate, MMN, and probiotics in reducing the risk of PTB. Ongoing studies will elucidate the role of magnesium supplementation and probiotics on reducing risk for PTB. Large-scale clinical trials of promising interventions are needed to provide sound evidence-based recommendations for clinical practice. Due to the heterogeneity in the etiology of PTB, we hypothesize that differential responses to treatment will be identified. Thus, it will be important to include a sufficiently wide and deep selection of high-throughput and comprehensive analyses of the host (e.g., genomics, metabolomics) as well as gut and vaginal microbiome (metagenomics, metabolomics) to allow for the identification of subpopulations and individual responses. If successful, it will be of utmost importance to develop implementation of targeted strategies that enable both practical and affordable scaling-up to cover gaps as well as evidence-based precision nutrition in antenatal care. This is central considering that PTB is a public health problem in both high- and low-income countries.

Table 3. Nutrients with known efficacy to reduce the risk of PTB.

Nutrient	Evidence for Efficacy	Dose	Duration	Comments
n−3 LC-PUFA (combinations of EPA and DHA)	26–61% reduction in the risk of early PTB	DHA: 133 to 2100 mg DHA/day EPA: 100 to 3000 mg EPA/day	Supplementation started between 12 to 30 weeks of gestation	Eight trials supplementing either DHA or EPA alone or using varying combinations of both (five trials in healthy pregnancies and three in at-risk pregnancies), two food-based interventions and 6 meta-analyses
DHA (predominantly DHA)	51.6% to 87.5% reduction in the risk of early PTB (<34 weeks)	600 to 800 mg DHA/day	Supplementation started <20 to 21 weeks of gestation	Two large RCTs available where PTB and EPTB were secondary outcomes and not the primary outcome.
Zinc	14% reduction in PTB	5 mg/day to 44 mg/day	Supplementations started from as early as before conception (one study) to at least starting before 26 weeks	Most studies were conducted in low income countries among women with poor nutritional status and likely to have low zinc concentrations. The reduction in PTB was not accompanied by reduction in LBW or a difference in the gestational age at birth.
Vitamin D	64% reduction in PTB	400 to 1000 IU/day (two trials), 60000–12000 IU (depending on baseline serum 25 (OH)D (one trial) cholecalciferol D3	Supplementation started between 20–30 weeks of gestation	The trials available were all of low quality.

DHA: docosahexaenoic acid, EPA: eicosapentanoic acid, EPTB: early PTB, PTB: preterm Birth, LBW: low birth weight.

Author Contributions: Conceptualization, T.M.S., O.S., I.S.-Z.; Investigation, T.M.S., O.S., K.M., I.S.-Z.; Original draft preparation, T.M.S., O.S., K.M., I.S.-Z.; Methodology, T.M.S., O.S.; Supervision, G.C.B., K.M.G., I.S.-Z.; critical appraisal, G.C.B. and K.M.G.; writing—review and editing, all authors.

References

1. Blencowe, H.; Cousens, S.; Chou, D.; Oestergaard, M.; Say, L.; Moller, A.B.; Kinney, M.; Lawn, J. Born Too Soon: The global epidemiology of 15 million preterm births. *Reprod. Health* **2013**, *10*, S2. [CrossRef] [PubMed]
2. Liu, L.; Johnson, H.L.; Cousens, S.; Perin, J.; Scott, S.; Lawn, J.E.; Rudan, I.; Campbell, H.; Cibulskis, R.; Li, M.; et al. Global, regional, and national causes of child mortality: An updated systematic analysis for 2010 with time trends since 2000. *Lancet* **2012**, *379*, 2151–2161. [CrossRef]
3. Raju, T.N.K.; Pemberton, V.L.; Saigal, S.; Blaisdell, C.J.; Moxey-Mims, M.; Buist, S. Long-Term Healthcare Outcomes of Preterm Birth: An Executive Summary of a Conference Sponsored by the National Institutes of Health. *J. Pediatr.* **2017**, *181*, 309–318. [CrossRef] [PubMed]
4. Luu, T.M.; Rehman Mian, M.O.; Nuyt, A.M. Long-Term Impact of Preterm Birth: Neurodevelopmental and Physical Health Outcomes. *Clin. Perinatol.* **2017**, *44*, 305–314. [CrossRef] [PubMed]
5. Jacob, J.; Lehne, M.; Mischker, A.; Klinger, N.; Zickermann, C.; Walker, J. Cost effects of preterm birth: A comparison of health care costs associated with early preterm, late preterm, and full-term birth in the first 3 years after birth. *Eur. J. Health* **2016**, *18*, 1041–1046. [CrossRef]
6. Heinonen, K.; Eriksson, J.G.; Kajantie, E.; Pesonen, A.K.; Barker, D.J.; Osmond, C.; Räikkönen, K. Late-Preterm Birth and Lifetime Socioeconomic Attainments: The Helsinki Birth Cohort Study. *Pediatrics* **2013**, *132*, 647–655. [CrossRef] [PubMed]
7. Chawanpaiboon, S.; Vogel, J.P.; Moller, A.-B.; Lumbiganon, P.; Petzold, M.; Hogan, D.; Landoulsi, S.; Jampathong, N.; Kongwattanakul, K.; Laopaiboon, M.; et al. Global, regional, and national estimates of levels of preterm birth in 2014, a systematic review and modelling analysis. *Lancet Glob. Health* **2018**, *7*, e37–e46. [CrossRef]
8. Blencowe, H.; Cousens, S.; Oestergaard, M.Z.; Chou, D.; Moller, A.B.; Narwal, R.; Adler, A.; Garcia, C.V.; Rohde, S.; Say, L.; et al. National, regional, and worldwide estimates of preterm birth rates in the year 2010 with time trends since 1990 for selected countries: A systematic analysis and implications. *Lancet* **2012**, *379*, 2162–2172. [CrossRef]

9. Van Zijl, M.D.; Koullali, B.; Mol, B.W.; Pajkrt, E.; Oudijk, M.A. Prevention of preterm delivery: Current challenges and future prospects. *Int. J. Womens Health* **2016**, *8*, 633–645. [CrossRef]
10. Leader, J.; Bajwa, A.; Lanes, A.; Hua, X.; White, R.R.; Rybak, N.; Walker, M. The Effect of Very Advanced Maternal Age on Maternal and Neonatal Outcomes: A Systematic Review. *J. Obstet. Gynaecol. Can.* **2018**, *40*, 1208–1218. [CrossRef]
11. Mayo, J.A.; Shachar, B.Z.; Stevenson, D.K.; Shaw, G.M. Nulliparous teenagers and preterm birth in California. *J. Périnat. Med.* **2017**, *45*, 959–967. [CrossRef] [PubMed]
12. Fuchs, F.; Senat, M.V. Multiple gestations and preterm birth. *Semin. Fetal Neonatal Med.* **2016**, *21*, 113–120. [CrossRef] [PubMed]
13. Berghella, V. Universal Cervical Length Screening for Prediction and Prevention of Preterm Birth. *Obstet. Gynecol. Surv.* **2012**, *67*, 653–657. [CrossRef] [PubMed]
14. Kyrgiou, M.; Koliopoulos, G.; Martin-Hirsch, P.; Arbyn, M.; Prendiville, W.; Paraskevaidis, E. Obstetric outcomes after conservative treatment for intraepithelial or early invasive cervical lesions: Systematic review and meta-analysis. *Lancet* **2006**, *367*, 489–498. [CrossRef]
15. Lemmers, M.; Verschoor, M.A.; Hooker, A.B.; Opmeer, B.C.; Limpens, J.; Huirne, J.A.; Ankum, W.M.; Mol, B.W. Dilatation and curettage increases the risk of subsequent preterm birth: A systematic review and meta-analysis. *Hum. Reprod. (Oxf. Engl.)* **2016**, *31*, 34–45. [CrossRef] [PubMed]
16. Smid, M.C.; Lee, J.H.; Grant, J.H.; Miles, G.; Stoddard, G.J.; Chapman, D.A.; Manuck, T.A. Maternal race and intergenerational preterm birth recurrence. *Am. J. Obstet. Gynecol.* **2017**, *217*, 480.e1–480.e9. [CrossRef] [PubMed]
17. Manuck, T.A. The genomics of prematurity in an era of more precise clinical phenotyping: A review. *Semin. Fetal Neonatal Med.* **2016**, *21*, 89–93. [CrossRef] [PubMed]
18. Strauss, J.F., 3rd; Romero, R.; Gomez-Lopez, N.; Haymond-Thornburg, H.; Modi, B.P.; Teves, M.E.; Pearson, L.N.; York, T.P.; Schenkein, H.A. Spontaneous Preterm Birth: Advances Toward the Discovery of Genetic Predisposition. *Am. J. Obstet. Gynecol.* **2017**, *218*, 294–314. [CrossRef] [PubMed]
19. Manuck, T.A. Racial and ethnic differences in preterm birth: A complex, multifactorial problem. *Semin. Perinatol.* **2017**, *41*, 511–518. [CrossRef]
20. Zhang, G.; Feenstra, B.; Bacelis, J.; Liu, X.; Muglia, L.M.; Juodakis, J.; Miller, D.E.; Litterman, N.; Jiang, P.P.; Russell, L.; et al. Genetic Associations with Gestational Duration and Spontaneous Preterm Birth. *N. Engl. J. Med.* **2017**, *377*, 1156–1167. [CrossRef]
21. Jarde, A.; Morais, M.; Kingston, D.; Giallo, R.; MacQueen, G.M.; Giglia, L.; Beyene, J.; Wang, Y.; McDonald, S.D. Neonatal Outcomes in Women With Untreated Antenatal Depression Compared With Women Without Depression. *JAMA Psychiatry* **2016**, *73*, 826–837. [CrossRef] [PubMed]
22. Rubens, C.E.; Sadovsky, Y.; Muglia, L.; Gravett, M.G.; Lackritz, E.; Gravett, C. Prevention of preterm birth: Harnessing science to address the global epidemic. *Sci. Transl. Med.* **2014**, *6*, 262sr5. [CrossRef] [PubMed]
23. Frey, H.A.; Klebanoff, M.A. The epidemiology, etiology, and costs of preterm birth. *Semin. Fetal Neonatal Med.* **2016**, *21*, 68–73. [CrossRef] [PubMed]
24. Nijman, T.A.; van Vliet, E.O.; Benders, M.J.; Mol, B.W.; Franx, A.; Nikkels, P.G.; Oudijk, M.A. Placental histology in spontaneous and indicated preterm birth: A case control study. *Placenta* **2016**, *48*, 56–62. [CrossRef] [PubMed]
25. Norman, S.M.; Odibo, A.O.; Macones, G.A.; Dicke, J.M.; Crane, J.P.; Cahill, A.G. Ultrasound-detected subchorionic hemorrhage and the obstetric implications. *Obstet. Gynecol.* **2010**, *116*, 311–315. [CrossRef] [PubMed]
26. Nagy, S.; Bush, M.; Stone, J.; Lapinski, R.H.; Gardo, S. Clinical significance of subchorionic and retroplacental hematomas detected in the first trimester of pregnancy. *Obstet. Gynecol.* **2003**, *102*, 94–100. [PubMed]
27. Vink, J.; Feltovich, H. Cervical etiology of spontaneous preterm birth. *Semin. Fetal Neonatal Med.* **2016**, *21*, 106–112. [CrossRef] [PubMed]
28. Staneva, A.; Bogossian, F.; Pritchard, M.; Wittkowski, A. The effects of maternal depression, anxiety, and perceived stress during pregnancy on preterm birth: A systematic review. *Women Birth* **2015**, *28*, 179–193. [CrossRef]
29. Robinson, B.G.; Emanuel, R.L.; Frim, D.M.; Majzoub, J.A. Glucocorticoid stimulates expression of corticotropin-releasing hormone gene in human placenta. *Proc. Natl. Acad. Sci. USA* **1988**, *85*, 5244–5248. [CrossRef]

30. Howland, M.A.; Sandman, C.A.; Glynn, L.M.; Crippen, C.; Davis, E.P. Fetal exposure to placental corticotropin-releasing hormone is associated with child self-reported internalizing symptoms. *Psychoneuroendocrinology* **2016**, *67*, 10–17. [CrossRef]
31. Sun, K.; Ma, R.; Cui, X.; Campos, B.; Webster, R.; Brockman, D.; Myatt, L. Glucocorticoids Induce Cytosolic Phospholipase A2 and Prostaglandin H Synthase Type 2 But Not Microsomal Prostaglandin E Synthase (PGES) and Cytosolic PGES Expression in Cultured Primary Human Amnion Cells. *J. Clin. Endocrinol. Metab.* **2003**, *88*, 5564–5571. [CrossRef] [PubMed]
32. Zhu, X.O.; Yang, Z.; Guo, C.M.; Ni, X.T.; Li, J.N.; Ge, Y.C.; Myatt, L.; Sun, K. Paradoxical stimulation of cyclooxygenase-2 expression by glucocorticoids via a cyclic AMP response element in human amnion fibroblasts. *Mol. Endocrinol.* **2009**, *23*, 1839–1849. [CrossRef] [PubMed]
33. Dunn, A.B.; Dunlop, A.L.; Hogue, C.J.; Miller, A.; Corwin, E.J. The Microbiome and Complement Activation: A Mechanistic Model for Preterm Birth. *Boil. Res. Nurs.* **2017**, *19*, 295–307. [CrossRef] [PubMed]
34. Romero, R.; Dey, S.K.; Fisher, S.J. Preterm Labor: One Syndrome, Many Causes. *Science* **2014**, *345*, 760–765. [CrossRef] [PubMed]
35. Kim, C.J.; Romero, R.; Chaemsaithong, P.; Chaiyasit, N.; Yoon, B.H.; Kim, Y.M. Acute chorioamnionitis and funisitis: Definition, pathologic features, and clinical significance. *Am. J. Obstet. Gynecol.* **2015**, *213*, S29–S52. [CrossRef] [PubMed]
36. Cappelletti, M.; Della Bella, S.; Ferrazzi, E.; Mavilio, D.; Divanovic, S. Inflammation and preterm birth. *J. Leukoc. Biol.* **2016**, *99*, 67–78. [CrossRef] [PubMed]
37. Romero, R.; Chaiworapongsa, T.; Alpay Savasan, Z.; Xu, Y.; Hussein, Y.; Dong, Z.; Kusanovic, J.P.; Kim, C.J.; Hassan, S.S. Damage-associated molecular patterns (DAMPs) in preterm labor with intact membranes and preterm PROM: A study of the alarmin HMGB1. *J. Matern. Fetal Neonatal Med.* **2011**, *24*, 1444–1455. [CrossRef] [PubMed]
38. Goldenberg, R.L.; Culhane, J.F.; Iams, J.D.; Romero, R. Epidemiology and causes of preterm birth. *Lancet* **2008**, *371*, 75–84. [CrossRef]
39. Lannon, S.M.R.; Vanderhoeven, J.P.; Eschenbach, D.A.; Gravett, M.G.; Waldorf, K.M.A. Synergy and Interactions Among Biological Pathways Leading to Preterm Premature Rupture of Membranes. *Reprod. Sci.* **2014**, *21*, 1215–1227. [CrossRef]
40. Norwitz, E.R.; Bonney, E.A.; Snegovskikh, V.V.; Williams, M.A.; Phillippe, M.; Park, J.S.; Abrahams, V.M. Molecular Regulation of Parturition: The Role of the Decidual Clock. *Cold Spring Harb. Perspect. Med.* **2015**, *5*, a023143. [CrossRef]
41. Menon, R.; Bonney, E.A.; Condon, J.; Mesiano, S.; Taylor, R.N. Novel concepts on pregnancy clocks and alarms: Redundancy and synergy in human parturition. *Hum. Reprod. Updat.* **2016**, *22*, 535–560. [CrossRef] [PubMed]
42. Navathe, R.; Berghella, V. Tocolysis for Acute Preterm Labor: Where Have We Been, Where Are We Now, and Where are We Going? *Am. J. Perinatol.* **2016**, *33*, 229–235. [PubMed]
43. Son, M.; Miller, E.S. Predicting preterm birth: Cervical length and fetal fibronectin. *Semin. Perinatol.* **2017**, *41*, 445–451. [CrossRef] [PubMed]
44. Koullali, B.; Oudijk, M.A.; Nijman, T.A.; Mol, B.W.; Pajkrt, E. Risk assessment and management to prevent preterm birth. *Semin. Fetal Neonatal Med.* **2016**, *21*, 80–88. [CrossRef] [PubMed]
45. Romero, R.; Conde-Agudelo, A.; El-Refaie, W.; Rode, L.; Brizot, M.L.; Cetingoz, E.; Serra, V.; Da Fonseca, E.; Abdelhafez, M.S.; Tabor, A.; et al. Vaginal progesterone decreases preterm birth and neonatal morbidity and mortality in women with a twin gestation and a short cervix: An updated meta-analysis of individual patient data. *Ultrasound Obstet. Gynecol.* **2017**, *49*, 303–314. [CrossRef]
46. Romero, R.; Nicolaides, K.H.; Conde-Agudelo, A.; O'Brien, J.M.; Cetingoz, E.; Da Fonseca, E.; Creasy, G.W.; Hassan, S.S. Vaginal progesterone decreases preterm birth birth </=34 weeks of gestation in women with a singleton pregnancy and a short cervix: an updated meta-analysis including data from the OPPTIMUM study. *Ultrasound Obstet. Gynecol.* **2016**, *48*, 308–317. [CrossRef] [PubMed]
47. Jarde, A.; Lutsiv, O.; Beyene, J.; McDonald, S.D. Vaginal progesterone, oral progesterone, 17-OHPC, cerclage and pessary for preventing preterm birth in singleton pregnancies: An updated systematic review and network meta-analysis. *BJOG Int. J. Obstet. Gynaecol.* **2019**, *126*, 556–567. [CrossRef]

48. Jarde, A.; Lutsiv, O.; Park, C.K.; Beyene, J.; Dodd, J.M.; Barrett, J.; Shah, P.S.; Cook, J.L.; Saito, S.; Biringer, A.B.; et al. Effectiveness of progesterone, cerclage and pessary for preventing preterm birth in singleton pregnancies: A systematic review and network meta-analysis. *BJOG Int. J. Obstet. Gynaecol.* **2017**, *124*, 1176–1189. [CrossRef]
49. Newnham, J.P.; Kemp, M.W.; White, S.W.; Arrese, C.A.; Hart, R.J.; Keelan, J.A. Applying Precision Public Health to Prevent Preterm Birth. *Front. Public Health* **2017**, *5*, 66. [CrossRef]
50. Bloomfield, F.H. How is maternal nutrition related to preterm birth? *Annu. Rev. Nutr.* **2011**, *31*, 235–261. [CrossRef]
51. Romero, R.; Espinoza, J.; Goncalves, L.F.; Kusanovic, J.P.; Friel, L.; Hassan, S. The role of inflammation and infection in preterm birth. *Semin. Reprod. Med.* **2007**, *25*, 21–39. [CrossRef] [PubMed]
52. Englund-Ögge, L.; Brantsæter, A.L.; Haugen, M.; Sengpiel, V.; Khatibi, A.; Myhre, R.; Myking, S.; Meltzer, H.M.; Kacerovsky, M.; Nilsen, R.M.; et al. Association between intake of artificially sweetened and sugar-sweetened beverages and preterm delivery: A large prospective cohort study123. *Am. J. Clin. Nutr.* **2012**, *96*, 552–559. [CrossRef] [PubMed]
53. Englund-Ögge, L.; Birgisdóttir, B.E.; Sengpiel, V.; Brantsæter, A.L.; Haugen, M.; Myhre, R.; Meltzer, H.M.; Jacobsson, B. Meal frequency patterns and glycemic properties of maternal diet in relation to preterm delivery: Results from a large prospective cohort study. *PLoS ONE* **2017**, *12*, e0172896. [CrossRef] [PubMed]
54. Englund-Ögge, L.; Brantsæter, A.L.; Sengpiel, V.; Haugen, M.; Birgisdottir, B.E.; Myhre, R.; Meltzer, H.M.; Jacobsson, B. Maternal dietary patterns and preterm delivery: Results from large prospective cohort study. *BMJ* **2014**, *348*, g1446. [CrossRef] [PubMed]
55. Mikkelsen, T.B.; Osterdal, M.L.; Knudsen, V.K.; Haugen, M.; Meltzer, H.M.; Bakketeig, L.; Olsen, S.F. Association between a Mediterranean-type diet and risk of preterm birth among Danish women: A prospective cohort study. *Acta Obstet. Gynecol. Scand.* **2008**, *87*, 325–330. [CrossRef] [PubMed]
56. Saunders, L.; Guldner, L.; Costet, N.; Kadhel, P.; Rouget, F.; Monfort, C.; Thomé, J.-P.; Multigner, L.; Cordier, S. Effect of a Mediterranean Diet during Pregnancy on Fetal Growth and Preterm Delivery: Results From a French Caribbean Mother-Child Cohort Study (TIMOUN). *Paediatr. Périnat. Epidemiol.* **2014**, *28*, 235–244. [CrossRef] [PubMed]
57. Khoury, J.; Henriksen, T.; Christophersen, B.; Tonstad, S. Effect of a cholesterol-lowering diet on maternal, cord, and neonatal lipids, and pregnancy outcome: A randomized clinical trial. *Am. J. Obstet. Gynecol.* **2005**, *193*, 1292–1301. [CrossRef] [PubMed]
58. Haugen, M.; Meltzer, H.M.; Brantsaeter, A.L.; Mikkelsen, T.; Osterdal, M.L.; Alexander, J.; Olsen, S.F.; Bakketeig, L. Mediterranean-type diet and risk of preterm birth among women in the Norwegian Mother and Child Cohort Study (MoBa): A prospective cohort study. *Acta Obstet. Gynecol. Scand.* **2008**, *87*, 319–324. [CrossRef]
59. Position of the American Dietetic Association and Dietitians of Canada: Vegetarian diets. *J. Am. Diet. Assoc.* **2003**, *103*, 748–765. [CrossRef]
60. Burdge, G.C.; Tan, S.Y.; Henry, C.J. Long-chain n-3 PUFA in vegetarian women: A metabolic perspective. *J. Nutr. Sci.* **2017**, *6*, e58. [CrossRef]
61. Rogne, T.; Tielemans, M.J.; Chong, M.F.; Yajnik, C.S.; Krishnaveni, G.V.; Poston, L.; Jaddoe, V.W.; Steegers, E.A.; Joshi, S.; Chong, Y.S.; et al. Associations of Maternal Vitamin B12 Concentration in Pregnancy With the Risks of Preterm Birth and Low Birth Weight: A Systematic Review and Meta-Analysis of Individual Participant Data. *Am. J. Epidemiol.* **2017**, *185*, 212–223. [CrossRef] [PubMed]
62. Raghavan, R.; Dreibelbis, C.; Kingshipp, B.L.; Wong, Y.P.; Abrams, B.; Gernand, A.D.; Rasmussen, K.M.; Siega-Riz, A.M.; Stang, J.O.; Casavale, K.; et al. Dietary patterns before and during pregnancy and birth outcomes: A systematic review. *Am. J. Clin. Nutr.* **2019**, *109*, 729S–756S. [CrossRef] [PubMed]
63. Chia, A.R.; Chen, L.W.; Lai, J.S.; Wong, C.H.; Neelakantan, N.; Van Dam, R.M.; Chong, M.F.F. Maternal Dietary Patterns and Birth Outcomes: A Systematic Review and Meta-Analysis. *Adv. Nutr.* **2019**, *10*, 685–695. [CrossRef] [PubMed]
64. Kibret, K.T.; Chojenta, C.; Gresham, E.; Tegegne, T.K.; Loxton, D. Maternal dietary patterns and risk of adverse pregnancy (hypertensive disorders of pregnancy and gestational diabetes mellitus) and birth (preterm birth and low birth weight) outcomes: A systematic review and meta-analysis. *Public Health Nutr.* **2018**, *22*, 506–520. [CrossRef] [PubMed]

65. Burdge, G.C.; Calder, P.C. Conversion of alpha-linolenic acid to longer-chain polyunsaturated fatty acids in human adults. *Reprod. Nutr. Dev.* **2005**, *45*, 581–597. [CrossRef] [PubMed]
66. Burdge, G.C.; Jones, A.E.; Wootton, S.A. Eicosapentaenoic and docosapentaenoic acids are the principal products of α-linolenic acid metabolism in young men. *Br. J. Nutr.* **2002**, *88*, 355–363. [CrossRef] [PubMed]
67. Baker, E.J.; Miles, E.A.; Burdge, G.C.; Yaqoob, P.; Calder, P.C. Metabolism and functional effects of plant-derived omega-3 fatty acids in humans. *Prog. Lipid Res.* **2016**, *64*, 30–56. [CrossRef] [PubMed]
68. Papanikolaou, Y.; Brooks, J.; Reider, C.; Fulgoni, V.L., 3rd. U.S. adults are not meeting recommended levels for fish and omega-3 fatty acid intake: Results of an analysis using observational data from NHANES 2003–2008. *Nutr. J.* **2014**, *13*, 31. [CrossRef]
69. Kuriki, K.; Nagaya, T.; Imaeda, N.; Tokudome, Y.; Fujiwara, N.; Sato, J.; Ikeda, M.; Maki, S.; Tokudome, S. Discrepancies in dietary intakes and plasma concentrations of fatty acids according to age among Japanese female dietitians. *Eur. J. Clin. Nutr.* **2002**, *56*, 524–531. [CrossRef]
70. Olsen, S.F.; Hansen, H.S.; Sorensen, T.I.; Jensen, B.; Secher, N.J.; Sommer, S.; Knudsen, L.B. Intake of marine fat, rich in (n-3)-polyunsaturated fatty acids, may increase birthweight by prolonging gestation. *Lancet (Lond. Engl.)* **1986**, *2*, 367–369. [CrossRef]
71. Olsen, S.F.; Østerdal, M.L.; Salvig, J.D.; Kesmodel, U.; Henriksen, T.B.; Hedegaard, M.; Secher, N.J. Duration of pregnancy in relation to seafood intake during early and mid pregnancy: Prospective cohort. *Eur. J. Epidemiol.* **2006**, *21*, 749–758. [CrossRef] [PubMed]
72. Brantsæter, A.L.; Englund-Ögge, L.; Haugen, M.; Birgisdottir, B.E.; Knutsen, H.K.; Sengpiel, V.; Myhre, R.; Alexander, J.; Nilsen, R.M.; Jacobsson, B.; et al. Maternal intake of seafood and supplementary long chain n-3 poly-unsaturated fatty acids and preterm delivery. *BMC Pregnancy Childbirth* **2017**, *17*, 61.
73. Olsen, S.F.; Secher, N.J. Low Consumption of Seafood in Early Pregnancy as a Risk Factor for Preterm Delivery: Prospective Cohort Study. *Obstet. Gynecol. Surv.* **2002**, *57*, 651–652. [CrossRef]
74. Oken, E.; Kleinman, K.P.; Olsen, S.F.; Rich-Edwards, J.W.; Gillman, M.W. Associations of Seafood and Elongated n-3 Fatty Acid Intake with Fetal Growth and Length of Gestation: Results from a US Pregnancy Cohort. *Am. J. Epidemiol.* **2004**, *160*, 774–783. [CrossRef] [PubMed]
75. Rogers, I.; Emmett, P.; Ness, A.; Golding, J. Maternal fish intake in late pregnancy and the frequency of low birth weight and intrauterine growth retardation in a cohort of British infants. *J. Epidemiol. Community Health* **2004**, *58*, 486–492. [CrossRef] [PubMed]
76. Carlson, S.E.; Colombo, J.; Gajewski, B.J.; Gustafson, K.M.; Mundy, D.; Yeast, J.; Georgieff, M.K.; Markley, L.A.; Kerling, E.H.; Shaddy, D.J. DHA supplementation and pregnancy outcomes. *Am. J. Clin. Nutr.* **2013**, *97*, 808–815. [CrossRef] [PubMed]
77. Makrides, M.; Gibson, R.A.; McPhee, A.J.; Yelland, L.; Quinlivan, J.; Ryan, P. Effect of DHA supplementation during pregnancy on maternal depression and neurodevelopment of young children: A randomized controlled trial. *JAMA* **2010**, *304*, 1675–1683. [CrossRef] [PubMed]
78. Ramakrishnan, U.; Stein, A.D.; Parra-Cabrera, S.; Wang, M.; Imhoff-Kunsch, B.; Juarez-Marquez, S.; Rivera, J.; Martorell, R. Effects of docosahexaenoic acid supplementation during pregnancy on gestational age and size at birth: Randomized, double-blind, placebo-controlled trial in Mexico. *Food Nutr. Bull.* **2010**, *31*, S108–S116. [CrossRef]
79. Helland, I.B.; Saugstad, O.D.; Smith, L.; Saarem, K.; Solvoll, K.; Ganes, T.; Drevon, C.A. Similar Effects on Infants of n-3 and n-6 Fatty Acids Supplementation to Pregnant and Lactating Women. *Pediatrics* **2001**, *108*, e82. [CrossRef]
80. Olsen, S.F.; Secher, N.J.; Tabor, A.; Weber, T.; Walker, J.J.; Gluud, C. Randomised clinical trials of fish oil supplementation in high risk pregnancies. Fish Oil Trials in Pregnancy (FOTIP) Team. *BJOG Int. J. Obstet. Gynaecol.* **2000**, *107*, 382–395. [CrossRef]
81. Onwude, J.L.; Lilford, R.J.; Hjartardottir, H.; Staines, A.; Tuffnell, D. A randomised double blind placebo controlled trial of fish oil in high risk pregnancy. *BJOG: Int. J. Obstet. Gynaecol.* **1995**, *102*, 95–100. [CrossRef] [PubMed]
82. Huisjes, H.J.; Visser, G.H.A.; Bulstra-Ramakers, M.T.E.W.; Bulstra-Ramakers, M.T.E.W. The effects of 3g eicosapentaenoic acid daily on recurrence of intrauterine growth retardation and pregnancy induced hypertension. *BJOG: Int. J. Obstet. Gynaecol.* **1995**, *102*, 123–126.

83. Olsen, S.; Sorensen, J.; Secher, N.; Hedegaard, M.; Henriksen, T.; Hansen, H.; Grant, A. Randomised controlled trial of effect of fish-oil supplementation on pregnancy duration. *Int. J. Gynecol. Obstet.* **1992**, *39*, 365–366. [CrossRef]
84. Mardones, F.; Urrutia, M.T.; Villarroel, L.; Rioseco, A.; Castillo, O.; Rozowski, J.; Tapia, J.L.; Bastias, G.; Bacallao, J.; Rojas, I. Effects of a dairy product fortified with multiple micronutrients and omega-3 fatty acids on birth weight and gestation duration in pregnant Chilean women. *Public Health Nutr.* **2008**, *11*, 30–40. [CrossRef] [PubMed]
85. Smuts, C.M.; Huang, M.; Mundy, D.; Plasse, T.; Major, S.; Carlson, S.E. A randomized trial of docosahexaenoic acid supplementation during the third trimester of pregnancy. *Obstet. Gynecol.* **2003**, *101*, 469–479. [PubMed]
86. Glaser, C.; Heinrich, J.; Koletzko, B. Role of FADS1 and FADS2 polymorphisms in polyunsaturated fatty acid metabolism. *Metabolism* **2010**, *59*, 993–999. [CrossRef] [PubMed]
87. Moltó-Puigmartí, C.; Van Dongen, M.C.J.M.; Dagnelie, P.C.; Plat, J.; Mensink, R.P.; Tan, F.E.S.; Heinrich, J.; Thijs, C. Maternal but Not Fetal FADS Gene Variants Modify the Association between Maternal Long-Chain PUFA Intake in Pregnancy and Birth Weight. *J. Nutr.* **2014**, *144*, 1430–1437. [CrossRef] [PubMed]
88. Carlson, S.E.; Gajewski, B.J.; Valentine, C.J.; Rogers, L.K.; Weiner, C.P.; DeFranco, E.A.; Buhimschi, C.S. Assessment of DHA on reducing early preterm birth: The ADORE randomized controlled trial protocol. *BMC Pregnancy Childbirth* **2017**, *17*, 62. [CrossRef]
89. Zhou, S.J.; Best, K.; Gibson, R.; McPhee, A.; Yelland, L.; Quinlivan, J.; Makrides, M. Study protocol for a randomised controlled trial evaluating the effect of prenatal omega-3 LCPUFA supplementation to reduce the incidence of preterm birth: The ORIP trial. *BMJ Open* **2017**, *7*, e018360. [CrossRef]
90. Briggs, V.; Goldenberg, T.; Ramakrishnan, U.; Imhoff-Kunsch, B.; Imhoff-Kunsch, B. Effect of n-3 Long-chain Polyunsaturated Fatty Acid Intake during Pregnancy on Maternal, Infant, and Child Health Outcomes: A Systematic Review. *Paediatr. Périnat. Epidemiol.* **2012**, *26*, 91–107.
91. Szajewska, H.; Horvath, A.; Koletzko, B. Effect of n-3 long-chain polyunsaturated fatty acid supplementation of women with low-risk pregnancies on pregnancy outcomes and growth measures at birth: A meta-analysis of randomized controlled trials. *Am. J. Clin. Nutr.* **2006**, *83*, 1337–1344. [CrossRef] [PubMed]
92. Makrides, M.; Duley, L.; Olsen, S.F. Marine oil, and other prostaglandin precursor, supplementation for pregnancy uncomplicated by pre-eclampsia or intrauterine growth restriction. *Cochrane Database Syst. Rev.* **2006**, *3*, CD003402. [CrossRef] [PubMed]
93. Horvath, A.; Koletzko, B.; Szajewska, H. Effect of supplementation of women in high-risk pregnancies with long-chain polyunsaturated fatty acids on pregnancy outcomes and growth measures at birth: A meta-analysis of randomized controlled trials. *Br. J. Nutr.* **2007**, *98*, 253–259. [CrossRef] [PubMed]
94. Kar, S.; Wong, M.; Rogozinska, E.; Thangaratinam, S. Effects of omega-3 fatty acids in prevention of early preterm delivery: A systematic review and meta-analysis of randomized studies. *Eur. J. Obstet. Gynecol. Reprod. Biol.* **2016**, *198*, 40–46. [CrossRef] [PubMed]
95. Middleton, P.; Gomersall, J.C.; Gould, J.F.; Shepherd, E.; Olsen, S.F.; Makrides, M. Omega-3 fatty acid addition during pregnancy. *Cochrane Database Syst. Rev.* **2018**, *11*, CD003402. [CrossRef] [PubMed]
96. Park, H.G.; Lawrence, P.; Engel, M.G.; Kothapalli, K.; Brenna, J.T. Metabolic fate of docosahexaenoic acid (DHA; 22:6n-3) in human cells: Direct retroconversion of DHA to eicosapentaenoic acid (20:5n-3) dominates over elongation to tetracosahexaenoic acid (24:6n-3). *FEBS Lett.* **2016**, *590*, 3188–3194. [CrossRef] [PubMed]
97. Olsen, S.F.; Secher, N.J.; Bjornsson, S.; Weber, T.; Atke, A. The potential benefits of using fish oil in relation to preterm labor: The case for a randomized controlled trial? *Acta Obstet. Gynecol. Scand.* **2003**, *82*, 978–982. [CrossRef] [PubMed]
98. Calder, P.C. The role of marine omega-3 (n-3) fatty acids in inflammatory processes, atherosclerosis and plaque stability. *Mol. Nutr. Food Res.* **2012**, *56*, 1073–1080. [CrossRef] [PubMed]
99. MacDonald, R.S. The role of zinc in growth and cell proliferation. *J. Nutr.* **2000**, *130*, 1500s–1508s. [CrossRef]
100. Black, R.E.; Allen, L.H.A.; Bhutta, Z.; Caulfield, L.E.; De Onis, M.; Ezzati, M.; Mathers, C.; Rivera, J. Maternal and child undernutrition: Global and regional exposures and health consequences. *Lancet* **2008**, *371*, 243–260. [CrossRef]
101. Keen, C.L.; Uriu-Adams, J.Y.; Uriu-Adams, J.Y. Zinc and reproduction: Effects of zinc deficiency on prenatal and early postnatal development. *Birth Defects Res. Part B Dev. Reprod. Toxicol.* **2010**, *89*, 313–325.

102. Chaffee, B.W.; King, J.C. Effect of Zinc Supplementation on Pregnancy and Infant Outcomes: A Systematic Review. *Paediatr. Périnat. Epidemiol.* **2012**, *26*, 118–137. [CrossRef] [PubMed]
103. Ota, E.; Mori, R.; Middleton, P.; Tobe-Gai, R.; Mahomed, K.; Miyazaki, C.A.; Bhutta, Z. Zinc supplementation for improving pregnancy and infant outcome. *Cochrane Database Syst. Rev.* **2015**, *2*, CD000230. [CrossRef] [PubMed]
104. Wilson, R.L.; Grieger, J.A.; Bianco-Miotto, T.; Roberts, C.T. Association between Maternal Zinc Status, Dietary Zinc Intake and Pregnancy Complications: A Systematic Review. *Nutrients* **2016**, *8*, 641. [CrossRef] [PubMed]
105. DeLuca, H.F. Overview of general physiologic features and functions of vitamin D. *Am. J. Clin. Nutr.* **2004**, *80*, 1689s–1696s. [CrossRef] [PubMed]
106. Mithal, A.; Wahl, D.A.; Bonjour, J.P.; Burckhardt, P.; Dawson-Hughes, B.; Eisman, J.A.; El-Hajj Fuleihan, G.; Josse, R.G.; Lips, P.; Morales-Torres, J. Global vitamin D status and determinants of hypovitaminosis D. *Osteoporos. Int.* **2009**, *20*, 1807–1820. [CrossRef] [PubMed]
107. Liu, N.Q.; Hewison, M. Vitamin D, the placenta and pregnancy. *Arch. Biochem. Biophys.* **2012**, *523*, 37–47. [CrossRef] [PubMed]
108. Liu, N.Q.; Kaplan, A.T.; Lagishetty, V.; Ouyang, Y.B.; Ouyang, Y.; Simmons, C.F.; Equils, O.; Hewison, M. Vitamin D and the Regulation of Placental Inflammation. *J. Immunol.* **2011**, *186*, 5968–5974. [CrossRef]
109. Zhou, S.; Tao, Y.; Huang, K.; Zhu, B. Vitamin D and risk of preterm birth: Up-to-date meta-analysis of randomized controlled trials and observational studies. *J. Obstet. Gynaecol. Res.* **2017**, *43*, 247–256. [CrossRef] [PubMed]
110. Qin, L.L.; Lu, F.G.; Yang, S.H.; Xu, H.L.; Luo, B.A. Does Maternal Vitamin D Deficiency Increase the Risk of Preterm Birth: A Meta-Analysis of Observational Studies. *Nutrients* **2016**, *8*, 301. [CrossRef] [PubMed]
111. Thorne-Lyman, A.; Fawzi, W.W. Vitamin D during pregnancy and maternal, neonatal and infant health outcomes: A systematic review and meta-analysis. *Paediatr. Périnat. Epidemiol.* **2012**, *26*, 75–90. [CrossRef] [PubMed]
112. De-Regil, L.M.; Palacios, C.; Lombardo, L.K.; Peña-Rosas, J.P. Vitamin D supplementation for women during pregnancy. *Cochrane Database Syst. Rev.* **2016**, *1*, CD008873.
113. Cooper, C.; Harvey, N.C.; Bishop, N.J.; Kennedy, S.; Papageorghiou, A.T.; Schoenmakers, I.; Fraser, R.; Gandhi, S.V.; Carr, A.; D'Angelo, S.; et al. Maternal gestational vitamin D supplementation and offspring bone health (MAVIDOS): A multicentre, double-blind, randomised placebo-controlled trial. *Lancet Diabetes Endocrinol.* **2016**, *4*, 393–402. [CrossRef]
114. Arikan, G.M.; Panzitt, T.; Gücer, F.; Scholz, H.S.; Reinisch, S.; Haas, J.; Weiss, P.A. Course of Maternal Serum Magnesium Levels in Low-Risk Gestations and in Preterm Labor and Delivery. *Fetal Diagn. Ther.* **1999**, *14*, 332–336. [CrossRef] [PubMed]
115. King, D.E.; Mainous, A.G., 3rd; Geesey, M.E.; Woolson, R.F. Dietary magnesium and C-reactive protein levels. *J. Am. Coll. Nutr.* **2005**, *24*, 166–171. [CrossRef] [PubMed]
116. Wynn, A.; Wynn, M. Magnesium and Other Nutrient Deficiencies as Possible Causes of Hypertension and Low Birthweight. *Nutr. Health* **1988**, *6*, 69–88. [CrossRef] [PubMed]
117. Lopez Bernal, A. The regulation of uterine relaxation. *Semin. Cell Dev. Biol.* **2007**, *18*, 340–347. [CrossRef] [PubMed]
118. Makrides, M.A.; Crowther, C. Magnesium supplementation in pregnancy. *Cochrane Database Syst. Rev.* **2001**, CD000937. [CrossRef]
119. Crosby, D.D.; Shepherd, E.A.; Crowther, C.; Makrides, M. Magnesium supplementation in pregnancy. *Cochrane Database Syst. Rev.* **2014**, *4*, CD000937.
120. Crowther, C.A.; Brown, J.; McKinlay, C.J.D.; Middleton, P. Magnesium sulphate for preventing preterm birth in threatened preterm labour. *Cochrane Database Syst. Rev.* **2014**, *8*, CD001060. [CrossRef]
121. Alves, J.G.B.; De Araújo, C.A.F.L.; Pontes, I.E.; Guimarães, A.C.; Ray, J.G. The BRAzil MAGnesium (BRAMAG) trial: A randomized clinical trial of oral magnesium supplementation in pregnancy for the prevention of preterm birth and perinatal and maternal morbidity. *BMC Pregnancy Childbirth* **2014**, *14*, 222. [CrossRef] [PubMed]
122. Buppasiri, P.; Lumbiganon, P.; Thinkhamrop, J.; Ngamjarus, C.; Laopaiboon, M.; Medley, N. Calcium supplementation (other than for preventing or treating hypertension) for improving pregnancy and infant outcomes. *Cochrane Database Syst. Rev.* **2015**, CD007079. [CrossRef] [PubMed]

123. Villar, J.; Merialdi, M.; Gulmezoglu, A.M.; Abalos, E.; Carroli, G.; Kulier, R.; de Onis, M. Nutritional interventions during pregnancy for the prevention or treatment of maternal morbidity and preterm delivery: An overview of randomized controlled trials. *J. Nutr.* **2003**, *133*, 1606s–1625s. [CrossRef] [PubMed]
124. Peña-Rosas, J.P.; Dowswell, T.; Peña-Rosas, J.P.; De-Regil, L.M.; Garcia-Casal, M.N.; Pena-Rosas, J.P.; De-Regil, L.M.; Garcia-Casal, M.N. Daily oral iron supplementation during pregnancy. *Cochrane Database Syst. Rev.* **2015**, CD004736. [CrossRef] [PubMed]
125. De-Regil, L.M.; Peña-Rosas, J.P.; Fernández-Gaxiola, A.C.; Rayco-Solon, P. Effects and safety of periconceptional oral folate supplementation for preventing birth defects. *Cochrane Database Syst. Rev.* **2015**, CD007950. [CrossRef] [PubMed]
126. Klebanoff, M.; Shiono, P.; Selby, J.; Trachtenberg, A.; Graubard, B. Anemia and spontaneous preterm birth. *Int. J. Gynecol. Obstet.* **1991**, *164*, 59–63.
127. Scholl, T.O.; Hediger, M.L.; Fischer, R.L.; Shearer, J.W. Anemia vs. iron deficiency: Increased risk of preterm delivery in a prospective study. *Am. J. Clin. Nutr.* **1992**, *55*, 985–988. [CrossRef]
128. Lassi, Z.S.; Salam, R.A.; Haider, B.A.; Bhutta, Z. Folic acid supplementation during pregnancy for maternal health and pregnancy outcomes. *Cochrane Database Syst. Rev.* **2013**, *3*, CD006896. [CrossRef]
129. West, K.P., Jr. Extent of vitamin A deficiency among preschool children and women of reproductive age. *J. Nutr.* **2002**, *132*, 2857s–2866s. [CrossRef]
130. Thorne-Lyman, A.L.; Fawzi, W.W. Vitamin A and carotenoids during pregnancy and maternal, neonatal and infant health outcomes: A systematic review and meta-analysis. *Paediatr. Périnat. Epidemiol.* **2012**, *26*, 36–54. [CrossRef]
131. West, K.P., Jr.; Katz, J.; Khatry, S.K.; LeClerq, S.C.; Pradhan, E.K.; Shrestha, S.R.; Connor, P.B.; Dali, S.M.; Christian, P.; Pokhrel, R.P.; et al. Double blind, cluster randomised trial of low dose supplementation with vitamin A or beta carotene on mortality related to pregnancy in Nepal. The NNIPS-2 Study Group. *BMJ* **1999**, *318*, 570–575. [CrossRef]
132. Mistry, H.D.; Williams, P.J. The importance of antioxidant micronutrients in pregnancy. *Oxid. Med. Cell. Longev.* **2011**, *2011*, 841749. [CrossRef] [PubMed]
133. Ray, J.G.; Laskin, C.A. Folic acid and homocyst(e)ine metabolic defects and the risk of placental abruption, pre-eclampsia and spontaneous pregnancy loss: A systematic review. *Placenta* **1999**, *20*, 519–529. [CrossRef] [PubMed]
134. Himes, K.P.; Simhan, H.N. Risk of recurrent preterm birth and placental pathology. *Obstet. Gynecol.* **2008**, *112*, 121–126. [CrossRef] [PubMed]
135. Catov, J.M.; Bodnar, L.M.; Olsen, J.; Olsen, S.A.; Nohr, E. Periconceptional multivitamin use and risk of preterm or small-for-gestational-age births in the Danish National Birth Cohort1234. *Am. J. Clin. Nutr.* **2011**, *94*, 906–912. [CrossRef] [PubMed]
136. Haider, B.A.; Bhutta, Z.A. Multiple-micronutrient supplementation for women during pregnancy. *Cochrane Database Syst. Rev.* **2015**, *11*, CD004905.
137. de Onis, M.; Villar, J.; Gulmezoglu, M. Nutritional interventions to prevent intrauterine growth retardation: Evidence from randomized controlled trials. *Eur. J. Clin. Nutr.* **1998**, *52*, S83–S93.
138. Kramer, M.S.; Kakuma, R. Energy and protein intake in pregnancy. *Cochrane Database Syst. Rev.* **2003**, *4*, CD000032.
139. Hillier, S.L.; Martin, D.H.; Pastorek, J.G.; Rao, A.V.; McNellis, D.; Regan, J.A.; Nugent, R.P.; Eschenbach, D.A.; Krohn, M.A.; Gibbs, R.S.; et al. Association between Bacterial Vaginosis and Preterm Delivery of a Low-Birth-Weight Infant. *N. Engl. J. Med.* **1995**, *333*, 1737–1742. [CrossRef]
140. Brocklehurst, P.; Gordon, A.; Heatley, E.; Milan, S.J. Antibiotics for treating bacterial vaginosis in pregnancy. *Cochrane Database Syst. Rev.* **2013**. [CrossRef]
141. Al-Ghazzewi, F.H.; Tester, R.F. Biotherapeutic agents and vaginal health. *J. Appl. Microbiol.* **2016**, *121*, 18–27. [CrossRef] [PubMed]
142. Hemarajata, P.; Versalovic, J. Effects of probiotics on gut microbiota: Mechanisms of intestinal immunomodulation and neuromodulation. *Ther. Adv. Gastroenterol.* **2013**, *6*, 39–51. [CrossRef] [PubMed]
143. Krauss-Silva, L.; Moreira, M.E.L.; Alves, M.B.; Rezende, M.R.; Braga, A.; Camacho, K.G.; Batista, M.R.R.; Savastano, C.; Almada-Horta, A.; Guerra, F. Randomized controlled trial of probiotics for the prevention of spontaneous preterm delivery associated with intrauterine infection: Study protocol. *Reprod. Health* **2010**, *7*, 14. [CrossRef] [PubMed]

144. Krauss-Silva, L.; Moreira, M.E.L.; Alves, M.B.; Braga, A.; Camacho, K.G.; Batista, M.R.R.; Almada-Horta, A.; Rebello, M.R.; Guerra, F. A randomised controlled trial of probiotics for the prevention of spontaneous preterm delivery associated with bacterial vaginosis: Preliminary results. *Trials* **2011**, *12*, 239. [CrossRef] [PubMed]
145. Gille, C.; Böer, B.; Marschal, M.; Urschitz, M.S.; Heinecke, V.; Hund, V.; Speidel, S.; Tarnow, I.; Mylonas, I.; Franz, A.; et al. Effect of probiotics on vaginal health in pregnancy. EFFPRO, a randomized controlled trial. *Am. J. Obstet. Gynecol.* **2016**, *215*, 608.e1–608.e7. [CrossRef] [PubMed]
146. Luoto, R.; Laitinen, K.; Nermes, M.; Isolauri, E. Impact of maternal probiotic-supplemented dietary counselling on pregnancy outcome and prenatal and postnatal growth: A double-blind, placebo-controlled study. *Br. J. Nutr.* **2010**, *103*, 1792–1799. [CrossRef]
147. Mantaring, J.; Benyacoub, J.; Destura, R.; Pecquet, S.; Vidal, K.; Volger, S.; Guinto, V. Effect of maternal supplement beverage with and without probiotics during pregnancy and lactation on maternal and infant health: A randomized controlled trial in the Philippines. *BMC Pregnancy Childbirth* **2018**, *18*, 193. [CrossRef]
148. Rautava, S.; Collado, M.C.; Salminen, S.; Isolauri, E. Probiotics modulate host-microbe interaction in the placenta and fetal gut: A randomized, double-blind, placebo-controlled trial. *Neonatology* **2012**, *102*, 178–184. [CrossRef]
149. Nordqvist, M.; Jacobsson, B.; Brantsæter, A.-L.; Myhre, R.; Nilsson, S.; Sengpiel, V. Timing of probiotic milk consumption during pregnancy and effects on the incidence of preeclampsia and preterm delivery: A prospective observational cohort study in Norway. *BMJ Open* **2018**, *8*, e018021. [CrossRef]
150. Myhre, R.; Brantsaeter, A.L.; Myking, S.; Gjessing, H.K.; Sengpiel, V.; Meltzer, H.M.; Haugen, M.; Jacobsson, B. Intake of probiotic food and risk of spontaneous preterm delivery. *Am. J. Clin. Nutr.* **2011**, *93*, 151–157. [CrossRef]
151. Othman, M.; Neilson, J.P.; Alfirevic, Z. Probiotics for preventing preterm labour. *Cochrane Database Syst. Rev.* **2007**, *1*, CD005941. [CrossRef] [PubMed]
152. Jarde, A.; Lewis-Mikhael, A.-M.; Moayyedi, P.; Stearns, J.C.; Collins, S.M.; Beyene, J.; McDonald, S.D. Pregnancy outcomes in women taking probiotics or prebiotics: A systematic review and meta-analysis. *BMC Pregnancy Childbirth* **2018**, *18*, 14. [CrossRef] [PubMed]
153. Grev, J.; Berg, M.; Soll, R. Maternal probiotic supplementation for prevention of morbidity and mortality in preterm infants. *Cochrane Database Syst. Rev.* **2018**, *12*, CD012519. [CrossRef] [PubMed]
154. Stojanovic, N.; Plecas, D.; Plesinac, S. Normal vaginal flora, disorders and application of probiotics in pregnancy. *Arch. Gynecol. Obstet.* **2012**, *286*, 325–332. [CrossRef] [PubMed]
155. Jespers, V.; van de Wijgert, J.; Cools, P.; Verhelst, R.; Verstraelen, H.; Delany-Moretlwe, S.; Mwaura, M.; Ndayisaba, G.F.; Mandaliya, K.; Menten, J.; et al. The significance of Lactobacillus crispatus and L. vaginalis for vaginal health and the negative effect of recent sex: A cross-sectional descriptive study across groups of African women. *BMC Infect. Dis.* **2015**, *15*, 115. [CrossRef]
156. Srinivasan, S.; Morgan, M.T.; Fiedler, T.L.; Djukovic, D.; Hoffman, N.G.; Raftery, D.; Marrazzo, J.M.; Fredricks, D.N. Metabolic signatures of bacterial vaginosis. *MBio* **2015**, *6*, e00204–e00215. [CrossRef]
157. Kim, J.Y.; Kwon, J.H.; Ahn, S.H.; Lee, S.I.; Han, Y.S.; Choi, Y.O.; Lee, S.Y.; Ahn, K.M.; Ji, G.E. Effect of probiotic mix (Bifidobacterium bifidum, Bifidobacterium lactis, Lactobacillus acidophilus) in the primary prevention of eczema: A double-blind, randomized, placebo-controlled trial. *Pediatr. Allergy Immunol.* **2010**, *21*, e386–e393. [CrossRef]
158. Ou, C.Y.; Kuo, H.C.; Wang, L.; Hsu, T.Y.; Chuang, H.; Liu, C.A.; Chang, J.C.; Yu, H.R.; Yang, K.D. Prenatal and postnatal probiotics reduces maternal but not childhood allergic diseases: A randomized, double-blind, placebo-controlled trial. *Clin. Exp. Allergy* **2012**, *42*, 1386–1396. [CrossRef]
159. Vitali, B.; Cruciani, F.; Baldassarre, M.E.; Capursi, T.; Spisni, E.; Valerii, M.C.; Candela, M.; Turroni, S.; Brigidi, P. Dietary supplementation with probiotics during late pregnancy: Outcome on vaginal microbiota and cytokine secretion. *BMC Microbiol.* **2012**, *12*, 236. [CrossRef]

9

Uncontrolled Eating during Pregnancy Predicts Fetal Growth: The Healthy Mom Zone Trial

Jennifer S. Savage [1,2,*], Emily E. Hohman [1], Katherine M. McNitt [1,2], Abigail M. Pauley [3], Krista S. Leonard [3], Tricia Turner [4], Jaimey M. Pauli [5,6], Alison D. Gernand [2], Daniel E. Rivera [7] and Danielle Symons Downs [3,5]

1 Center for Childhood Obesity Research, The Pennsylvania State University, University Park, State College, PA 16802, USA; eeh12@psu.edu (E.E.H.); kmm6054@psu.edu (K.M.M.)
2 Department of Nutritional Sciences, The Pennsylvania State University, University Park, State College, PA 16802, USA; adg14@psu.edu
3 Exercise Psychology Laboratory, Department of Kinesiology, The Pennsylvania State University, University Park, State College, PA 16802, USA; amp34@psu.edu (A.M.P.); kbl5167@psu.edu (K.S.L.); dsd11@psu.edu (D.S.D.)
4 Diagnostic Medical Sonography, South Hills School of Business and Technology, State College, PA 16801, USA; tslturner3@gmail.com
5 Department of Obstetrics and Gynecology, Penn State College of Medicine, Hershey, PA 17033, USA; jpauli@pennstatehealth.psu.edu
6 Department of Maternal & Fetal Medicine, Penn State College of Medicine, Hershey, PA 17033, USA
7 Control Systems Engineering Laboratory, School for Engineering of Matter, Transport, and Energy, Arizona State University, Tempe, AZ 85287, USA; daniel.rivera@asu.edu
* Correspondence: jfs195@psu.edu

Abstract: Excess maternal weight gain during pregnancy elevates infants' risk for macrosomia and early-onset obesity. Eating behavior is also related to weight gain, but the relationship to fetal growth is unclear. We examined whether Healthy Mom Zone, an individually tailored, adaptive gestational weight gain intervention, and maternal eating behaviors affected fetal growth in pregnant women (n = 27) with a BMI > 24. At study enrollment (6–13 weeks gestation) and monthly thereafter, the Three-Factor Eating Questionnaire was completed. Ultrasounds were obtained monthly from 14–34 weeks gestation. Data were analyzed using multilevel modeling. Higher baseline levels of uncontrolled eating predicted faster rates of fetal growth in late gestation. Cognitive restraint was not associated with fetal growth, but moderated the effect of uncontrolled eating on fetal growth. Emotional eating was not associated with fetal growth. Among women with higher baseline levels of uncontrolled eating, fetuses of women in the control group grew faster and were larger in later gestation than those in the intervention group (study group × baseline uncontrolled eating × gestational week interaction, p = 0.03). This is one of the first intervention studies to use an individually tailored, adaptive design to manage weight gain in pregnancy to demonstrate potential effects on fetal growth. Results also suggest that it may be important to develop intervention content and strategies specific to pregnant women with high vs. low levels of disinhibited eating.

Keywords: pregnancy; gestational weight gain intervention; eating behavior; restraint; disinhibition; uncontrolled and emotional eating; fetal growth; overweight and obesity; generalized linear models

---

1. Introduction

Over 50% of women in the United States enter pregnancy already having overweight or obesity; the majority of these women (60%) gain more weight in pregnancy than is recommended by the Institute of Medicine (IOM) [1]. Data also indicate that 23% of US 2–5-year-olds have overweight [2] and 9%–14%

have obesity [3,4], underscoring the need for research on early obesity prevention. The prenatal period may be an opportune time to intervene and break the intergenerational cycle of obesity by reducing fetal exposure to an "obesogenic" intrauterine environment [5,6] through promoting maternal energy balance (EB) (i.e., a nutrient-rich, low-energy dense diet and physical activity) [7]. Infant birth weight is commonly used as a surrogate marker for intrauterine growth and as an indicator of the conditions experienced in utero [8]. Maternal weight gain during pregnancy is necessary for healthy fetal development, but high gestational weight gain elevates infant risk for macrosomia and early onset obesity [1]. Further, infant birth weight is a positive, independent predictor of obesity during later childhood [9–11], and high birth weight is associated with increased risk for adult-onset obesity and diabetes [12].

Behavioral interventions have effectively managed weight among normal weight women, but similar interventions have had mixed effects among women with overweight or obesity [13]. Together, these data indicate the need for effective interventions that promote healthy gestational weight gain and are able to influence the etiology of obesity for offspring at a critical time in development. Based on past research and our own pilot data [7,14–17], we developed Healthy Mom Zone [18], an individually tailored and "intensively adaptive" intervention to effectively manage gestational weight gain and promote optimal maternal and child health in women with overweight or obesity. This novel intervention provides each woman with the support needed to manage her gestational weight gain, while adapting the dose and intensity of the intervention to her unique needs across pregnancy. Healthy Mom Zone is also innovative, applying principles/methods from systems science and engineering [19] including dynamical modeling, simulation, and controller design to optimize the intervention. Intensive longitudinal data (e.g., weight, energy intake, eating behavior, physical activity, and psychosocial factors) were collected and used in making decisions about adapting the intervention.

Throughout pregnancy, maternal nutritional status and dietary intake are key factors influencing the health of both the child and mother [20]. However, misreporting of dietary intake is common, making it difficult to identify how dietary intake patterns, macronutrient intakes, or even energy density are associated with gestational weight gain and fetal programming [21]. Among pregnant women with overweight or obesity, as many as one-third to one-half under-report dietary intake, with rates higher in late compared to early pregnancy [22], a finding supported by our own Healthy Mom Zone data [23].

Moreover, an individual's eating behavior and attitudes influence food choices, impact the regulation of food intake, and ultimately affect weight. Given the recall bias of self-reported dietary intake, alternative modifiable factors such as eating behavior (e.g., restrained eating, uncontrolled eating, emotional eating) that are relatively easy to measure may be amenable to intervention during pregnancy. Dietary restraint and disinhibited eating (emotional and uncontrolled), as measured by the Eating Inventory (EI) (also referred to as the Three Factor Eating Questionnaire [24,25]), are psychological constructs that assess behavioral control and attitudes toward food and eating. Cognitive dietary restraint is defined as a tendency to consciously restrict or control food intake, regardless of physiological signs of hunger and satiety. Uncontrolled eating is defined as a tendency to overeat relative to physiologic need and feeling of lack of control, whereas emotional eating is the tendency to overeat during depressed and melancholic states [26].

Eating behaviors may be a "proxy" for dietary intake in lieu of accurate, self-reported dietary intake [27]. In the general population, disinhibited eating is positively associated with food intake and weight [28–32], but the association between dietary restraint and emotional eating with these outcomes remains unclear [29–31,33–37]. In our current obesogenic environment, cognitive controls of eating may be necessary to prevent overeating and moderate weight gain [38]. For example, a randomized weight loss study reported that cognitive restrained eating was associated with lower energy intakes [39]. In pregnant women, restrained eating and emotional eating have been positively associated with poorer diet quality and greater overall weight gain [40–43]. However, cross-sectional studies [30,31,44] and longitudinal data [45] in nonpregnant individuals have revealed that it is not the independent effects of restraint and disinhibition but their interaction that predicts food intake and ultimately body weight, with restraint moderating the impact of uncontrolled eating. No study, to our knowledge, has examined the long-term effects of the interaction between restrained and disinhibited eating (uncontrolled or emotional) in pregnant women with overweight/obesity on fetal growth.

The primary aim of this study was to determine the effect of an individually tailored, adaptive intervention designed to help pregnant women with overweight and obesity to manage their gestational weight gain within the IOM guidelines on fetal growth, compared to a standard of care control. A secondary aim was to explore the interactive effects of maternal cognitive restraint, with uncontrolled and emotional eating during pregnancy, on fetal growth. Based on previous data [27,32,36,40,41,45], we expect that: (1) fetuses of women receiving the treatment would gain weight slower on average compared to control fetuses; (2) higher levels of emotional and uncontrolled eating will predict faster fetal weight gain; and (3) cognitive restraint will attenuate the positive relationship between emotional and uncontrolled eating and fetal weight gain. Findings from this study may inform counseling during pregnancy.

2. Methods

2.1. Study Design and Participants

Data for this analysis were collected as part of an ancillary study to measure fetal growth in women participating in Healthy Mom Zone, an optimization trial within the multiphase optimization strategy (MOST) framework [46], of an adaptive intervention to manage gestational weight gain among pregnant women with overweight or obesity [18]. This study was approved by the Pennsylvania State University Institutional Review Board (study ID #00003752, initial approval date 12/1/2015), and participants provided written consent for their participation. Women were eligible if they were 6–13 weeks pregnant with a single fetus, English-speaking, non-smoking, had a prepregnancy BMI > 24, and were free of significant pregnancy complications or medical conditions. The study was powered on the primary outcome of gestational weight gain; a sample size of 24 participants (12 per group) was determined to yield 80% power to detect a standardized effect size for gestational weight gain of 1.2 using a two-sided test with a significance level of $p = 0.05$. We aimed to recruit 30 participants, accounting for up to 25% drop out [18]. Participants ($n = 31$) were randomized to the intervention or a standard care control group. From this initial group, three women had a miscarriage at <12 weeks gestation, and one woman dropped out of the study at 22 weeks gestation, representing 87.1% sample retention (9.7% miscarriage rate and 3.2% drop rate). For the purpose of analysis, women with a prepregnancy BMI 24.1–29.9 were classified as having overweight (OW) and those with BMI ≥ 30 were classified as having obesity (OB). Fetal growth data were collected on a total of 27 women (intervention: 9 OW/4 OB; control: 7 OW/7 OB). One woman (control group, OW) did not complete the baseline survey measure of eating behavior, resulting in a sample of $n = 26$ women for those analyses.

2.2. Intervention

Healthy Mom Zone is an individually tailored, adaptive intervention to optimize gestational weight gain among pregnant women with overweight and obesity. This optimization trial was built within the multiphase optimization strategy (MOST) framework [46] with the aim of developing an intervention to efficiently and effectively manage weight gain over pregnancy. Details of the Healthy Mom Zone intervention are published elsewhere [18], but in short, principles from the theory of planned behavior (TPB) [47] and self-regulation [48] provide the conceptual framework for the intervention. The key intervention components include education, goal-setting/action plans, self-monitoring, and active learning. Participants in the intervention group met weekly with a study dietitian and were given customized calorie and physical activity goals. Plots of each woman's weight, physical activity, and dietary intake via real-time data collection procedures were plotted to generate a report illustrating gestational weight gain in the context of the IOM guidelines. This report was discussed by the dietitian.

In addition, emails were sent discussing maternal behaviors that impact baby health and growth. Lastly, gestational weight gain was evaluated weekly and decision rules were used in 3–4 week cycles to decide when and how the intervention may be adapted for an individual. When a participant's weight gain trajectory exceeded the recommended rate, they received an intervention step-up consisting of additional healthy eating active learning sessions (e.g., cooking demonstrations, grocery store tours) and onsite physical activity sessions with a fitness instructor. All women in the study received standard prenatal care (e.g., regular visits, prenatal counseling) with their personal healthcare provider.

2.3. Measures

At study enrollment, height and weight were measured by clinical research center staff. Participants completed a baseline background questionnaire that assessed prepregnancy weight, height, age, years of education, combined family income, and general health. At study enrollment and every four weeks thereafter, women completed the three-factor eating questionnaire (TFEQ-21) [24] via online survey through REDCap [49]. This 21-item scale, with a four point response scale ranging from (1) definitely true to (4) definitely false, measures three subscales: cognitive restraint (e.g., "I consciously hold back on how much I eat at meals to keep from gaining weight."), uncontrolled eating (e.g., "Sometimes when I start eating, I just can't seem to stop."), and emotional eating (e.g., "I start to eat when I feel anxious."). Scores for each subscale were calculated by averaging respective items.

Standard ultrasounds were obtained at approximately 14, 18, 22, 26, 30, and 34 weeks gestation by a sonographer using the same ultrasound machine (Philips iU22 MATRIX, Philips Healthcare, Andover, MA, USA). Standard fetal biometry measures including biparietal diameter (BPD), head circumference (HC), abdominal (AC), and femur length (FL), were assessed. Estimated fetal weight was calculated using a validated equation [50]. Gestational age was calculated using the date of last menstrual period. All ultrasounds were reviewed by a study physician, and any concerns identified were communicated to the participant's personal physician. Birth weight and gestational age at birth were abstracted from medical records or reported by participants if medical records were not available. Sex-specific birth weight-for-gestational age percentiles were determined using the INTERGROWTH-21st standards [51].

2.4. Analysis

Eating behavior variables were centered to disaggregate within- and between-person effects and to aid interpretation. Between-person effects were assessed using baseline levels of each eating behavior centered on the population mean, so that the centered baseline values represented each individual's deviation from the average baseline level across all women in the study. Within-person effects were assessed using change scores, such that each monthly eating behavior score represented a woman's change from her own baseline. Though survey data (i.e., eating behavior) and fetal ultrasounds were collected monthly, the timing of these measurements relative to one another was variable due to variation in gestational age at enrollment. For the purpose of this analysis, ultrasound data was paired with the most recent eating behavior survey completed prior to the scan. In seven instances across four participants, no eating behavior data preceded the scan, thus, survey data completed within seven days after the scan were used. The mean (SD) time between survey completion and ultrasound scan was 12.2 (8.9) days.

Statistical analysis was performed in SAS 9.4 (SAS Institute, Cary, NC, USA). Data were analyzed using multilevel modeling (PROC MIXED). All models utilized the restricted maximum likelihood (REML) estimation method, Satterthwaite method for computing df, and an unstructured covariance structure. Determination of model fit was based on several criteria including model convergence, a positive definite G matrix, and Akaike information criteria. Intraclass correlation coefficients (ICCs) were calculated as the ratio of between-subjects variance to total variance. Change over time in each of the three eating behavior subscales was modeled as a linear function of gestational week with a random intercept and slope. For cognitive restraint, the random gestational week slope term resulted in a nonpositive definite G matrix, so it was removed from the model. Interactions of gestational week with study group and prepregnancy BMI were tested to determine if the rate of change over time differed by these variables.

Estimated fetal weight was also modeled using multilevel modeling. Linear, quadratic, and cubic effects of gestational week were considered. Once the model describing fetal weight over time was finalized, study group and maternal prepregnancy BMI were added, and interactions with gestational week were tested. Next, a set of models were run for each of the three eating behavior constructs. These models tested (a) main effect of the baseline eating behavior, (b) interaction between baseline eating behavior and gestational week, (c) main effect of change in eating behavior, (d) interaction between change in eating behavior and gestational week, (e) interaction between baseline and change in eating behavior, and (f) three-way interaction between baseline and change in eating behavior and gestational week. For all interactions with gestational week, interactions with both the linear and quadratic gestational week terms were tested; the interaction with the quadratic term was dropped when not significant and was not reported here. Finally, two sets of models were tested to evaluate interactions between cognitive restraint and each of the two disinhibited eating behavior constructs (uncontrolled eating and emotional eating). These models tested (a) interaction between baseline cognitive restraint and baseline disinhibited eating; (b) three-way interactions between baseline cognitive restraint, baseline disinhibited eating, and gestational week; (c) interactions of baseline cognitive restraint and disinhibited eating with change in cognitive restraint and disinhibited eating; (d) three-way interactions between change in cognitive restraint, change in disinhibited eating, and gestational week; and (e) interactions described in (a)–(d) but with the quadratic gestational age term in place of the linear term. Two final models, one including cognitive restraint × uncontrolled eating and one including cognitive restraint × emotional eating, were evaluated using backward and forward selections.

3. Results

3.1. Descriptive Characteristics

Descriptive statistics are located in Table 1. Mean age of women at study entry was 30.6 (SD = 2.9) ranging from 24 to 37 years. Mean gestational age at the start of the study was 10.6 weeks (median 10.7 weeks). The majority of women were married and pregnant with their first baby (66.7% no prior live births; 33.3% had 1 previous live birth). Women were, on average, well-educated and fairly affluent. Moreover, the majority (81.5%) of women were employed full-time. Forty-one percent of women had obesity prior to pregnancy. Infants were born at a mean of 39.5 (1.4) weeks gestation. Mean birth weight was 3381 g (SD 617, range 2050–4570), reflecting an average birth weight for gestational age percentile of 56.6 (SD 31.9, range 2.6–99.4). Three infants (11.1%, 2 intervention, 1 control) were macrosomic (birth weight > 4000 g), and four infants (14.8%, 2 intervention, 2 control) were small for gestational age (SGA, <10th percentile) at birth. Out of 162 ultrasound scans, eight (4.9%) were flagged by the study physician, including five for growth restriction concerns. For two of these participants (both intervention), the concern resolved on its own at subsequent scans.

Mean (SD) baseline values were 2.79 (0.47) for cognitive restraint (range = 2.00–3.67), 2.15 (0.39) for uncontrolled eating (range = 1.33–3.00), and 2.14 (0.59) for emotional eating (range = 1.00–3.33). Baseline values did not differ by study group. Baseline cognitive restraint and uncontrolled eating did not differ by prepregnancy BMI status, but women with obesity had significantly higher baseline emotional eating than those with overweight (2.41 (0.52) vs. 1.95 (0.57), $p = 0.047$). Cognitive restraint significantly decreased across gestation (restraint = 2.90–0.014 × gestational age in weeks, $p = 0.0008$), as did uncontrolled eating (uncontrolled eating = 2.25–0.007 × gestational age in weeks, $p = 0.006$). Emotional eating did not significantly change across gestation (emotional eating = 2.10–0.006 × gestational age in weeks, $p = 0.14$), and there were no differences in rate of change by study group or prepregnancy BMI status for any of the eating behavior subscales. Baseline cognitive restraint was negatively associated with change in cognitive restraint ($p = 0.03$), such that women with higher baseline restraint experienced greater decreases in restraint across pregnancy. However, there was no association between baseline scores and change scores for uncontrolled eating and emotional eating. Intraclass correlations were 0.59 for cognitive restraint, 0.85 for uncontrolled eating, and 0.79 for emotional eating, suggesting that the majority of variance in all three constructs was between individuals rather than within individuals.

Table 1. Characteristics of women at baseline (n = 27).

	Overall (n = 27)	**Intervention (n = 13)**	**Control (n = 14)**
	M (SD) Range	**M (SD) Range**	**M (SD) Range**
Age (years)	30.6 (2.9) 24–37	30.3 (2.8) 24–35	30.9 (3.2) 27–37
Gestational Age at Study Start (weeks)	10.6 (1.6) 7.3–13.0	10.5 (1.7) 7.3–13.0	10.6 (1.6) 7.9–12.9
Weight at Study Start (lbs.)	190.4 (46.8) 134–294	182.2 (40.5) 145–294	197.9 (52.3) 134–292
Body Mass Index	31.6 (7.0) 24.1–48.9	30.7 (6.7) 24.1–48.9	32.4 (7.5) 24.5–42.8
	%	%	%
% BMI = 24.1–29.9 % Obese (BMI ≥ 30)	59.3 40.7	69.2 30.8	50 50
Parity Primiparous (no prior live birth) Multiparous: 1 previous live birth	 66.7 33.3	 53.9 46.2	 78.6 21.4
Education Graduate/professional College High school	 48.2 48.2 3.7	 38.5 61.5 0	 57.1 35.7 7.1
Marital Status Married Single Divorced	 92.6 3.7 3.7	 92.3 0 7.7	 92.9 7.1 0
Race Non-Hispanic White Asian	 96.3 3.7	 92.3 7.7	 100 0
Family Income >$100,000 $40–$100,000 $20–$40,000 $10–$20,000	 33.3 44.4 18.5 3.7	 30.8 61.5 0 7.7	 35.7 28.6 35.7 0
Employment Full-time Part-time Self-employed Other	 81.5 11.1 3.7 3.7	 84.6 15.4 0 0	 78.6 7.1 7.1 7.1

Abbreviations: M = Mean; SD = Standard deviation; BMI = body mass index.

3.2. *Unconditional Polynomial Models for Fetal Weight Change*

Fetal growth from 14–34 weeks was modeled using a multilevel model. The first model included a random intercept and random and fixed linear effects of gestational week. The random intercept resulted in a nonpositive definite G matrix and was removed from the model. Next, a quadratic fixed effect of gestational week was added, which improved the fit of the model (likelihood ratio test $p < 0.0001$). Quadratic random effects and cubic fixed and random effects were tested but did not improve model fit.

3.3. *Conditional Polynomial Models for Fetal Weight Change*

3.3.1. Treatment Effect of Intervention and Fetal Growth

For Model 1, there was no significant main effect of study group on fetal weight. There was a trend for an interaction between study group and gestational week ($p = 0.095$, Model 1, Table 2), such that fetuses of women in the control group tended to grow faster and be larger in later gestation than those in the intervention group (Figure 1), before and after adjusting for prepregnancy BMI.

Table 2. Multilevel model parameter estimates predicting change in fetal weight (g) based on randomized intervention vs. control and interactions with eating ($n = 27$).

	Model 1: Study Group		
Term	**Est**	**SE**	***p***
Intercept	1232.8	151.2	<0.0001
Gestational week	−161.9	10.34	<0.0001
Gestational week^2	5.80	0.21	<0.0001
Prepregnancy BMI	0.30	2.74	0.91
Study group: Intervention *	89.46	61.56	0.14
Study group * × gestational week	−4.94	2.93	0.095

* Study group reference level is control. Abbreviations: Est = estimate; SE = standard error; BMI = body mass index.

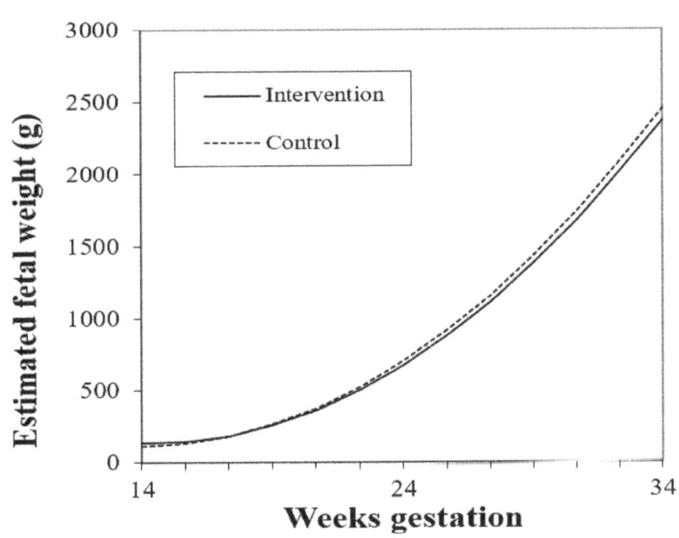

Figure 1. Estimated fetal weight trajectory in intervention and control group (study group × gestational week, $p = 0.095$). Estimates were generated using multilevel modeling (SAS PROC MIXED).

3.3.2. Individual Eating Behaviors and Fetal Growth

Eating characteristics (uncontrolled eating, emotional eating, and cognitive restraint) were each added, individually, to Model 1 to test higher order interactions and main effects. When higher-order interactions were not significant, models were simplified. For uncontrolled eating, there was a significant two-way interaction between baseline uncontrolled eating and gestational age^2 (Table 3, Model 2, $p = 0.03$). As shown in Figure 2, women with higher baseline levels of uncontrolled eating had faster rates of fetal growth in late gestation. Next, change in uncontrolled eating from baseline was added to the model. There was a significant interaction between change in uncontrolled eating and gestational age (Table 4, Model 3, $p = 0.04$). In contrast to the effect of baseline uncontrolled eating, women who experienced greater decreases in uncontrolled eating had faster rates of fetal growth. In both Models 2 and 3, the gestational week × study group effect was statistically significant. In addition, the interaction between baseline uncontrolled eating and gestational week^2 from Model 2 remained statistically significant with the addition of change in uncontrolled eating, suggesting independent effects of baseline and change in this eating behavior. Neither baseline levels nor change across gestation in cognitive restraint or emotional eating were associated with fetal growth.

Table 3. Multilevel model parameter estimates predicting change in fetal weight (g) based on randomized intervention vs. control and baseline uncontrolled eating ($n = 26$).

	Model 2: Study group + Baseline Uncontrolled Eating		
Term	**Est**	**SE**	***p***
Intercept	1195.7	154.5	<0.0001
Gestational week	−160.9	10.34	<0.0001
Gestational week^2	5.80	0.21	<0.0001
Prepregnancy BMI	0.89	2.86	0.76
Study group: Intervention *	122.0	63.02	0.06
Study group * × gestational week	−6.59	3.03	0.03
Baseline uncontrolled eating	475.3	330.5	0.15
Baseline uncontrolled eating × gestational week	−49.04	28.21	0.08
Baseline uncontrolled eating × gestational week^2	1.21	0.57	0.03

* Study group reference level is control. Abbreviations: Est = estimate; SE = standard error; BMI = body mass index.

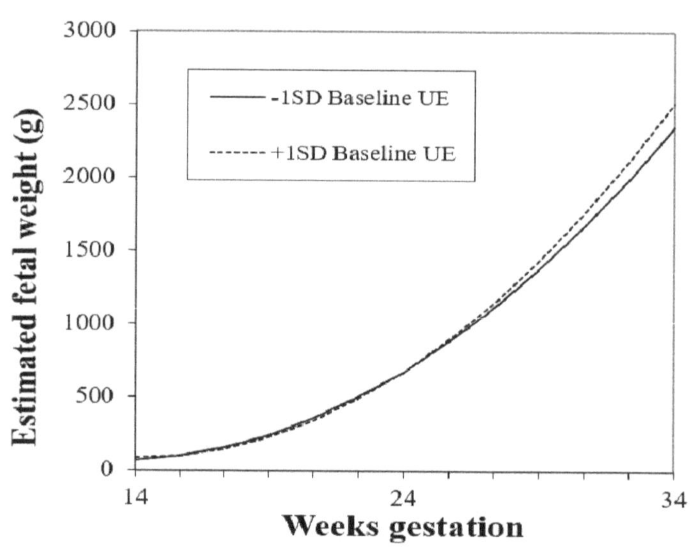

Figure 2. Estimated fetal weight trajectory at higher (mean + 1 SD) and lower (mean − 1 SD) levels of baseline uncontrolled eating (UE), (baseline uncontrolled eating × gestational age^2, $p = 0.03$). Estimates were generated using multilevel modeling (SAS PROC MIXED).

Table 4. Multilevel model parameter estimates predicting change in fetal weight (g) based on randomized intervention vs. control, baseline uncontrolled eating, and change in uncontrolled eating ($n = 26$).

	Model 3: Study group + Baseline Uncontrolled Eating + Change in Uncontrolled Eating		
Term	**Est**	**SE**	***p***
Intercept	1270.8	154.3	<0.0001
Gestational week	−159.6	10.63	<0.0001
Gestational week^2	5.74	0.21	<0.0001
Prepregnancy BMI	−1.45	2.71	0.60
Study group: Intervention *	110.3	64.65	0.09
Study group * × gestational week	−6.56	2.96	0.03
Baseline uncontrolled eating	532.6	330.8	0.11
Baseline uncontrolled eating × gestational week	−53.72	28.26	0.06
Baseline uncontrolled eating × gestational week^2	1.32	0.57	0.02
Change in uncontrolled eating	252.1	181.0	0.17
Change in uncontrolled eating × gestational week	−13.94	6.74	0.04

* Study group reference level is control. Abbreviations: Est = estimate; SE = standard error; BMI = body mass index.

3.3.3. Cognitive Restraint × Disinhibited Eating and Fetal Growth

Lastly, backward and forward selection were used to estimate a final model that included interactions between cognitive restraint and disinhibited eating (i.e., emotional eating and uncontrolled eating). All potential three-way interactions were considered. For cognitive restraint × uncontrolled eating (Table 5, Model 4), there were no significant three-way interactions. Baseline cognitive restraint × change in uncontrolled eating emerged as significant ($p = 0.02$). In women who experienced increases in uncontrolled eating across pregnancy, baseline cognitive restraint was negatively associated with fetal weight. This interaction was not specific to a particular time in gestation (i.e., there was no significant three-way interaction between baseline cognitive restraint, change in uncontrolled eating, and gestational week). The interaction between baseline uncontrolled eating and gestational age^2 remained significant, such that women with higher baseline levels of uncontrolled eating had faster rates of fetal growth in late gestation. However, the interaction between change in uncontrolled eating and gestational age observed in Model 3 did not emerge as significant in this final model. Lastly, the effect of study group on change in fetal growth remained significant (study group × gestational week $p = 0.02$).

For cognitive restraint × emotional eating, there were no statistically significant main effects or interactions between restraint and emotional eating.

3.3.4. Post-hoc Analysis: Study Group × Uncontrolled Eating Interaction

Although neither baseline nor change in uncontrolled eating differed by study group, inclusion of uncontrolled eating in Models 2–4 resulted in a statistically significant interaction between study group and gestational age. To further investigate why this relationship might emerge after accounting for baseline uncontrolled eating, we explored adding interactions between uncontrolled eating and study group to Model 4. A two-way interaction between uncontrolled eating and study group was not statistically significant, but there was evidence for a three-way interaction between baseline uncontrolled eating, study group, and gestational age ($p = 0.02$, Model 5, Table 6). Higher baseline level of uncontrolled eating was associated with faster fetal growth among control group participants but not among those receiving the intervention (Figure 3). Similar results were observed when these interactions were added to Models 2 and 3.

Table 5. Multilevel model parameter estimates predicting change in fetal weight (g) based on randomized intervention vs. control, uncontrolled eating, and cognitive restraint (n = 26).

	Model 4: Study Group + Uncontrolled Eating + Cognitive Restraint		
Term	**Est**	**SE**	***p***
Intercept	1283.4	156.4	<0.0001
Gestational week	−161.4	10.49	<0.0001
Gestational week^2	5.80	0.21	<0.0001
Prepregnancy BMI	−1.28	2.92	0.66
Study group: Intervention *	113.2	64.17	0.08
Study group * × gestational week	−7.45	3.05	0.02
Baseline uncontrolled eating	501.5	328.3	0.13
Baseline uncontrolled eating × gestational week	−49.78	28.03	0.08
Baseline uncontrolled eating × gestational week^2	1.25	0.56	0.03
Change in uncontrolled eating	−116.4	52.68	0.03
Baseline cognitive restraint	11.18	42.88	0.80
Baseline cognitive restraint × change in uncontrolled eating	−272.3	116.9	0.02

* Study group reference level is control. Abbreviations: Est = estimate; SE = standard error; BMI = body mass index.

Table 6. Multilevel model parameter estimates predicting change in fetal weight (g) including interactions between study group and uncontrolled eating (n = 26).

	Model 5: Study Group × Uncontrolled Eating + Cognitive Restraint		
Term	**Est**	**SE**	***p***
Intercept	1267.4	155.7	<0.0001
Gestational week	−160.6	10.40	<0.0001
Gestational week^2	5.80	0.21	<0.0001
Prepregnancy BMI	−1.21	2.93	0.68
Study group: Intervention *	117.0	63.58	0.07
Study group * × gestational week	−7.67	3.03	0.01
Baseline uncontrolled eating	256.8	352.8	0.47
Baseline uncontrolled eating × gestational week	−35.22	28.64	0.22
Baseline uncontrolled eating × gestational week^2	1.18	0.56	0.04
Change in uncontrolled eating	−111.3	52.60	0.04
Baseline cognitive restraint	10.36	42.70	0.81
Baseline cognitive restraint × change in uncontrolled eating	−259.0	116.1	0.03
Study group × baseline uncontrolled eating	310.6	175.3	0.08
Study group × baseline uncontrolled eating × gestational week	−17.00	8.25	0.04

* Study group reference level is control. Abbreviations: Est = estimate; SE = standard error; BMI = body mass index.

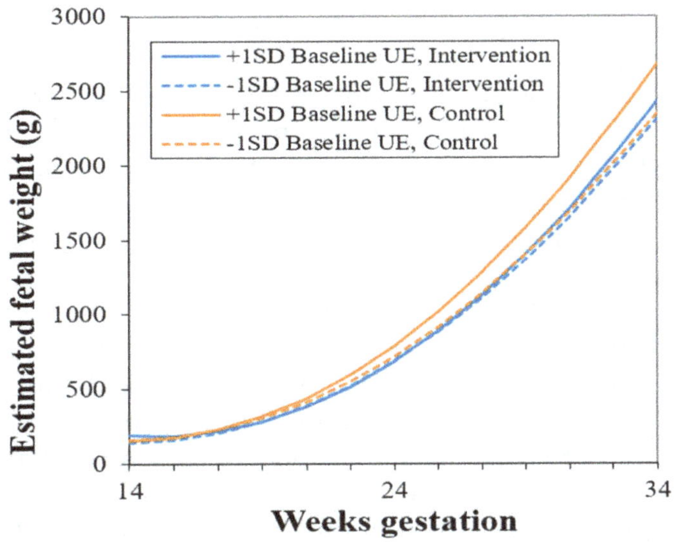

Figure 3. Estimated fetal weight trajectory at higher (mean + 1 SD) and lower (mean − 1 SD) levels of baseline uncontrolled eating (UE) in intervention and control group participants, (baseline uncontrolled eating × study group × gestational age, $p = 0.04$). Estimates were generated using multilevel modeling (SAS PROC MIXED).

4. Discussion

Healthy Mom Zone, an individually tailored, adaptive intervention designed to effectively manage gestational weight gain among women with overweight or obesity tended to result in a slower rate of fetal growth compared to fetuses of control women, with significant effects emerging in models that accounted for uncontrolled eating. Higher uncontrolled eating at study entry was associated with faster fetal growth. Findings also suggest that cognitive restraint on its own appears to have little effect on fetal growth, but may help moderate fetal growth among women who experience increases in uncontrolled eating during pregnancy. Several of these findings warrant discussion.

Though not statistically significant in Model 1, the Healthy Mom Zone intervention had a protective effect on fetal growth once uncontrolled eating was added (Models 2–4); intervention fetuses gained weight at a slower rate on average compared to control fetuses. It is important to note that the intervention did not increase risk for an infant being born small for gestational age. This finding has clinical relevance for several reasons. Women who are overweight or obese are 65% and 163% more likely, respectively, to deliver babies who are large for their gestational age, regardless of whether the mother develops gestational diabetes during pregnancy [52]. In addition, risk of fetal macrosomia, having a birth weight of more than 8 pounds or 4000 grams regardless of gestational age, is more likely among women with obesity. This is important because women with overweight or obesity are also more likely to exceed gestational weight gain guidelines, further elevating infant risk for macrosomia. The clinical relevance is that decreasing risk for faster weight gain may decrease health risks for the mother (e.g., labor and delivery complications) and the infant (e.g., childhood obesity, metabolic syndrome) both during pregnancy and after childbirth. Thus, our behavioral intervention has the potential to mediate this risk, in particular among pregnant women with overweight or obesity.

In the current study, both cognitive restraint and uncontrolled eating decreased on average across gestation, and there was no change in emotional eating. Similarly, previous studies have found that cognitive restraint is lower during pregnancy compared to prepregnancy levels or non-pregnant women [53,54]. Research on changes in disinhibition across pregnancy is scant. We did not observe any association between prepregnancy BMI and cognitive restraint or uncontrolled eating; however, this may be because our sample was limited to women with BMI > 24. Two previous studies have found that pregnant women with obesity tend to report higher levels of disinhibited eating [55,56] than their normal weight counterparts. Further research is needed to evaluate how these eating behaviors change throughout pregnancy.

As hypothesized, greater uncontrolled eating in late first trimester was associated with faster fetal growth in late pregnancy. However, there was no association between emotional eating and fetal growth. To our knowledge, this study is the first to describe relationships between maternal disinhibited eating during pregnancy and fetal growth in utero in a non-eating disorder population. One previous study has examined the relationship between maternal eating behavior and postnatal growth. Mothers' emotional eating, assessed at infant age 12 months, was positively associated with infant weight gain through 12 months, while external eating was negatively associated with infant weight gain. Maternal restraint was not associated with infant weight gain [57]. Further research is needed to clarify the relationship between maternal disinhibited eating and fetal/infant weight gain, and to determine the extent to which this relationship is reflective of modifiable factors, such as maternal diet, weight gain, and feeding practices, as opposed to nonmodifiable factors such as genetics.

Emotional eating and external eating have been associated with excess gestational weight gain [42]. Qualitative studies of pregnant women have found that emotional and external eating are often described as a barrier to healthy eating and management of gestational weight gain [58–60]. Our finding that uncontrolled eating is associated with fetal weight gain adds to this literature, suggesting that disinhibited eating behaviors may be an ideal target for gestational weight gain management interventions. Our Healthy Mom Zone intervention focused primarily on dietary intake, physical activity, and self-monitoring of weight. Expansion of intervention content focused on mindfulness, stress reduction, and emotion regulation, strategies that have been shown to reduce disinhibited eating in nonpregnant populations [61–63], may further benefit pregnant women with overweight or obesity.

Similar to the uncertain relationship between restraint and weight in nonpregnant adults, mixed findings have been reported for restraint and gestational weight gain [41,42,64,65]. Previous work in nonpregnant populations suggests that restraint may not be directly associated with weight but rather as a moderator of the effect of disinhibition [30,31,44,45]. A similar interaction effect may be involved in fetal growth. We observed a significant interaction between baseline cognitive restraint and change in uncontrolled eating, where among women who experienced increases in uncontrolled eating during pregnancy, those with higher baseline cognitive restraint had smaller fetuses than those with lower baseline cognitive restraint [31,44,45]. This suggests that a greater ability to consciously control food intake may help protect against adverse effects of increases in uncontrolled eating on fetal weight gain.

We did not have an a priori hypothesis about differential effects of the intervention on fetal growth by baseline eating behavior, but our post-hoc analysis of the interaction between study group and baseline uncontrolled eating suggests that the intervention may have been beneficial, particularly for women with higher baseline uncontrolled eating. It is possible that the intervention provided women who were already prone to uncontrolled eating with strategies to cope with inclinations to overeat, providing a buffering effect against excess fetal growth. Future analyses will examine whether baseline levels of eating behavior predict differential response to the Healthy Mom Zone intervention for other outcomes including maternal weight gain. Factors such as eating behavior that predict intervention response may be used to identify patients that are most likely to benefit from an intensive intervention.

There are also some limitations of this research. The small sample size, although adequate for an optimization trial within the MOST framework [46], precludes the ability to make assumptions at a population level. The intervention and control groups were unbalanced in terms of the proportion of women with obesity; however, all analyses controlled for prepregnancy BMI. In addition, the target population was a homogenous sample of women (e.g., married, middle to upper class, Caucasian) from largely rural and suburban areas in central Pennsylvania, thus limiting the extension of the study findings to more culturally diverse and urban populations of pregnant women with overweight or obesity. Future research will aim to broaden generalizability of our study findings. In addition, we do plan to understand the application of Healthy Mom Zone to a more diverse sample of pregnant women in the future, including those who are normal weight, more culturally diverse, and reside in varied communities across the US. Lastly, intensive longitudinal data collection may have affected behavior, and responses may have become biased due to repeated assessments throughout gestation. However, this longitudinal design is also a strength of this study, allowing us to better understand how individual differences in eating behavior are related to fetal growth.

5. Conclusions

Healthy Mom Zone, an individually tailored, intensive behavioral intervention designed to help women with overweight or obesity manage gestational weight gain shows promise for preventing rapid fetal growth, particularly for women prone to uncontrolled eating, though these findings must be replicated in a larger and more diverse sample. Our results also suggest that uncontrolled eating may increase risk for faster fetal growth, and that restraint on its own seems to have little influence. However, among women who experience increases in uncontrolled eating during pregnancy, higher restraint may help moderate fetal growth. Implications for these findings include that understanding participant eating behaviors at baseline may be important for future gestational weight gain interventions. Lastly, findings illustrate a need to develop intervention content and strategies specific to women with high vs. low levels of disinhibited eating.

Author Contributions: J.S.S. lead the fetal growth ancillary project, contributed to study conception and design, contributed to data analysis, interpreted results, and drafted the manuscript. E.E.H. contributed to study design, analyzed the data, interpreted results, and aided in drafting the manuscript. K.M.M., A.M.P., K.S.L., T.T., and J.M.P. contributed to study design and data collection. A.D.G. and D.E.R. contributed to study design and interpretation of results. D.S.D. lead the intervention study, contributed to study conception and design, and interpretation of results. All authors participated in critical revision of the manuscript and approved the final version.

Acknowledgments: We would like to acknowledge the assistance of the Healthy Mom Zone team who assisted with participant recruitment and data collection for this study. Support for this work has been provided by the National Heart, Lung, and Blood Institute (NHLBI) of the National Institutes of Health (NIH) through grants R56-HL126799 and R01-HL119245. REDCap support was received from the Penn State Clinical & Translational Sciences Institute through the National Center for Advancing Translational Sciences (NCATS) NIH grant UL1 TR002014. The opinions expressed in this article are the authors' own and do not necessarily reflect the views of NIH.

References

1. Institute of Medicine (US) and National Research Council (US) Committee to Reexamine IOM Pregnancy Weight Guidelines. *Weight Gain during Pregnancy: Reexamining the Guidelines*; National Academies Press (US): Washington, DC, USA, 2009.
2. Ogden, C.L.; Carroll, M.D.; Kit, B.K.; Flegal, K.M. Prevalence of childhood and adult obesity in the United States, 2011–2012. *JAMA* **2014**, *311*, 806–814. [CrossRef]
3. Ogden, C.L.; Carroll, M.D.; Lawman, H.G.; Fryar, C.D.; Kruszon-Moran, D.; Kit, B.K.; Flegal, K.M. Trends in Obesity Prevalence Among Children and Adolescents in the United States, 1988–1994 through 2013–2014. *JAMA* **2016**, *315*, 2292–2299. [PubMed]
4. Hales, C.M.; Fryar, C.D.; Carroll, M.D.; Freedman, D.S.; Ogden, C.L. Trends in Obesity and Severe Obesity Prevalence in US Youth and Adults by Sex and Age, 2007–2008 to 2015–2016. *JAMA* **2018**, *319*, 1723–1725. [CrossRef] [PubMed]
5. Patti, M.E. Intergenerational programming of metabolic disease: Evidence from human populations and experimental animal models. *Cell. Mol. Life Sci.* **2013**, *70*, 1597–1608. [CrossRef]
6. Adamo, K.B.; Ferraro, Z.M.; Brett, K.E. Can we modify the intrauterine environment to halt the intergenerational cycle of obesity? *Int. J. Environ. Res. Public Health* **2012**, *9*, 1263–1307. [CrossRef] [PubMed]
7. Dong, Y.; Rivera, D.E.; Thomas, D.M.; Navarro-Barrientos, J.E.; Downs, D.S.; Savage, J.S.; Collins, L.M. A Dynamical Systems Model for Improving Gestational Weight Gain Behavioral Interventions. In Proceedings of the American Control Conference, Montreal, QC, Canada, 27–29 June 2012; pp. 4059–4064.

8. Fallucca, S.; Vasta, M.; Sciullo, E.; Balducci, S.; Fallucca, F. Birth weight: Genetic and intrauterine environment in normal pregnancy. *Diabetes Care* **2009**, *32*, e149. [CrossRef] [PubMed]
9. Reilly, J.J.; Armstrong, J.; Dorosty, A.R.; Emmett, P.M.; Ness, A.; Rogers, I.; Steer, C.; Sherriff, A. Early life risk factors for obesity in childhood: Cohort study. *BMJ* **2005**, *330*, 1357. [CrossRef]
10. Martin, J.A.; Hamilton, B.E.; Ventura, S.J.; Osterman, M.J.; Kirmeyer, S.; Mathews, T.J.; Wilson, E.C. Births: Final data for 2009. *Natl. Vital Stat. Rep.* **2011**, *60*, 1–70.
11. Nohr, E.A.; Vaeth, M.; Baker, J.L.; Sorensen, T.I.; Olsen, J.; Rasmussen, K.M. Pregnancy outcomes related to gestational weight gain in women defined by their body mass index, parity, height, and smoking status. *Am. J. Clin. Nutr.* **2009**, *90*, 1288–1294. [CrossRef] [PubMed]
12. Wei, J.-N.; Sung, F.-C.; Li, C.-Y.; Chang, C.-H.; Lin, R.-S.; Lin, C.-C.; Chiang, C.-C.; Chuang, L.-M. Low birth weight and high birth weight infants are both at an increased risk to have type 2 diabetes among schoolchildren in Taiwan. *Diabetes Care* **2003**, *26*, 343–348. [CrossRef]
13. Muktabhant, B.; Lawrie, T.A.; Lumbiganon, P.; Laopaiboon, M. Diet or exercise, or both, for preventing excessive weight gain in pregnancy. *Cochrane Database Syst. Rev.* **2015**. [CrossRef] [PubMed]
14. Pauley, A.M.; Hohman, E.; Savage, J.S.; Rivera, D.E.; Guo, P.; Leonard, K.S.; Downs, D.S. Gestational Weight Gain Intervention Impacts Determinants of Healthy Eating and Exercise in Overweight/Obese Pregnant Women. *J. Obes.* **2018**, *2018*, 6469170. [CrossRef]
15. Downs, D.S. Obesity in Special Populations: Pregnancy. *Prim. Care* **2016**, *43*, 109–120. [CrossRef] [PubMed]
16. Downs, D.S.; Savage, J.S.; Rauff, E.L. Falling Short of Guidelines? Nutrition and Weight Gain Knowledge in Pregnancy. *J. Women's Heal. Care* **2014**, *3*, 1–6.
17. Dong, Y.; Rivera, D.E.; Downs, D.S.; Savage, J.S.; Thomas, D.M.; Collins, L.M. Hybrid Model Predictive Control for Optimizing Gestational Weight Gain Behavioral Interventions. In Proceedings of the American Control Conference, Washington, DC, USA, 17–19 June 2013; pp. 1970–1975.
18. Symons Downs, D.; Savage, J.S.; Rivera, D.E.; Smyth, J.M.; Rolls, B.J.; Hohman, E.E.; McNitt, K.M.; Kunselman, A.R.; Stetter, C.; Pauley, A.M.; et al. Individually Tailored, Adaptive Intervention to Manage Gestational Weight Gain: Protocol for a Randomized Controlled Trial in Women with Overweight and Obesity. *JMIR Res. Protoc.* **2018**, *7*, e150. [CrossRef] [PubMed]
19. Collins, L.M.; Murphy, S.A.; Strecher, V. The multiphase optimization strategy (MOST) and the sequential multiple assignment randomized trial (SMART): New methods for more potent eHealth interventions. *Am. J. Prevent. Med.* **2007**, *32* (Suppl. 5), S112–S118. [CrossRef] [PubMed]
20. Christian, P.; Mullany, L.C.; Hurley, K.M.; Katz, J.; Black, R.E. Nutrition and maternal, neonatal, and child health. *Semin. Perinatol.* **2015**, *39*, 361–372. [CrossRef] [PubMed]
21. Livingstone, M.B.; Black, A.E. Markers of the validity of reported energy intake. *J. Nutr.* **2003**, *133* (Suppl. 3), 895S–920S. [CrossRef]
22. Sui, Z.; Cramp, C.; Moran, L.J.; McNaughton, S.A.; Deussen, A.R.; Grivell, R.M.; Dodd, J.M. The characterisation of overweight and obese women who are under reporting energy intake during pregnancy. *BMC Pregnancy Childbirth* **2018**, *18*, 204.
23. Guo, P.; Rivera, D.E.; Savage, J.S.; Hohman, E.E.; Pauley, A.M.; Leonard, K.S.; Symons Downs, D. System identification approaches for energy intake estimation: Enhancing interventions for managing gestational weight gain. *IEEE Trans. Control Syst. Technol.* **2018**. [CrossRef]
24. Cappelleri, J.C.; Bushmakin, A.G.; Gerber, R.; Leidy, N.K.; Sexton, C.C.; Lowe, M.R.; Karlsson, J. Psychometric analysis of the Three-Factor Eating Questionnaire-R21: Results from a large diverse sample of obese and non-obese participants. *Int. J. Obes.* **2009**, *33*, 611–620. [CrossRef] [PubMed]
25. Stunkard, A.J.; Messick, S. The three-factor eating questionnaire to measure dietary restraint, disinhibition and hunger. *J. Psychosom. Res.* **1985**, *29*, 71–83. [CrossRef]
26. Stunkard, A.J.; Messick, S. *Eating Inventory Manual*; The Psychological Corporation: San Antonio, TX, USA, 1988.
27. Lowe, M.R.; Kral, T.V. Stress-induced eating in restrained eaters may not be caused by stress or restraint. *Appetite* **2006**, *46*, 16–21. [CrossRef] [PubMed]
28. Lindroos, A.-K.; Mathiassen, M.E.; Bengtsson, C.; Lindroos, A.; Lissner, L.; Karlsson, J.; Sullivan, M.; Sjöström, L. Dietary intake in relation to restrained eating, disinhibition, and hunger in obese and nonobese Swedish women. *Obes. Res.* **1997**, *5*, 175–185. [CrossRef] [PubMed]

29. Hainer, V.; Kunešová, M.; Bellisle, F.; Parizkova, J.; Braunerova, R.; Wagenknecht, M.; Lajka, J.; Hill, M.; Stunkard, A. The eating inventory, body adiposity and prevalence of disease in a quota sample of Czech adults. *Int. J. Obesity (Lond.)* **2006**, *30*, 830–836. [CrossRef]
30. Williamson, D.A.; Lawson, O.J.; Brooks, E.R.; Wozniak, P.J.; Ryan, D.H.; Bray, G.A.; Duchmann, E.G. Association of body mass with dietary restraint and disinhibition. *Appetite* **1995**, *25*, 31–41. [CrossRef]
31. Hays, N.P.; Bathalon, G.P.; McCrory, M.A.; Roubenoff, R.; Lipman, R.; Roberts, S.B. Eating behavior correlates of adult weight gain and obesity in healthy women aged 55–65 y. *Am. J. Clin. Nutr.* **2002**, *75*, 476–483. [CrossRef]
32. Smith, C.F.; Geiselman, P.J.; Williamson, D.A.; Champagne, C.M.; Bray, G.A.; Ryan, D.H. Association of dietary restraint and disinhibition with eating behavior, body mass, and hunger. *Eat. Weight Disord. Ewd* **1998**, *3*, 7–15. [CrossRef]
33. Foster, G.D.; Wadden, T.A.; Swain, R.M.; Stunkard, A.J.; Platte, P.; Vogt, R.A. The eating inventory in obese women: Clinical correlates and relationship to weight loss. *Int. J. Obes.* **1998**, *22*, 778–785. [CrossRef]
34. Lauzon-Guillain, B.; Basdevant, A.; Romon, M.; Karlsson, J.; Borys, J.M.; Charles, M.A. Is restraint eating a risk factor for weight gain in a general population? *Am. J. Clin. Nutr.* **2006**, *83*, 132–138. [CrossRef]
35. Lowe, M.R.; Annunziato, R.A.; Markowitz, J.T.; Didie, E.; Bellace, D.L.; Riddell, L.; Maille, C.; McKinney, S.; Stice, E. Multiple types of dieting prospectively predict weight gain during the freshman year of college. *Appetite* **2006**, *47*, 83–90. [CrossRef]
36. Olea Lopez, A.L.; Johnson, L. Associations between Restrained Eating and the Size and Frequency of Overall Intake, Meal, Snack and Drink Occasions in the UK Adult National Diet and Nutrition Survey. *PLoS ONE* **2016**, *11*, e0156320. [CrossRef] [PubMed]
37. Bongers, P.; Jansen, A. Emotional Eating Is Not What You Think It Is and Emotional Eating Scales Do Not Measure What You Think They Measure. *Front. Psychol.* **2016**, *7*, 1932. [CrossRef] [PubMed]
38. Hill, J.O.; Wyatt, H.R.; Reed, G.W.; Peters, J.C. Obesity and the environment: Where do we go from here? *Science* **2003**, *299*, 853–855. [CrossRef] [PubMed]
39. Keränen, A.-M.; Savolainen, M.J.; Reponen, A.H.; Kujari, M.-L.; Lindeman, S.M.; Bloigu, R.S.; Laitinen, J.H.; Teeriniemi, A.-M. The effect of eating behavior on weight loss and maintenance during a lifestyle intervention. *Prev. Med.* **2009**, *49*, 32–38. [CrossRef] [PubMed]
40. Mumford, S.L.; Siega-Riz, A.M.; Herring, A.; Evenson, K.R. Dietary restraint and gestational weight gain. *J. Am. Diet. Assoc.* **2008**, *108*, 1646–1653. [CrossRef]
41. Heery, E.; Wall, P.G.; Kelleher, C.C.; McAuliffe, F.M. Effects of dietary restraint and weight gain attitudes on gestational weight gain. *Appetite* **2016**, *107*, 501–510. [CrossRef]
42. Blau, L.E.; Orloff, N.C.; Flammer, A.; Slatch, C.; Hormes, J.M. Food craving frequency mediates the relationship between emotional eating and excess weight gain in pregnancy. *Eat. Behav.* **2018**, *31*, 120–124. [CrossRef]
43. Hutchinson, A.D.; Charters, M.; Prichard, I.; Fletcher, C.; Wilson, C. Understanding maternal dietary choices during pregnancy: The role of social norms and mindful eating. *Appetite* **2017**, *112*, 227–234. [CrossRef]
44. Lawson, O.J.; Champagne, C.M.; Brooks, E.R.; Howat, P.M.; Wozniak, P.J.; Williamson, D.A.; Delany, J.P.; Bray, G.A.; Ryan, D.H. The association of body weight, dietary intake, and energy expenditure with dietary restraint and disinhibition. *Obes. Res.* **1995**, *3*, 153–161. [CrossRef]
45. Savage, J.S.; Hoffman, L.; Birch, L.L. Dieting, restraint, and disinhibition predict women's weight change over 6 y. *Am. J. Clin. Nutr.* **2009**, *90*, 33–40. [CrossRef]
46. Rivera, D.E.; Hekler, E.; Savage, J.S.; Symons Downs, D. Intensively adaptive interventions using control systems engineering: Two illustrative examples. In *Optimization of Behavioral, Biobehavioral, and Biomedical Interventions*; Collins, L.M., Ed.; Springer: Cham, Switzerland, 2018; pp. 21–173.
47. Ajzen, I. The theory of planned behavior. *Organ. Behav. Hum. Decis. Process.* **1991**, *50*, 179–211. [CrossRef]
48. Carver, C.; Scheier, M. *On the Self-Regulation of Behavior*; Cambridge University Press: Cambridge, UK, 1998.
49. Harris, P.A.; Taylor, R.; Thielke, R.; Payne, J.; Gonzalez, N.; Conde, J.G. Research electronic data capture (REDCap)—A metadata-driven methodology and workflow process for providing translational research informatics support. *J. Biomed. Inf.* **2009**, *42*, 377–381. [CrossRef]
50. Hadlock, F.P.; Harrist, R.B.; Carpenter, R.J.; Deter, R.L.; Park, S.K. Sonographic estimation of fetal weight. The value of femur length in addition to head and abdomen measurements. *Radiology* **1984**, *150*, 535–540. [CrossRef]

51. Villar, J.; Ismail, L.C.; Victora, C.G.; Ohuma, E.; Bertino, E.; Altman, D.G.; Lambert, A.; Papageorghiou, A.T.; Carvalho, M.; Jaffer, Y.; et al. International standards for newborn weight, length, and head circumference by gestational age and sex: The Newborn Cross-Sectional Study of the INTERGROWTH-21st Project. *Lancet* **2014**, *384*, 857–868. [CrossRef]
52. Black, M.H.; Sacks, D.A.; Xiang, A.H.; Lawrence, J.M. The relative contribution of prepregnancy overweight and obesity, gestational weight gain, and IADPSG-defined gestational diabetes mellitus to fetal overgrowth. *Diabetes Care* **2013**, *36*, 56–62. [CrossRef]
53. Clark, M.; Ogden, J. The impact of pregnancy on eating behaviour and aspects of weight concern. *Int. J. Obes. Relat. Metab. Disord.* **1999**, *23*, 18–24. [CrossRef]
54. Fairburn, C.G.; Stein, A.; Jones, R. Eating habits and eating disorders during pregnancy. *Psychosom. Med.* **1992**, *54*, 665–672. [CrossRef] [PubMed]
55. Shloim, N.; Hetherington, M.M.; Rudolf, M.; Feltbower, R.G. Relationship between body mass index and women's body image, self-esteem and eating behaviours in pregnancy: A cross-cultural study. *J. Health Psychol.* **2015**, *20*, 413–426. [CrossRef] [PubMed]
56. Slane, J.D.; Levine, M.D. Association of Restraint and Disinhibition to Gestational Weight Gain among Pregnant Former Smokers. *Women's Health Issues* **2015**, *25*, 390–395. [CrossRef]
57. Wright, C.M.; Parkinson, K.N.; Drewett, R.F. The influence of maternal socioeconomic and emotional factors on infant weight gain and weight faltering (failure to thrive): Data from a prospective birth cohort. *Arch. Dis. Child.* **2006**, *91*, 312–317. [CrossRef] [PubMed]
58. Wang, M.L.; Arroyo, J.; Druker, S.; Sankey, H.Z.; Rosal, M.C. Knowledge, Attitudes and Provider Advice by Pre-Pregnancy Weight Status: A Qualitative Study of Pregnant Latinas with Excessive Gestational Weight Gain. *Women Health* **2015**, *55*, 805–828. [CrossRef] [PubMed]
59. Chang, M.W.; Nitzke, S.; Buist, D.; Cain, D.; Horning, S.; Eghtedary, K. I am pregnant and want to do better but I can't: Focus groups with low-income overweight and obese pregnant women. *Matern. Child Health J.* **2015**, *19*, 1060–1070. [CrossRef] [PubMed]
60. Chang, M.W.; Nitzke, S.; Guilford, E.; Adair, C.H.; Hazard, D.L. Motivators and barriers to healthful eating and physical activity among low-income overweight and obese mothers. *J. Am. Diet Assoc.* **2008**, *108*, 1023–1028. [CrossRef] [PubMed]
61. Levoy, E.; Lazaridou, A.; Brewer, J.; Fulwiler, C. An exploratory study of Mindfulness Based Stress Reduction for emotional eating. *Appetite* **2017**, *109*, 124–130. [CrossRef]
62. Armitage, C.J. Randomized test of a brief psychological intervention to reduce and prevent emotional eating in a community sample. *J. Public Health (Oxf.)* **2015**, *37*, 438–444. [CrossRef]
63. Katterman, S.N.; Kleinman, B.M.; Hood, M.M.; Nackers, L.M.; Corsica, J.A. Mindfulness meditation as an intervention for binge eating, emotional eating, and weight loss: A systematic review. *Eat. Behav.* **2014**, *15*, 197–204. [CrossRef]
64. Conway, R.; Reddy, S.; Davies, J. Dietary restraint and weight gain during pregnancy. *Eur. J. Clin. Nutr.* **1999**, *53*, 849–853. [CrossRef]
65. Laraia, B.; Epel, E.; Siega-Riz, A.M. Food insecurity with past experience of restrained eating is a recipe for increased gestational weight gain. *Appetite* **2013**, *65*, 178–184. [CrossRef] [PubMed]

10

Dysregulation of Neuronal Genes by Fetal-Neonatal Iron Deficiency Anemia is Associated with Altered DNA Methylation in the Rat Hippocampus

Yu-Chin Lien [1], David E Condon [1], Michael K Georgieff [2], Rebecca A Simmons [1,3,*] and Phu V Tran [2,*]

1 Center for Research on Reproduction and Women's Health, Perelman School of Medicine, The University of Pennsylvania, Philadelphia, PA 19104, USA; ylien@pennmedicine.upenn.edu (Y.-C.L.); dec986@gmail.com (D.E.C.)

2 Department of Pediatrics, University of Minnesota School of Medicine, Minneapolis, MN 55455, USA; georg001@umn.edu

3 Children's Hospital of Philadelphia, Philadelphia, PA 19104, USA

* Correspondence: rsimmons@pennmedicine.upenn.edu (R.A.S.); tranx271@umn.edu (P.V.T.)

Abstract: Early-life iron deficiency results in long-term abnormalities in cognitive function and affective behavior in adulthood. In preclinical models, these effects have been associated with long-term dysregulation of key neuronal genes. While limited evidence suggests histone methylation as an epigenetic mechanism underlying gene dysregulation, the role of DNA methylation remains unknown. To determine whether DNA methylation is a potential mechanism by which early-life iron deficiency induces gene dysregulation, we performed whole genome bisulfite sequencing to identify loci with altered DNA methylation in the postnatal day (P) 15 iron-deficient (ID) rat hippocampus, a time point at which the highest level of hippocampal iron deficiency is concurrent with peak iron demand for axonal and dendritic growth. We identified 229 differentially methylated loci and they were mapped within 108 genes. Among them, 63 and 45 genes showed significantly increased and decreased DNA methylation in the P15 ID hippocampus, respectively. To establish a correlation between differentially methylated loci and gene dysregulation, the methylome data were compared to our published P15 hippocampal transcriptome. Both datasets showed alteration of similar functional networks regulating nervous system development and cell-to-cell signaling that are critical for learning and behavior. Collectively, the present findings support a role for DNA methylation in neural gene dysregulation following early-life iron deficiency.

Keywords: hippocampus; DNA methylation; DNA sequencing; iron; neurobiology; transcriptome; micronutrient deficiency; neuroplasticity

1. Introduction

Fetal and neonatal (early-life) iron deficiency with or without anemia affects more than 30% of pregnant women and preschool age children worldwide, and results in long-term cognitive and behavioral abnormalities [1–8]. We have previously investigated the effects of early-life iron deficiency using a rat model, whereby pups were made iron-deficient (ID) from gestational day 2 through postnatal day (P) 7 by providing pregnant and nursing dams with an ID diet, after which they were rescued with an iron-sufficient (IS) diet. This model of maternal-fetal iron deficiency results in a 50% reduction in brain iron concentration by P7 [9], the age at which rat brain development approximates that of a full-term human newborn [10,11]. The deficit in brain iron content is similar to the degree of brain iron deficiency observed in full-term newborn humans [12,13]. Similar cognitive and behavioral abnormalities are observed in our rat model [14–16] and are accompanied by abnormal neuronal morphology [17,18] and glutamatergic neurotransmission [19] in the hippocampus. Iron treatment starting at P7 resolves brain iron deficiency by P56 [20]. Despite this resolution, the formerly iron-deficient (FID) rats show persistent cognitive impairment accompanied by abnormal neuronal morphology [17,18], glutamatergic neurotransmission [19], and lower expression of genes critical for neural plasticity in the hippocampus [21–23]. The persistent dysregulation of hippocampal gene expression in the adult FID rat hippocampus [22] suggests a possible role for epigenetic regulation. Indeed, in a previous study we showed that early-life iron deficiency induced epigenetic modifications at the *Bdnf* locus, a critically important gene coding for a growth factor that regulates brain development and adult synaptic plasticity [24]. As such, comprehensive genome-wide analyses of DNA and histone methylation remain uninvestigated as iron is a critical cofactor for DNA and histone modifying proteins, such as the ten-eleven translocation (TET) enzymes and the Jumonji C-terminal domain (JmjC) family of histone demethylases [25,26].

DNA methylation is essential for neuronal differentiation and maturation in the developing central nervous system and plays a critical role in learning and memory in the adult brain [27]. Altered DNA methylation patterns are associated with many neurological and psychiatric disorders [27]. While DNA methylation at promoter regions is relatively well studied and strongly associated with transcriptional silencing [28], methylation in intergenic regions and gene bodies has been less characterized and may have different functions [27]. Whole genome bisulfite sequencing (WGBS) is the most comprehensive method to analyze 5-methyl cytosine (5mC) at a single-nucleotide resolution [29]. In our previously published methodological paper, a novel method to identify differentially methylated regions (DMRs), namely the Defiant program, was developed. Here, using the same WGBS dataset [30], we present the first genome-wide assessment of DNA methylation in the developing postnatal day 15 (P15) rat hippocampus, during a period of peak iron deficiency and robust axonal growth and dendritic branching [18,31]. In addition to confirming previously reported individual genes and loci that were altered epigenetically due to iron deficiency, we identify novel loci critical to neural function that are epigenetically modified by early-life iron deficiency.

2. Materials and Methods

2.1. Animals

The University of Minnesota Institutional Animal Care and Use Committee approved all experiments in this study. Gestational day 2 (G2) pregnant Sprague-Dawley rats were purchased from Charles Rivers (Wilmington, MA). Rats were kept in a 12 h:12 h light:dark cycle with ad lib food and water. Fetal-neonatal iron deficiency was induced by dietary manipulation as described previously [32]. In brief, pregnant dams were given a purified ID diet (4 mg Fe/kg, TD 80396, Harlan Teklad, Madison, WI) from G2 to P7, at which time nursing dams were given a purified iron sufficient (IS) diet (200 mg Fe/kg, TD 01583, Harlan Teklad) to generate ID pups. Both ID and IS diets were similar in all contents with the exception of iron (ferric citrate) content. Control IS pups were generated from pregnant dams maintained on a purified IS diet. All litters were culled to eight pups with six males and two females at birth. Only male offspring were used in experiments.

2.2. Hippocampal Dissection

P15 male rats were sacrificed by an intraperitoneal injection of Pentobarbital (100 mg/kg). The brains were removed and bisected along the midline on an ice-cold metal block. Each hippocampus was dissected and immediately flash-frozen in liquid N_2 and stored at −80 °C.

2.3. *Whole Genome Bisulfite Sequencing and Library Preparation*

Genomic DNA from IS and ID hippocampi was isolated using an AllPrep DNA/RNA Mini Kit (Qiagen). WGBS was performed using a previously published protocol [33]. Briefly, 1 µg of genomic DNA was fragmented into ~300 bp fragments using a M220 Covaris Ultrasonicator (Covaris, Woburn, MA, USA). Sequencing libraries were generated using a NEBNext genomic sequencing kit (New England Biolabs, Ipswich, MA, USA) and ligated with Illumina methylated paired end adaptors. Libraries were bisulfite-converted using an Imprint DNA modification kit (MilliporeSigma, St. Louis, MO, USA), and the size of 300–600 bp was selected using the Pippin Prep DNA size selection system (Sage Science, Beverly, MA, USA). Libraries were then amplified using Pfu-Turbo Cx Hotstart DNA polymerase (Agilent Technologies, Santa Clara, CA, USA). Paired-end libraries were sequenced to 100 bp on an Illumina hiSeq2000. Three biological replicates for each group were performed in WGBS. WGBS data are available on the Gene Expression Omnibus under GSE98064.

2.4. *Identification of DMRs Using the Defiant Program*

DMRs were identified by our in-house developed Defiant (DMRs: Easy, Fast, Identification and ANnoTation) program based on five criteria, as described previously [30]. Briefly, adapters were trimmed from the reads using a custom C language program. Trimmed reads were aligned against the rat genome (rn4). When reads overlapped at a base, the methylation status from read 1 was used. Methylation data at the C and G in a CpG pair were merged to produce the estimate for that locus. DMRs were defined with a minimum coverage of 10 in all six samples, p-value < 0.05, and a minimum methylation percentage change of 10%. Since the Defiant program did not use a pre-defined border to identify DMRs, the p-value < 0.05 cutoff only influenced the widths and quantity of DMRs. The Benjamini–Hochberg approach was applied for multiple testing to obtain false discovery rate (FDR, q-values). Genes were assigned to the DMRs based on a promoter cutoff of 15 kb to the transcription start site, with the direction of transcription taken into account.

2.5. *Bioinformatics*

The knowledge-based Ingenuity Pathway Analysis® (IPA, Qiagen, Germantown, MD, USA) was employed to identify networks, canonical pathways, molecular and cellular functions, and behavioral and neurological dysfunctions using a P15 DNA methylation dataset from WGBS. The microarray dataset from a prior study [34] was also analyzed by IPA. IPA maps gene networks using an algorithm based on molecular function, cellular function, and functional group. Fisher's exact test was used to calculate the significance of the association between genes in the datasets and the analyzed pathways or functions.

3. Results

3.1. *Early-Life Iron Deficiency Induced Differential DNA Methylation in the Rat Hippocampus*

We performed whole genome cytosine methylation bisulfite sequencing on P15 ID (n = 3) and IS (n = 3) rat hippocampi. To determine whether iron deficiency alters the genome-wide pattern of DNA methylation in the developing hippocampus, DNA methylation at 1000 randomly selected loci were compared between ID and IS samples to generate a representative heat map. This unsupervised clustering approach showed consistent patterns of methylation across all samples, without an overall shift toward hypo- or hypermethylation in the ID group (Figure 1a). To determine whether iron deficiency induces changes in DNA methylation at a locus-specific level, a ≥ 10% methylation change with p-value < 0.05 was used as an inclusion criterion [30]. We identified 229 DMRs (Figure 1b and Table S1), including 58% intergenic, 26% intronic, and 11% exonic regions (Figure 1c). Approximately 4% of DMRs were located in promoter regions. These DMRs mapped to within 15 kb of the transcription start site of 108 genes with 63 hypermethylated and 45 hypomethylated loci in ID compared to IS hippocampi (Table 1).

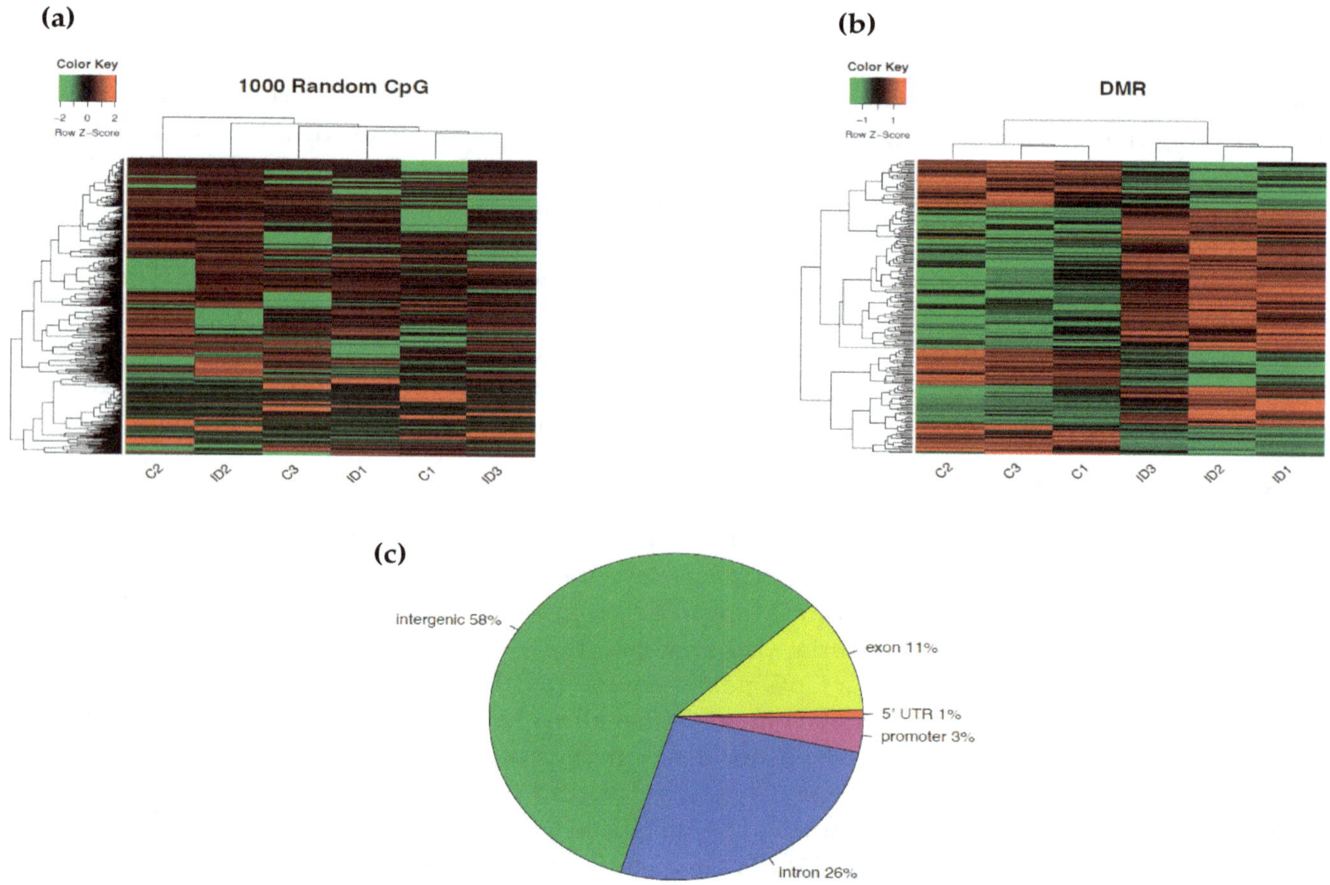

Figure 1. DNA methylome of the postnatal day (P) 15 rat hippocampus. (**a**) An unsupervised clustering heat map of 1000 randomly selected loci showing an absence of bias in global methylation between iron-sufficient (IS) and iron-deficient (ID) hippocampi. Each row in the heat map corresponds to data from a single locus. The branching dendrogram at the top corresponds to the relationships among samples. Hyper- and hypomethylation are shown on a continuum from red to green, respectively. (**b**) Heat map of differentially methylated regions (DMRs) showing significant differences in cytosine methylation between IS (labeled C1-3) and ID (labeled ID1-3) hippocampi. Each row in the heat map corresponds to data point from a single locus, whereas columns correspond to individual samples. The branching dendrogram corresponds to the relationships among samples, as determined by clustering using the 229 identified DMRs. Hyper- and hypomethylation are shown on a continuum from red to green, respectively. (**c**) Pie chart representing the location and proportion of DMRs. The gene body included exons and introns. The promoter was limited to 15 kb upstream from the transcriptional start site. The 5′-untranslated region began at the transcription start site and ended before the initiation sequence. The intergenic region is comprised of the regions not included in the above defined regions.

Table 1. CpG methylation within the 15 kb promoter region of genes in the P15 iron-deficient rat hippocampus.

Hypermethylation				Hypomethylation			
Gene Name	**#CpG**	**DMethylation(%)**	***q*-value**	**Gene Name**	**#CpG**	**DMethylation(%)**	***q*-value**
Adamts19	5	58.5	0.016	*Abhd11*	5	−36.6	0.032
Aebp1	5	10.5	0.118	*Adarb2*	6	−19.7	0.031
Ak4	6	56.0	0.016	*Arhgap28*	5	−21.2	0.026
Ankrd13a	5	26.8	0.024	*Arhgef15*	5	−41.6	0.025
Arf1	6	17.8	0.026	*Arhgef3*	6	−19.8	0.048
Arhgap31	5	36.8	0.035	*Armc8*	9	−10.7	0.041
Armc3	8	43.1	0.031	*Bag2*	6	−21.8	0.059
B4galnt3	5	31.8	0.040	*Cds1*	6	−27.8	0.047

Table 1. *Cont.*

Hypermethylation				Hypomethylation			
Gene Name	#CpG	DMethylation(%)	*q*-value	Gene Name	#CpG	DMethylation(%)	*q*-value
Bcl11b	6	44.7	0.035	*Commd1*	6	−40.4	0.016
Btbd9	5	23.6	0.039	*Dip2a*	10	−57.3	0.039
Cacna1c	5	27.9	0.032	*Dnaja2*	6	−39.0	0.037
Camk2b	9	19.3	0.032	*Dnpep*	5	−14.3	0.051
Capn12	7	21.5	0.024	*Dpf1*	10	−20.6	0.039
Chd2	7	59.7	0.031	*Dpf3*	6	−13.3	0.018
Clvs1	11	26.5	0.031	*Fkrp*	10	−77.7	0.018
Cog3	5	27.4	0.032	*Guca1a*	6	−29.0	0.032
Dgki	5	51.3	0.026	*Hint1*	8	−25.1	0.025
Ephb1	5	33.2	0.040	*Jak3*	8	−20.4	0.023
Ezr	5	51.9	0.018	*Kif26b*	6	−44.2	0.031
Fat3	9	50.1	0.018	*Klhl40*	5	−25.0	0.028
Fig4	5	47.9	0.016	*Lims2*	10	−11.6	0.016
Foxb2	5	32.6	0.039	*LOC691083*	5	−45.6	0.045
Gucy2c	9	86.6	0.016	*Mknk1*	5	−56.8	0.025
Hip1r	5	56.4	0.034	*Mobp*	5	−48.9	0.048
Iqcg	9	52.6	0.020	*Ncf1*	9	−38.4	0.032
Itsn1	5	29.8	0.032	*Pck1*	5	−48.2	0.023
Jph3	8	25.1	0.024	*Pgm3*	5	−69.0	0.024
Kank3	5	28.7	0.031	*Pon2*	6	−10.0	0.029
Kctd15	6	55.1	0.032	*Ppp1r3b*	7	−19.4	0.031
Kctd6	7	27.3	0.016	*Rasd2*	5	−22.4	0.016
Macrod1	5	35.4	0.033	*RGD735029*	5	−17.2	0.032
Map3k11	10	12.9	0.016	*Sardh*	5	−42.9	0.022
Marveld2	6	17.9	0.018	*Sh3pxd2a*	5	−39.4	0.016
Mc3r	5	42.2	0.016	*Slit3*	5	−41.5	0.029
Mib1	6	48.9	0.032	*Smyd3*	6	−28.2	0.112
Mogat1	5	27.4	0.035	*Ss18l1*	6	−18.6	0.042
Mrpl19	6	23.9	0.059	*St8sia1*	6	−20.1	0.016
Myo3b	5	17.1	0.024	*Tal1*	7	−35.1	0.024
Neto2	6	24.3	0.031	*Tmem120b*	5	−37.7	0.024
Olr987	5	21.1	0.016	*Tmem181*	5	−47.1	0.018
Pabpn1l	5	33.3	0.016	*Trrap*	5	−28.2	0.023
Pde2a	5	28.6	0.025	*Usf2*	10	−18.3	0.016
Pde6c	6	46.1	0.024	*Ush1g*	9	−17.2	0.037
Ppp1r21	15	24.9	0.030	*Ust*	5	−54.1	0.037
Prkar1b	5	40.2	0.024	*Wiz*	5	−45.3	0.034
Ptpn14	5	30.1	0.016				
Rev3l	5	16.7	0.023				
Ric8b	6	42.0	0.025				
Riok2	5	48.0	0.031				
Sbk1	6	39.5	0.026				
Scrt2	6	36.8	0.038				
Slc38a1	5	38.2	0.029				
Slc5a1	7	37.4	0.026				
Snurf	5	34.7	0.001				
Spon1	8	73.6	0.031				
Srgap2	5	28.6	0.026				
Tbc1d20	6	13.5	0.042				
Tenm2	5	42.5	0.016				
Tfap2b	5	22.6	0.035				
Tgif2	5	32.2	0.017				
Tnni1	31	29.8	0.016				
Unc93b1	5	54.8	0.020				
Usp36	21	28.8	0.043				

3.2. Early-Life Iron Deficiency Altered the Methylation Status of Genes Regulating Neuronal Development and Function

To identify potential molecular pathways disrupted in the ID hippocampus, IPA was used to map DMRs onto functional networks. The top 10 canonical pathways are shown for DMRs from ID hippocampi (Table 2). Notable pathways critical for neuronal differentiation and function include β-adrenergic signaling, axonal guidance signaling, reelin signaling, Rho family GTPase signaling, cAMP-mediated signaling, and synaptic long-term potentiation.

Table 2. Top 10 canonical pathways implicated by DMRs in the P15 iron-deficient rat hippocampus.

Ingenuity Canonical Pathways	*p*-Value	Differentially Methylated Genes in the Pathway
Nitric Oxide Signaling in the Cardiovascular System	0.002	*CACNA1C, PRKAR1B, PDE2A, GUCY2C*
Cardiac β-Adrenergic Signaling	0.005	*CACNA1C, PRKAR1B, PDE2A, PDE6C*
cAMP-Mediated Signaling	0.005	*CAMK2B, MC3R, PRKAR1B, PDE2A, PDE6C*
Axonal Guidance Signaling	0.006	*ARHGEF15, ITSN1, SLIT3, MKNK1, PRKAR1B, EPHB1, SRGAP2*
Relaxin Signaling	0.007	*PRKAR1B, PDE2A, GUCY2C, PDE6C*
Reelin Signaling in Neurons	0.010	*ARHGEF15, ARHGEF3, MAP3K11*
G-Protein Coupled Receptor Signaling	0.011	*CAMK2B, MC3R, PRKAR1B, PDE2A, PDE6C*
Protein Kinase A Signaling	0.013	*CAMK2B, PTPN14, TNNI1, PRKAR1B, PDE2A, PDE6C*
Synaptic Long-Term Potentiation	0.021	*CAMK2B, CACNA1C, PRKAR1B*
Signaling by Rho Family GTPases	0.034	*ARHGEF15, ARHGEF3, MAP3K11, EZR*

3.3. The Methylation Status of Genes Regulating Axonal Guidance Was Altered in the P15 ID Hippocampus

Neuronal connections are formed by the extension of axons to reach their synaptic targets. This process is controlled by ligands and their receptors at the axonal growth cone, which can sense attractive and repulsive guidance cues to help navigate an axon to its destination [35–39]. These guidance molecules include netrins, slits, semaphorins, and ephrins. Iron deficiency altered methylation at the genes regulating ephrin B signaling/ephrin receptor signaling (data not shown), including increased methylation at *Ephb1*, *Itsn1*, *Prkar1b*, and *Srgap2*, and decreased methylation at *Arhgef15*, *Mknk1*, and *Slit3* loci (Table 1). Decreased methylation at *Arhgef15* and *Arhgef3* and increased methylation at *Map3k11* and *Ezr* loci suggest altered Rho GTPase signaling (Table 2), which transduces guidance signals in the growth cone and regulates cytoskeletal dynamics, an important cellular process for the formation of long-term potentiation (LTP) [40], a cellular basis of learning and memory [41,42].

3.4. Differential DNA Methylation is a Potential Epigenetic Mechanism Contributing to Neural Gene Dysregulation in the P15 ID Hippocampus

To determine whether differential DNA methylation in the P15 ID hippocampus potentially contributes to neural gene dysregulation, we compared our WGBS methylomic dataset and the P15 ID hippocampal transcriptomic dataset [34]. IPA revealed that cAMP-mediated signaling, axonal guidance signaling, reelin signaling, synaptic long-term potentiation, Rho family GTPase signaling, and ephrin B signaling were among the 18 pathways that were altered in both datasets (Table 3). The top functional networks altered in the P15 ID hippocampal methylome (Table 4) were also observed in the P15 ID hippocampal transcriptome. These include cell-to-cell signaling, nervous system development and function, behavior, neurological disease, molecular transport, and lipid metabolism. The transcriptomic dataset corroborates the methylome data and further highlights the disruption of synaptic transmission (Figure 2a), neuritogenesis (Figure 2b), and movement disorders (Figure 2c,d).

Table 3. Overlapping canonical pathways of the P15 DNA methylome and P15 microarray datasets.

	Methylome Analysis		Microarray Analysis	
Ingenuity Canonical Pathways	***p*-value**	**Differentially Methylated Genes**	***p*-value**	**Differentially Expressed Genes**
Nitric Oxide Signaling in the Cardiovascular System	0.002	*CACNA1C, PRKAR1B, PDE2A, GUCY2C*	0.000	*ITPR2, PIK3R3, KDR, PTPN11, PRKAA1, GUCY2D, ITPR1, CAMK4, PRKAG1, PDE2A, PDGFC*
Cellular Effects of Sildenafil (Viagra)	0.004	*CACNA1C, PRKAR1B, PDE2A, GUCY2C*	0.000	*MYH3, CACNG8, ITPR2, ADCY3, GPR37, GUCY2D, ITPR1, ADCY2, PLCE1, CAMK4, PRKAG1, PDE2A*
Cardiac β-Adrenergic Signaling	0.005	*CACNA1C, PRKAR1B, PDE2A, PDE6C*	0.036	*ADCY3, PKIG, ADCY2, PRKAG1, PDE2A, PPP2R2A, PPP1R11*
cAMP-Mediated Signaling	0.005	*CAMK2B, MC3R, PRKAR1B, PDE2A, PDE6C*	0.000	*GABBR1, CHRM3, CAMK4, VIPR1, PDE2A, Htr5b, CHRM2, CNGA2, CAMK2A, GNAI3, ADCY3, HRH3, PKIG, ADCY2, LHCGR, OPRM1, GRM6*
Axonal Guidance Signaling	0.006	*ARHGEF15, ITSN1, SLIT3, MKNK1, PRKAR1B, EPHB1, SRGAP2*	0.003	*CXCL12, PIK3R3, TUBB, EPHA3, ROBO1, PLCE1, DPYSL5, RTN4R, RTN4, GNAI3, FZD4, PDGFC, BAIAP2, SEMA4F, CXCR4, NRAS, CFL1, PTPN11, NTRK2, PRKAG1*
Relaxin Signaling	0.007	*PRKAR1B, PDE2A, GUCY2C, PDE6C*	0.008	*PIK3R3, ADCY3, PTPN11, GUCY2D, ADCY2, PRKAG1, PDE2A, NFKBIA, GNAI3*
Reelin Signaling in Neurons	0.010	*ARHGEF15, ARHGEF3, MAP3K11*	0.004	*PAFAH1B1, PIK3R3, PTPN11, APP, MAPT, ARHGEF9, APBB1*
G-Protein Coupled Receptor Signaling	0.011	*CAMK2B, MC3R, PRKAR1B, PDE2A, PDE6C*	0.000	*PIK3R3, GABBR1, CHRM3, CAMK4, VIPR1, PDE2A, Htr5b, NFKBIA, CHRM2, CAMK2A, GNAI3, NRAS, PDPK1, ADCY3, HRH3, PTPN11, ADCY2, PRKAG1, GRM5, LHCGR, OPRM1, GRM6*
Protein Kinase A Signaling	0.013	*CAMK2B, Ptpn14, TNNI1, PRKAR1B, PDE2A, PDE6C*	0.000	*ITPR2, PLCE1, NFKBIA, CNGA2, GNAI3, PYGB, ADCY3, PTPN11, ITPR1, ADCY2, PTPRF, TGFBR1, PPP1R1B, YWHAB, PPP1R11, DUSP12, PTPRN, CDC25A, PTPN2, PTPRO, H3F3A/H3F3B, CAMK4, PDE2A, PTPN23, CAMK2A, BAD, DUSP5, PTPN12, PRKAG1*
Breast Cancer Regulation by Stathmin1	0.017	*CAMK2B, ARHGEF15, ARHGEF3, PRKAR1B*	0.000	*ITPR2, PIK3R3, TUBB, CAMK4, PPP2R2A, CAMK2A, GNAI3, STMN1, NRAS, ADCY3, PTPN11, ITPR1, ADCY2, ARHGEF9, PRKAG1, PPP1R11*
Synaptic Long-Term Potentiation	0.021	*CAMK2B, CACNA1C, PRKAR1B*	0.000	*NRAS, ITPR2, GRINA, ITPR1, PLCE1, CAMK4, PRKAG1, GRM5, GRIN1, CAMK2A, GRM6, PPP1R11*
Gustation Pathway	0.023	*PRKAR1B, PDE2A, PDE6C*	0.000	*CACNG8, ITPR2, ADCY3, CACNB4, CACNA2D1, P2RX5, ITPR1, ADCY2, PRKAG1, PDE2A, P2RY1, CACNA1H*
Sperm Motility	0.023	*MAP3K11, PRKAR1B, PDE2A*	0.002	*ITPR2, PAFAH1B1, ITPR1, PLCE1, CAMK4, PRKAG1, PDE2A, CNGA2, CACNA1H*
GNRH Signaling	0.032	*CAMK2B, MAP3K11, PRKAR1B*	0.000	*CACNG8, ITPR2, CACNB4, CAMK4, CAMK2A, GNAI3, CACNA1H, NRAS, ADCY3, CACNA2D1, GNRHR, ITPR1, ADCY2, PRKAG1*
Signaling by Rho Family GTPases	0.034	*ARHGEF15, ARHGEF3, MAP3K11, EZR*	0.010	*BAIAP2, CFL1, RHOT2, PIK3R3, PTPN11, RHOB, CDH1, ARHGEF9, PLD1, RHOV, GNAI3, STMN1*
Molecular Mechanisms of Cancer	0.042	*CAMK2B, ARHGEF15, ARHGEF3, JAK3, PRKAR1B*	0.000	*RASGRF1, RHOT2, PIK3R3, CDC25A, CASP9, NFKBIA, CAMK2A, BAD, GNAI3, FZD4, NCSTN, NRAS, RALBP1, ADCY3, PTPN11, RHOB, HIF1A, ADCY2, CASP3, TGFBR1, CDH1, ARHGEF9, PRKAG1, RHOV*
Melatonin Signaling	0.048	*CAMK2B, PRKAR1B*	0.021	*PLCE1, CAMK4, PRKAG1, CAMK2A, GNAI3*
Ephrin B Signaling	0.049	*ITSN1, EPHB1*	0.022	*CXCL12, CXCR4, CFL1, CAP1, GNAI3*

Table 4. IPA annotated functional similarity between the DNA methylome and transcriptome of the P15 ID rat hippocampus.

Category	Diseases or Functions Annotation	*p*-value	Differentially Methylated Genes	*p*-value	Number of Genes
Cell-To-Cell Signaling	Synaptic Depression/Neurotransmission	1.65E-04	*CAMK2B, ARF1, ITSN1, DGKI, PRKAR1B, EPHB1*	1.94E-10	21
Nervous System Development and Function	Neuritogenesis/Extension of Neurites	8.40E-03	*CAMK2B, ST8SIA1, ITSN1, SS18L1, BCL11B, EZR, SLIT3, UST, EPHB1, SRGAP2*	4.92E-16	62
Behavior	Locomotion	3.09E-04	*RASD2, HINT1, MC3R, BTBD9, NCF1, CACNA1C, JPH3, FIG4, TAL1*	1.08E-13	40
	Learning	2.22E-02	*CAMK2B, NCF1, BTBD9, DGKI, CACNA1C, PRKAR1B, JPH3*	3.51E-21	57
Neurological Disease	Cell Death of Cerebral Cortex Cells	1.33E-02	*ST8SIA1, ITSN1, MAP3K11, NCF1, SH3PXD2A*	8.55E-14	32
	Movement Disorder	4.68E-02	*CAMK2B, AEBP1, CDS1, ST8SIA1, HINT1, BCL11B, TFAP2B, PDE6C, USP36, RASD2, MC3R, BTBD9, CACNA1C*	5.58E-32	117
Lipid Metabolism	Quantity of Sphingolipid/Steroid	2.73E-03	*ST8SIA1, HINT1, BCL11B, PON2*	4.24E-09	40
Molecular Transport	Quantity of Heavy Metal	1.13E-02	*ARF1, USF2, COMMD1*	4.32E-19	58
	Transport of Molecule	1.92E-02	*SLC5A1, SLC38A1*	5.41E-31	144

Integrating the P15 ID WGBS methylome and microarray datasets led to the identification of three genes, including *Pde2a*, *Mobp*, and *Cds1* (Table 5). All three genes showed differential methylation in their intronic regions. *Pde2a* (+28.6%) was hypermethylated while *Mobp* (−48.9%) and *Cds1* (−27.8%) were hypomethylated in the P15 ID hippocampus. All three genes were upregulated in the P15 ID hippocampus. While DNA methylation at gene promoters is strongly associated with gene silencing [28], DNA methylation in intronic regions may mark enhancers or repressors and can be associated with changes in gene expression [43,44]. Phosphodiesterase 2A (Pde2a) is highly expressed in the brain and metabolizes cGMP and cAMP to regulate short-term synaptic plasticity, axonal excitability, and transmitter release in the hippocampal, cortical, and striatal networks [45,46]. Myelin-associated oligodendrocyte basic protein (Mobp) is the third most abundant protein in the central nervous system (CNS), and is exclusively expressed in oligodendrocytes, the myelinating glial cells of the CNS [47]. Mobp plays a role in compacting or stabilizing the myelin sheath and regulates the morphological differentiation of oligodendrocytes [48]. CDP-diacylglycerol synthase 1 (Cds1) is a key enzyme in regulating second messenger phosphatidylinositol 4,5-bisphosphate (PIP_2) levels. It is localized in the endoplasmic reticulum and mitochondria [49] and is involved in the synthesis of phosphatidylglycerol and cardiolipin, an important component of the inner mitochondrial membrane [50]. Cds1 is a novel regulator of lipid droplet formation, lipid storage, and adipocyte development [51], and plays a critical role in mammalian energy storage, which is compromised in developing iron-deficient neurons [52].

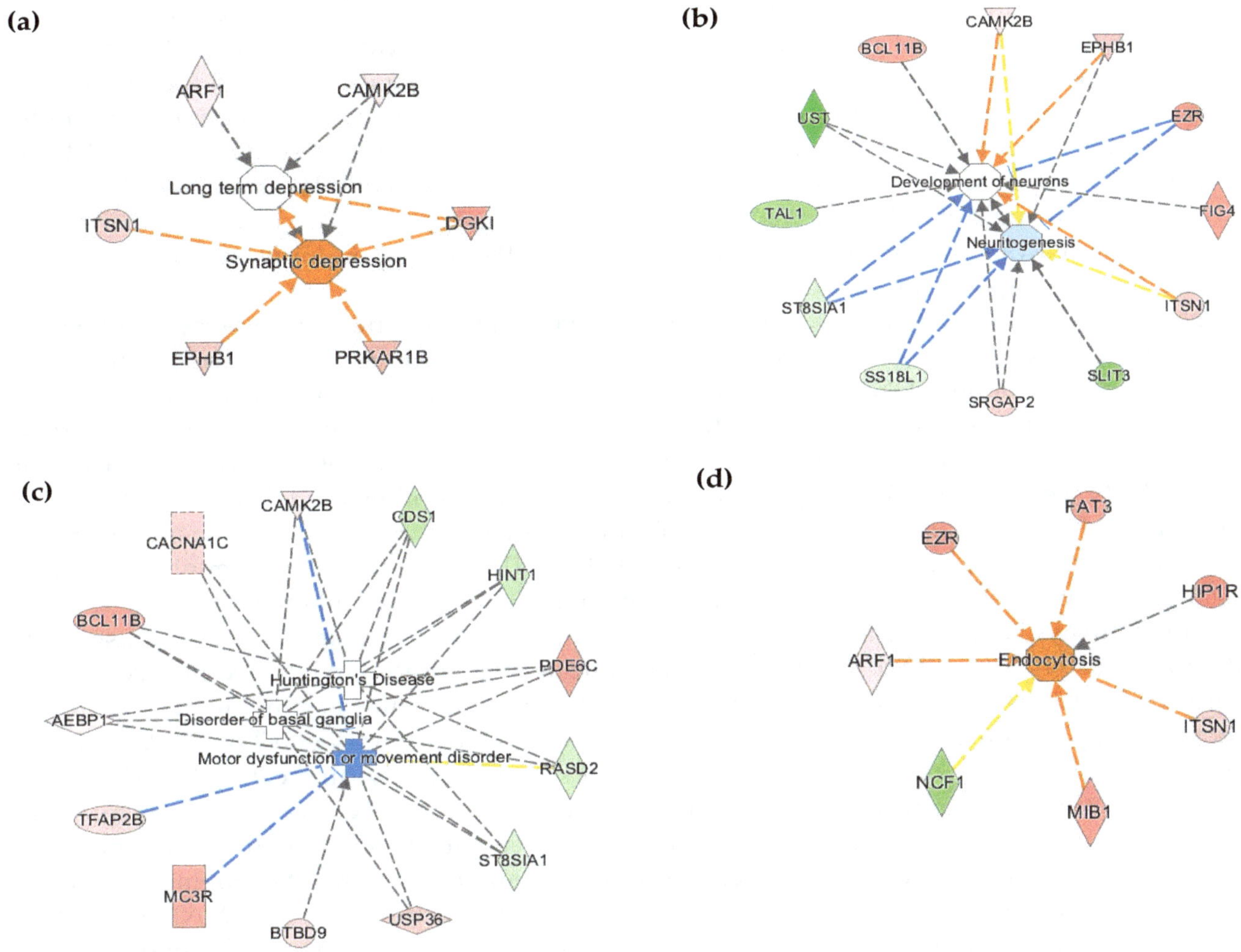

Figure 2. Ingenuity Pathway Analysis® (IPA) functional annotation of altered DNA methylation at loci that are involved in (**a**) synaptic depression, (**b**) neuritogenesis and neuronal development, (**c**) pathogenesis of neurological diseases, and (**d**) lipid metabolism and molecular transport, including endocytosis. Red-filled and green-filled shapes indicate increased and decreased methylation, respectively. Orange-red lines indicate activation; blue lines indicate inhibition; yellow lines indicate findings inconsistent with the state of downstream activity; grey lines indicate that the effect was not predicted.

Table 5. Overlapping genes of the P15 DNA methylome and microarray datasets.

Gene Name	Symbol	Δ Methylation (%)	CpGs Location	FC (ID/IS)	Location	Type(s)
Phosphodiesterase 2A	*Pde2a*	28.6	Intron 2	1.16	Plasma Membrane	enzyme
Myelin-associated oligodendrocyte basic protein	*Mobp*	−48.9	Intron 2	1.37	Cytoplasm	other
CDP-diacylglycerol synthase 1	*Cds1*	−27.8	Intron 11	1.23	Endoplasmic reticulum & mitochondria	enzyme

Δ Methylation values are means from DNA methylome, and FC (fold change) values are means from microarray.

4. Discussion

Fetal and early postnatal life iron deficiency causes long-lasting impairments in learning, memory, and socio-emotional behaviors [1,14–16,53], including an increased risk for autism, depression, and schizophrenia in humans [2,54,55]. These long-term neurobehavioral deficits occur despite early diagnosis and treatment, indicating the need for adequate iron during critical periods of brain development. In preclinical models, these effects have been ascribed in part to the persistence of abnormalities in monoamine signaling, myelination, neural metabolism, and the expression of neuroplasticity-associated proteins into adulthood [20,56–58]. The molecular mechanisms underlying these persistent changes have not been fully elucidated. The present study goes well beyond previous studies by systematically analyzing the alteration of DNA methylation induced by early-life iron deficiency using a whole genome bisulfite sequencing approach. Consistent with previous transcriptomic analysis, the changes in DNA methylation in the ID hippocampus mapped to functional networks that are important for neuronal plasticity.

DNA methylation is an important epigenetic mechanism regulating gene expression, often across the lifespan. Methylation at genomic regions has different influences on gene transcriptional activity depending on the location of DNA methylation. In the present study, differential methylation was highly enriched at intergenic regions (58%) in the ID hippocampus. This outcome is similar to our previous findings in pancreatic islets of an intrauterine growth restriction rat model [59], where approximately 65% of DMRs were located in intergenic regions, as well as to other models of early-life adverse environments [33,60–62]. These conserved intergenic regions may represent important enhancers or cis-regulatory sites in regulating gene expression [43,63,64]. Thus, these DMRs might account for a substantially fewer number of loci with DMRs compared to a number of differentially expressed genes in the microarray dataset and a small overlap between these two datasets. Our data also showed that approximately 37% of DMRs in the ID hippocampus were located in gene bodies (26% and 11% in introns and exons, respectively). DNA methylation in gene bodies is generally associated with higher gene expression in dividing cells [65], in contrast to the regulatory effect of DNA methylation in promoter regions. However, this association is not seen in non-dividing cells [27]. Although not many cells in the hippocampus are actively dividing at P15, these DNA modifications might have occurred during the period of active proliferation in the prenatal period when the pregnant dam and fetus were iron-deficient. Additional DMR analysis at a timepoint when the developing hippocampus undergoes active proliferation will provide further insight into this notion. DNA methylation in gene bodies may define the exon boundaries, regulate alternative promoters in gene bodies, and regulate mRNA splicing and alternative splicing [65–68]. Wan et al. (2013) showed that tissue-specific DMRs are preferentially located in exons and introns of protein-coding genes [69]. These biologically relevant DMRs are enriched in alternatively spliced genes and a subset of developmental genes. It is possible that the real effect of DNA methylation in the P15 ID hippocampus is within these domains. Our microarray analysis [34] was insufficient to probe such effects. Finally, iron deficiency-induced intragenic DMRs could modify potential gene enhancers [43,44,70,71]. The intragenic DMRs in the ID hippocampus may directly contribute to neural gene dysregulation by modifying the accessibility of alternative splice sites or promoters. These analyses constitute a potential direction for future study.

Our WGBS analysis of the ID hippocampus identified pertinent signaling pathways that could underlie the neurobehavioral abnormalities associated with early-life iron deficiency. The DNA methylome showed that DNA methylation at genes regulating cAMP-mediated signaling and protein kinase A signaling was significantly altered in the P15 ID rat hippocampus (Table 2). Both pathways play critical roles in regulating LTP, as well as the plasticity of axonal guidance responses [72,73]. In addition, the predicted changes to the β-adrenergic signaling and nitric oxide signaling pathways in the ID hippocampus would likely result in lower activities of cAMP, cGMP, protein kinase C (PKC), mitogen-activated protein kinase (MAPK), and N-methyl-D-aspartate (NMDA) receptors [74,75]. Likewise, altered Rho GTPase signaling could change the axonal responses to guidance cues and affect neuronal connections and LTP formation. The Rho family of GTPases plays a key role in the formation of LTP by regulating cellular processes, including axon outgrowth and growth cone dynamics [76,77]. This effect is consistent with and provides a molecular basis for our previous finding of abnormal dendritogenesis and synaptogenesis in these ID rats [17]. Our study also revealed the alteration of the reelin signaling pathway in the ID hippocampus. Reelin regulates neuronal migration and cell positioning in the developing neocortex and cerebellar cortex [78], and modulates synaptogenesis, synaptic plasticity, and LTP, which are necessary for learning and memory in the adult brain [79,80]. Reelin can bind to two lipoprotein receptors, apolipoprotein E receptor 2 (ApoER2) and very-low-density-lipoprotein receptor (VLDLR), and initiates signaling cascades, including NMDA receptor activity, that are critical for hippocampal-dependent learning and memory [79,81]. Altered reelin signaling has been implicated in the pathogenesis of schizophrenia, bipolar disorder, and autism [82,83], all which have been associated with early-life iron deficiency [2,54,55].

DNA methylation patterns are dynamically regulated by DNA methyltransferase (DNMT) and TET enzymes [84]. TET proteins are responsible for catalyzing the conversion of 5-methylcytosine (5mC) to 5-hydroxymethylcytosine (5hmC) and other oxidized methylcytosines, thereby initiating the active DNA demethylation process. TET enzymatic activity is iron-dependent [25,85]. Consequently, iron deficiency could decrease TET activity, leading to global DNA hypermethylation. However, our WGBS results did not show an overall shift toward hypermethylation, suggesting a minimal effect of potentially compromised TET activity in the P15 ID hippocampus. As such, 5hmC has been shown to be an important epigenetic modification for chromatin structure and transcriptional regulation [86–88]. TET proteins and 5hmC are highly enriched in the brain and play an important role in neuronal development and differentiation [87,89,90]. Changes to 5hmC levels are associated with neurodegenerative diseases, such as Alzheimer's disease, Huntington's disease, and Parkinson's disease [91]. Early-life iron deficiency may decrease TET activity and dynamically alter the DNA methylation pattern between 5mC and 5hmC, leading to the dysregulation of neuronal gene expression in the ID hippocampus. Due to methodological limitations, our current WGBS study could not distinguish 5mC and 5hmC levels. Investigations of loci-specific and genome-wide 5hmC alterations in the ID hippocampus are ongoing and will be presented in a future publication.

DNA methylation has been demonstrated to be an important factor in central nervous system development, the modulation of normal brain function, and the pathogenesis of neurological and psychiatric disorders [27]. Despite the limitations of our study, such as minimal biological replicates due to the high cost of WGBS and possible sex-dependent differences in ID rat brains, our current study is the first hippocampal methylome study on the developing rat brain, and provides evidence for DNA methylation as a potential epigenetic mechanism contributing to hippocampal gene dysregulation in early-life ID animals. Given that 95% of DMRs were found in the intergenic and intragenic regions, future studies will need to uncover the mechanisms by which DMRs reprogram gene regulation and mRNA splicing alteration in the ID hippocampus.

Author Contributions: Y.-C.L., P.V.T., R.A.S., and M.K.G. designed the study, which was conducted and analyzed by Y.-C.L. and P.V.T. D.E.C. developed the Defiant method for DMR analysis. This manuscript was written by Y.-C.L. together with P.V.T. and R.A.S. with input from all authors. All authors have read and approved the manuscript.

Acknowledgments: We thank Kyoung-Jae Won and Jonathan Schug for assisting in whole genome bisulfite-sequencing data analysis.

References

1. Lozoff, B.; Beard, J.; Connor, J.; Barbara, F.; Georgieff, M.; Schallert, T. Long-lasting neural and behavioral effects of iron deficiency in infancy. *Nutr. Rev.* **2006**, *64*, S34–S91. [CrossRef] [PubMed]
2. Insel, B.J.; Schaefer, C.A.; McKeague, I.W.; Susser, E.S.; Brown, A.S. Maternal iron deficiency and the risk of schizophrenia in offspring. *Arch. Gen. Psychiatry* **2008**, *65*, 1136–1144. [CrossRef]

3. Christian, P.; Murray-Kolb, L.E.; Khatry, S.K.; Katz, J.; Schaefer, B.A.; Cole, P.M.; Leclerq, S.C.; Tielsch, J.M. Prenatal micronutrient supplementation and intellectual and motor function in early school-aged children in Nepal. *JAMA* **2010**, *304*, 2716–2723. [CrossRef]
4. Li, Q.; Yan, H.; Zeng, L.; Cheng, Y.; Liang, W.; Dang, S.; Wang, Q.; Tsuji, I. Effects of maternal multimicronutrient supplementation on the mental development of infants in rural western China: Follow-up evaluation of a double-blind, randomized, controlled trial. *Pediatrics* **2009**, *123*, e685–e692. [CrossRef] [PubMed]
5. Schmidt, M.K.; Muslimatun, S.; West, C.E.; Schultink, W.; Hautvast, J.G. Mental and psychomotor development in Indonesian infants of mothers supplemented with vitamin A in addition to iron during pregnancy. *Br. J. Nutr.* **2004**, *91*, 279–286. [CrossRef] [PubMed]
6. Chang, S.; Zeng, L.; Brouwer, I.D.; Kok, F.J.; Yan, H. Effect of Iron Deficiency Anemia in Pregnancy on Child Mental Development in Rural China. *Pediatrics* **2013**. [CrossRef]
7. Siddappa, A.M.; Georgieff, M.K.; Wewerka, S.; Worwa, C.; Nelson, C.A.; Deregnier, R.A. Iron deficiency alters auditory recognition memory in newborn infants of diabetic mothers. *Pediatr. Res.* **2004**, *55*, 1034–1041. [CrossRef]
8. Rao, R.; Georgieff, M.K. Iron in fetal and neonatal nutrition. *Semin. Fetal Neonatal Med.* **2007**, *12*, 54–63. [CrossRef]
9. Rao, R.; Tkac, I.; Townsend, E.L.; Gruetter, R.; Georgieff, M.K. Perinatal iron deficiency alters the neurochemical profile of the developing rat hippocampus. *J. Nutr.* **2003**, *133*, 3215–3221. [PubMed]
10. Avishai-Eliner, S.; Brunson, K.L.; Sandman, C.A.; Baram, T.Z. Stressed-out, or in (utero)? *Trends Neurosci.* **2002**, *25*, 518–524. [PubMed]
11. Semple, B.D.; Blomgren, K.; Gimlin, K.; Ferriero, D.M.; Noble-Haeusslein, L.J. Brain development in rodents and humans: Identifying benchmarks of maturation and vulnerability to injury across species. *Prog. Neurobiol.* **2013**, *106–107*, 1–16. [CrossRef] [PubMed]
12. Petry, C.D.; Eaton, M.A.; Wobken, J.D.; Mills, M.M.; Johnson, D.E.; Georgieff, M.K. Iron deficiency of liver, heart, and brain in newborn infants of diabetic mothers. *J. Pediatr.* **1992**, *121*, 109–114. [CrossRef]
13. Georgieff, M.K.; Petry, C.D.; Wobken, J.D.; Oyer, C.E. Liver and brain iron deficiency in newborn infants with bilateral renal agenesis (Potter's syndrome). *Pediatr. Pathol. Lab. Med.* **1996**, *16*, 509–519. [CrossRef] [PubMed]
14. Unger, E.L.; Hurst, A.R.; Georgieff, M.K.; Schallert, T.; Rao, R.; Connor, J.R.; Kaciroti, N.; Lozoff, B.; Felt, B. Behavior and monoamine deficits in prenatal and perinatal iron deficiency are not corrected by early postnatal moderate-iron or high-iron diets in rats. *J. Nutr.* **2012**, *142*, 2040–2049. [CrossRef]
15. Schmidt, A.T.; Waldow, K.J.; Grove, W.M.; Salinas, J.A.; Georgieff, M.K. Dissociating the long-term effects of fetal/neonatal iron deficiency on three types of learning in the rat. *Behav. Neurosci.* **2007**, *121*, 475–482. [CrossRef] [PubMed]
16. Felt, B.T.; Beard, J.L.; Schallert, T.; Shao, J.; Aldridge, J.W.; Connor, J.R.; Georgieff, M.K.; Lozoff, B. Persistent neurochemical and behavioral abnormalities in adulthood despite early iron supplementation for perinatal iron deficiency anemia in rats. *Behav. Brain Res.* **2006**, *171*, 261–270. [CrossRef]
17. Brunette, K.E.; Tran, P.V.; Wobken, J.D.; Carlson, E.S.; Georgieff, M.K. Gestational and neonatal iron deficiency alters apical dendrite structure of CA1 pyramidal neurons in adult rat hippocampus. *Dev. Neurosci.* **2010**, *32*, 238–248. [CrossRef]
18. Jorgenson, L.A.; Wobken, J.D.; Georgieff, M.K. Perinatal iron deficiency alters apical dendritic growth in hippocampal CA1 pyramidal neurons. *Dev. Neurosci.* **2003**, *25*, 412–420. [CrossRef] [PubMed]
19. Jorgenson, L.A.; Sun, M.; O'Connor, M.; Georgieff, M.K. Fetal iron deficiency disrupts the maturation of synaptic function and efficacy in area CA1 of the developing rat hippocampus. *Hippocampus* **2005**, *15*, 1094–1102. [CrossRef]
20. Rao, R.; Tkac, I.; Schmidt, A.T.; Georgieff, M.K. Fetal and neonatal iron deficiency causes volume loss and alters the neurochemical profile of the adult rat hippocampus. *Nutr. Neurosci.* **2011**, *14*, 59–65. [CrossRef]
21. Clardy, S.L.; Wang, X.; Zhao, W.; Liu, W.; Chase, G.A.; Beard, J.L.; True Felt, B.; Connor, J.R. Acute and chronic effects of developmental iron deficiency on mRNA expression patterns in the brain. *J. Neural Transm. Suppl.* **2006**, 173–196.
22. Tran, P.V.; Kennedy, B.C.; Pisansky, M.T.; Won, K.; Gewirtz, J.C.; Simmons, R.A.; Georgieff, M.K. Prenatal choline supplementation diminishes early-life iron deficiency induced reprogramming of molecular networks associated with behavioral abnormalities in the adult rat hippocampus. *J. Nutr.* **2016**, *146*, 484–493. [CrossRef]

23. Tran, P.V.; Carlson, E.S.; Fretham, S.J.; Georgieff, M.K. Early-life iron deficiency anemia alters neurotrophic factor expression and hippocampal neuron differentiation in male rats. *J. Nutr.* **2008**, *138*, 2495–2501. [CrossRef]
24. Tran, P.V.; Kennedy, B.C.; Lien, Y.C.; Simmons, R.A.; Georgieff, M.K. Fetal iron deficiency induces chromatin remodeling at the Bdnf locus in adult rat hippocampus. *Am. J. Physiol. Regul. Integr. Comp. Physiol.* **2015**, *308*, R276–R282. [CrossRef]
25. Tahiliani, M.; Koh, K.P.; Shen, Y.; Pastor, W.A.; Bandukwala, H.; Brudno, Y.; Agarwal, S.; Iyer, L.M.; Liu, D.R.; Aravind, L.; et al. Conversion of 5-methylcytosine to 5-hydroxymethylcytosine in mammalian DNA by MLL partner TET1. *Science* **2009**, *324*, 930–935. [CrossRef]
26. Hou, H.; Yu, H. Structural insights into histone lysine demethylation. *Curr. Opin. Struct. Biol.* **2010**, *20*, 739–748. [CrossRef]
27. Moore, L.D.; Le, T.; Fan, G. DNA methylation and its basic function. *Neuropsychopharmacology* **2013**, *38*, 23–38. [CrossRef]
28. Weber, M.; Hellmann, I.; Stadler, M.B.; Ramos, L.; Pääbo, S.; Rebhan, M.; Schübeler, D. Distribution, silencing potential and evolutionary impact of promoter DNA methylation in the human genome. *Nat. Genet.* **2007**, *39*, 457–466. [CrossRef]
29. Stevens, M.; Cheng, J.B.; Li, D.; Xie, M.; Hong, C.; Maire, C.L.; Ligon, K.L.; Hirst, M.; Marra, M.A.; Costello, J.F.; et al. Estimating absolute methylation levels at single-CpG resolution from methylation enrichment and restriction enzyme sequencing methods. *Genome Res.* **2013**, *23*, 1541–1553. [CrossRef]
30. Condon, D.E.; Tran, P.V.; Lien, Y.C.; Schug, J.; Georgieff, M.K.; Simmons, R.A.; Won, K.J. Defiant: (DMRs: Easy, fast, identification and ANnoTation) identifies differentially Methylated regions from iron-deficient rat hippocampus. *BMC Bioinf.* **2018**, *19*, 31. [CrossRef]
31. Fretham, S.J.; Carlson, E.S.; Georgieff, M.K. The role of iron in learning and memory. *Adv. Nutr.* **2011**, *2*, 112–121. [CrossRef]
32. Tran, P.V.; Fretham, S.J.; Wobken, J.; Miller, B.S.; Georgieff, M.K. Gestational-neonatal iron deficiency suppresses and iron treatment reactivates IGF signaling in developing rat hippocampus. *Am. J. Physiol. Endocrinol. Metab.* **2012**, *302*, E316–E324. [CrossRef]
33. Sheaffer, K.L.; Kim, R.; Aoki, R.; Elliott, E.N.; Schug, J.; Burger, L.; Schübeler, D.; Kaestner, K.H. DNA methylation is required for the control of stem cell differentiation in the small intestine. *Genes Dev.* **2014**, *28*, 652–664. [CrossRef]
34. Carlson, E.S.; Stead, J.D.; Neal, C.R.; Petryk, A.; Georgieff, M.K. Perinatal iron deficiency results in altered developmental expression of genes mediating energy metabolism and neuronal morphogenesis in hippocampus. *Hippocampus* **2007**, *17*, 679–691. [CrossRef]
35. Chilton, J.K. Molecular mechanisms of axon guidance. *Dev. Biol.* **2006**, *292*, 13–24. [CrossRef]
36. Dickson, B.J. Molecular mechanisms of axon guidance. *Science* **2002**, *298*, 1959–1964. [CrossRef]
37. Egea, J.; Klein, R. Bidirectional Eph-ephrin signaling during axon guidance. *Trends Cell. Biol.* **2007**, *17*, 230–238. [CrossRef]
38. Rohani, N.; Canty, L.; Luu, O.; Fagotto, F.; Winklbauer, R. EphrinB/EphB signaling controls embryonic germ layer separation by contact-induced cell detachment. *PLoS Biol.* **2011**, *9*, e1000597. [CrossRef]
39. Shamah, S.M.; Lin, M.Z.; Goldberg, J.L.; Estrach, S.; Sahin, M.; Hu, L.; Bazalakova, M.; Neve, R.L.; Corfas, G.; Debant, A.; et al. EphA receptors regulate growth cone dynamics through the novel guanine nucleotide exchange factor ephexin. *Cell* **2001**, *105*, 233–244. [CrossRef]
40. Rex, C.S.; Chen, L.Y.; Sharma, A.; Liu, J.; Babayan, A.H.; Gall, C.M.; Lynch, G. Different Rho GTPase-dependent signaling pathways initiate sequential steps in the consolidation of long-term potentiation. *J. Cell. Biol.* **2009**, *186*, 85–97. [CrossRef]
41. Malenka, R.C.; Nicoll, R.A. Long-term potentiation—A decade of progress? *Science* **1999**, *285*, 1870–1874. [CrossRef]
42. Nicoll, R.A. A Brief History of Long-Term Potentiation. *Neuron* **2017**, *93*, 281–290. [CrossRef]
43. Blattler, A.; Yao, L.; Witt, H.; Guo, Y.; Nicolet, C.M.; Berman, B.P.; Farnham, P.J. Global loss of DNA methylation uncovers intronic enhancers in genes showing expression changes. *Genome Biol.* **2014**, *15*, 469. [CrossRef]
44. Singer, M.; Kosti, I.; Pachter, L.; Mandel-Gutfreund, Y. A diverse epigenetic landscape at human exons with implication for expression. *Nucleic Acids Res.* **2015**, *43*, 3498–3508. [CrossRef]

45. Stephenson, D.T.; Coskran, T.M.; Kelly, M.P.; Kleiman, R.J.; Morton, D.; O'Neill, S.M.; Schmidt, C.J.; Weinberg, R.J.; Menniti, F.S. The distribution of phosphodiesterase 2A in the rat brain. *Neuroscience* **2012**, *226*, 145–155. [CrossRef]
46. Fernández-Fernández, D.; Rosenbrock, H.; Kroker, K.S. Inhibition of PDE2A, but not PDE9A, modulates presynaptic short-term plasticity measured by paired-pulse facilitation in the CA1 region of the hippocampus. *Synapse* **2015**, *69*, 484–496. [CrossRef]
47. Montague, P.; McCallion, A.S.; Davies, R.W.; Griffiths, I.R. Myelin-associated oligodendrocytic basic protein: A family of abundant CNS myelin proteins in search of a function. *Dev. Neurosci.* **2006**, *28*, 479–487. [CrossRef]
48. Schäfer, I.; Müller, C.; Luhmann, H.J.; White, R. MOBP levels are regulated by Fyn kinase and affect the morphological differentiation of oligodendrocytes. *J. Cell Sci.* **2016**, *129*, 930–942. [CrossRef]
49. Kuchler, K.; Daum, G.; Paltauf, F. Subcellular and submitochondrial localization of phospholipid-synthesizing enzymes in Saccharomyces cerevisiae. *J. Bacteriol.* **1986**, *165*, 901–910. [CrossRef]
50. Nowicki, M.; Müller, F.; Frentzen, M. Cardiolipin synthase of Arabidopsis thaliana. *FEBS Lett.* **2005**, *579*, 2161–2165. [CrossRef]
51. Qi, Y.; Kapterian, T.S.; Du, X.; Ma, Q.; Fei, W.; Zhang, Y.; Huang, X.; Dawes, I.W.; Yang, H. CDP-diacylglycerol synthases regulate the growth of lipid droplets and adipocyte development. *J. Lipid Res.* **2016**, *57*, 767–780. [CrossRef]
52. Bastian, T.W.; von Hohenberg, W.C.; Georgieff, M.K.; Lanier, L.M. Chronic Energy Depletion due to Iron Deficiency Impairs Dendritic Mitochondrial Motility during Hippocampal Neuron Development. *J. Neurosci.* **2019**, *39*, 802–813. [CrossRef]
53. Corapci, F.; Calatroni, A.; Kaciroti, N.; Jimenez, E.; Lozoff, B. Longitudinal evaluation of externalizing and internalizing behavior problems following iron deficiency in infancy. *J. Pediatr. Psychol.* **2010**, *35*, 296–305. [CrossRef]
54. Lukowski, A.F.; Koss, M.; Burden, M.J.; Jonides, J.; Nelson, C.A.; Kaciroti, N.; Jimenez, E.; Lozoff, B. Iron deficiency in infancy and neurocognitive functioning at 19 years: Evidence of long-term deficits in executive function and recognition memory. *Nutr. Neurosci.* **2010**, *13*, 54–70. [CrossRef]
55. Schmidt, R.J.; Tancredi, D.J.; Krakowiak, P.; Hansen, R.L.; Ozonoff, S. Maternal intake of supplemental iron and risk of autism spectrum disorder. *Am. J. Epidemiol.* **2014**, *180*, 890–900. [CrossRef]
56. Connor, J.R.; Menzies, S.L. Relationship of iron to oligodendrocytes and myelination. *Glia* **1996**, *17*, 83–93. [CrossRef]
57. Beard, J.L.; Wiesinger, J.A.; Connor, J.R. Pre- and postweaning iron deficiency alters myelination in Sprague-Dawley rats. *Dev. Neurosci.* **2003**, *25*, 308–315. [CrossRef]
58. Tran, P.V.; Fretham, S.J.; Carlson, E.S.; Georgieff, M.K. Long-term reduction of hippocampal brain-derived neurotrophic factor activity after fetal-neonatal iron deficiency in adult rats. *Pediatr. Res.* **2009**, *65*, 493–498. [CrossRef]
59. Thompson, R.F.; Fazzari, M.J.; Niu, H.; Barzilai, N.; Simmons, R.A.; Greally, J.M. Experimental intrauterine growth restriction induces alterations in DNA methylation and gene expression in pancreatic islets of rats. *J. Biol. Chem.* **2010**, *285*, 15111–15118. [CrossRef]
60. Xiao, Y.; Camarillo, C.; Ping, Y.; Arana, T.B.; Zhao, H.; Thompson, P.M.; Xu, C.; Su, B.B.; Fan, H.; Ordonez, J.; et al. The DNA methylome and transcriptome of different brain regions in schizophrenia and bipolar disorder. *PLoS ONE* **2014**, *9*, e95875. [CrossRef]
61. Li, M.; Gao, F.; Xia, Y.; Tang, Y.; Zhao, W.; Jin, C.; Luo, H.; Wang, J.; Li, Q.; Wang, Y. Filtrating colorectal cancer associated genes by integrated analyses of global DNA methylation and hydroxymethylation in cancer and normal tissue. *Sci. Rep.* **2016**, *6*, 31826. [CrossRef]
62. Radford, E.J.; Ito, M.; Shi, H.; Corish, J.A.; Yamazawa, K.; Isganaitis, E.; Seisenberger, S.; Hore, T.A.; Reik, W.; Erkek, S.; et al. In utero effects. In utero undernourishment perturbs the adult sperm methylome and intergenerational metabolism. *Science* **2014**, *345*, 1255903. [CrossRef]
63. Consortium, E.P. An integrated encyclopedia of DNA elements in the human genome. *Nature* **2012**, *489*, 57–74. [CrossRef]
64. Pennacchio, L.A.; Ahituv, N.; Moses, A.M.; Prabhakar, S.; Nobrega, M.A.; Shoukry, M.; Minovitsky, S.; Dubchak, I.; Holt, A.; Lewis, K.D.; et al. In vivo enhancer analysis of human conserved non-coding sequences. *Nature* **2006**, *444*, 499–502. [CrossRef]

65. Lev Maor, G.; Yearim, A.; Ast, G. The alternative role of DNA methylation in splicing regulation. *Trends Genet.* **2015**, *31*, 274–280. [CrossRef]
66. Maunakea, A.K.; Nagarajan, R.P.; Bilenky, M.; Ballinger, T.J.; D'Souza, C.; Fouse, S.D.; Johnson, B.E.; Hong, C.; Nielsen, C.; Zhao, Y.; et al. Conserved role of intragenic DNA methylation in regulating alternative promoters. *Nature* **2010**, *466*, 253–257. [CrossRef]
67. Oberdoerffer, S. A conserved role for intragenic DNA methylation in alternative pre-mRNA splicing. *Transcription* **2012**, *3*, 106–109. [CrossRef]
68. Gelfman, S.; Cohen, N.; Yearim, A.; Ast, G. DNA-methylation effect on cotranscriptional splicing is dependent on GC architecture of the exon-intron structure. *Genome Res.* **2013**, *23*, 789–799. [CrossRef]
69. Wan, J.; Oliver, V.F.; Zhu, H.; Zack, D.J.; Qian, J.; Merbs, S.L. Integrative analysis of tissue-specific methylation and alternative splicing identifies conserved transcription factor binding motifs. *Nucleic Acids Res.* **2013**, *41*, 8503–8514. [CrossRef]
70. Ishihara, K.; Oshimura, M.; Nakao, M. CTCF-dependent chromatin insulator is linked to epigenetic remodeling. *Mol. Cell.* **2006**, *23*, 733–742. [CrossRef]
71. Pikaart, M.J.; Recillas-Targa, F.; Felsenfeld, G. Loss of transcriptional activity of a transgene is accompanied by DNA methylation and histone deacetylation and is prevented by insulators. *Genes Dev.* **1998**, *12*, 2852–2862. [CrossRef]
72. Ming, G.L.; Song, H.J.; Berninger, B.; Holt, C.E.; Tessier-Lavigne, M.; Poo, M.M. cAMP-dependent growth cone guidance by netrin-1. *Neuron* **1997**, *19*, 1225–1235. [CrossRef]
73. Moore, S.W.; Kennedy, T.E. Protein kinase A regulates the sensitivity of spinal commissural axon turning to netrin-1 but does not switch between chemoattraction and chemorepulsion. *J. Neurosci.* **2006**, *26*, 2419–2423. [CrossRef]
74. Sweatt, J.D. Toward a molecular explanation for long-term potentiation. *Learn. Mem.* **1999**, *6*, 399–416. [CrossRef]
75. Thomas, M.J.; Moody, T.D.; Makhinson, M.; O'Dell, T.J. Activity-dependent beta-adrenergic modulation of low frequency stimulation induced LTP in the hippocampal CA1 region. *Neuron* **1996**, *17*, 475–482. [CrossRef]
76. Bito, H.; Furuyashiki, T.; Ishihara, H.; Shibasaki, Y.; Ohashi, K.; Mizuno, K.; Maekawa, M.; Ishizaki, T.; Narumiya, S. A critical role for a Rho-associated kinase, p160ROCK, in determining axon outgrowth in mammalian CNS neurons. *Neuron* **2000**, *26*, 431–441. [CrossRef]
77. Heasman, S.J.; Ridley, A.J. Mammalian Rho GTPases: New insights into their functions from in vivo studies. *Nat. Rev. Mol. Cell. Biol.* **2008**, *9*, 690–701. [CrossRef]
78. Lakatosova, S.; Ostatnikova, D. Reelin and its complex involvement in brain development and function. *Int. J. Biochem. Cell. Biol.* **2012**, *44*, 1501–1504. [CrossRef]
79. Weeber, E.J.; Beffert, U.; Jones, C.; Christian, J.M.; Forster, E.; Sweatt, J.D.; Herz, J. Reelin and ApoE receptors cooperate to enhance hippocampal synaptic plasticity and learning. *J. Biol. Chem.* **2002**, *277*, 39944–39952. [CrossRef]
80. D'Arcangelo, G. Apoer2: A reelin receptor to remember. *Neuron* **2005**, *47*, 471–473. [CrossRef]
81. Chen, Y.; Beffert, U.; Ertunc, M.; Tang, T.S.; Kavalali, E.T.; Bezprozvanny, I.; Herz, J. Reelin modulates NMDA receptor activity in cortical neurons. *J. Neurosci.* **2005**, *25*, 8209–8216. [CrossRef]
82. Fatemi, S.H.; Kroll, J.L.; Stary, J.M. Altered levels of Reelin and its isoforms in schizophrenia and mood disorders. *Neuroreport* **2001**, *12*, 3209–3215. [CrossRef]
83. Fatemi, S.H.; Stary, J.M.; Halt, A.R.; Realmuto, G.R. Dysregulation of Reelin and Bcl-2 proteins in autistic cerebellum. *J. Autism Dev. Disord.* **2001**, *31*, 529–535. [CrossRef]
84. Li, E.; Zhang, Y. DNA methylation in mammals. *Cold Spring Harb. Perspect. Biol.* **2014**, *6*, a019133. [CrossRef]
85. Zhao, B.; Yang, Y.; Wang, X.; Chong, Z.; Yin, R.; Song, S.H.; Zhao, C.; Li, C.; Huang, H.; Sun, B.F.; et al. Redox-active quinones induces genome-wide DNA methylation changes by an iron-mediated and Tet-dependent mechanism. *Nucleic Acids Res.* **2014**, *42*, 1593–1605. [CrossRef]
86. Freudenberg, J.M.; Ghosh, S.; Lackford, B.L.; Yellaboina, S.; Zheng, X.; Li, R.; Cuddapah, S.; Wade, P.A.; Hu, G.; Jothi, R. Acute depletion of Tet1-dependent 5-hydroxymethylcytosine levels impairs LIF/Stat3 signaling and results in loss of embryonic stem cell identity. *Nucleic Acids Res.* **2012**, *40*, 3364–3377. [CrossRef]
87. Zhu, X.; Girardo, D.; Govek, E.E.; John, K.; Mellén, M.; Tamayo, P.; Mesirov, J.P.; Hatten, M.E. Role of Tet1/3 Genes and Chromatin Remodeling Genes in Cerebellar Circuit Formation. *Neuron* **2016**, *89*, 100–112. [CrossRef]

88. Branco, M.R.; Ficz, G.; Reik, W. Uncovering the role of 5-hydroxymethylcytosine in the epigenome. *Nat. Rev. Genet.* **2011**, *13*, 7–13. [CrossRef]
89. Szulwach, K.E.; Li, X.; Li, Y.; Song, C.X.; Wu, H.; Dai, Q.; Irier, H.; Upadhyay, A.K.; Gearing, M.; Levey, A.I.; et al. 5-hmC-mediated epigenetic dynamics during postnatal neurodevelopment and aging. *Nat. Neurosci.* **2011**, *14*, 1607–1616. [CrossRef]
90. Hahn, M.A.; Qiu, R.; Wu, X.; Li, A.X.; Zhang, H.; Wang, J.; Jui, J.; Jin, S.G.; Jiang, Y.; Pfeifer, G.P.; et al. Dynamics of 5-hydroxymethylcytosine and chromatin marks in Mammalian neurogenesis. *Cell. Rep.* **2013**, *3*, 291–300. [CrossRef]
91. Al-Mahdawi, S.; Virmouni, S.A.; Pook, M.A. The emerging role of 5-hydroxymethylcytosine in neurodegenerative diseases. *Front. Neurosci.* **2014**, *8*, 397. [CrossRef]

11

Behavioral Determinants of Objectively Assessed Diet Quality in Obese Pregnancy

Jasper Most [1], Candida J. Rebello [2], Abby D. Altazan [1], Corby K. Martin [3], Marshall St Amant [4] and Leanne M. Redman [1,*]

1 Reproductive Endocrinology and Women's Health, Pennington Biomedical Research Center, Baton Rouge, LA 70817, USA
2 Clinical Trials Unit, Pennington Biomedical Research Center, Baton Rouge, LA 70817, USA
3 Ingestive Behavior, Weight Management, and Health Promotion Laboratory, Pennington Biomedical Research Center, Baton Rouge, LA 70817, USA
4 Woman's Hospital, 100 Woman's Way, Baton Rouge, LA 70817, USA
* Correspondence: leanne.redman@pbrc.edu

Abstract: Interventions to promote healthy pregnancy in women with obesity by improving diet quality have been widely unsuccessful. We hypothesized that diet quality is determined by eating behaviors, but evidence in women with obesity is lacking. We evaluated diet quality and eating behavior in 56 women with obesity (mean ± SEM, 36.7 ± 0.7 kg/m^2, 46% White, 50% nulliparous) early in pregnancy (14.9 ± 0.1 weeks). Diet quality was objectively assessed with food photography over six days and defined by Healthy Eating Index. Eating behaviors were assessed by validated questionnaires. Women reported consuming diets high in fat (38 ± 1% of energy) and the HEI was considered "poor" on average (46.7 ± 1.3), and for 71% of women. Diet quality was independently associated with education level ($p = 0.01$), food cravings ($p < 0.01$), and awareness towards eating ($p = 0.01$). Cravings for sweets and fast foods were positively correlated with respective intakes of these foods ($p < 0.01$ and $p = 0.04$, respectively), whereas cravings for fruits and vegetables did not relate to diet intake. We provide evidence of the determinants of poor diet quality in pregnant women with obesity. Based on this observational study, strategies to improve diet quality and pregnancy outcomes are to satisfy cravings for healthy snacks and foods, and to promote awareness towards eating behaviors.

Keywords: Pregnancy; obesity; diet quality; Healthy Eating Index; food cravings; mindful eating; education; race; food photography

1. Introduction

Poor quality of maternal diet is considered one of the most significant predictors of adverse pregnancy outcomes [1–5] and poor infant health [5–9]. Both poor diet quality and adverse pregnancy outcomes are more frequent among women with obesity [10,11].

Among women with normal weight or who are overweight, improvements in maternal diet quality reduced the prevalence of adverse outcomes including excess gestational weight gain [12,13], gestational diabetes, and hypertensive disorders in mothers [2] and macrosomia in infants [14]. However, in women with obesity, successful dietary interventions are seldom reported, likely due to small effects on diet quality [14–17].

To develop more successful behavioral interventions for women with obesity requires an understanding of determinants of poor diet quality, i.e., consumption of specific food groups, mindful eating, or food cravings. Others have shown in 24 h recalls, that poor diet quality of women with obesity was determined by low intake of fruits [10], but not due to intake of other food groups. Eating behaviors such as mindful eating or food cravings associate with poor diet quality in nonpregnant subjects [18]. Women with obesity appear more likely to report indulgence in food cravings and less mindfulness towards eating, but such data has only been reported in women who were not pregnant [19]. Furthermore, the available evidence from these studies is limited by their use of self-reported diet data, varying metrics for diet quality, and lack of information on eating behaviors to understand how behaviors could be targeted to improve diet quality. To our knowledge, no study has defined the behavioral determinants of diet quality in pregnant women with obesity.

The aim of this study was to characterize diet quality in pregnant women with obesity and identify maternal eating patterns and behaviors that contribute to the quality of the diet in early pregnancy. In addition, we assessed if maternal eating attitudes and behaviors are influenced by race, education level, or nausea and vomiting. To this end, dietary intake, including diet quality and eating patterns, and eating attitudes and behaviors were simultaneously assessed between 13 and 16 weeks gestation. We hypothesized that maternal eating behavior such as food cravings and mindfulness would contribute to maternal diet quality objectively assessed by food photography.

2. Materials and Methods

2.1. Study Design

Participants were enrolled in a prospective observational study at the Pennington Biomedical Research Center to assess the determinants of gestational weight gain [20,21]. Between 13 and 16 weeks of gestation (14.9 ± 0.1 weeks), dietary intake and eating patterns were assessed over six consecutive days by a validated food photography method [22]. Eating behaviors were assessed with self-report questionnaires. The study was approved by the Pennington Biomedical Research Center Institutional Review Board and written informed consent was obtained from all participants prior to the initiation of procedures.

2.2. Participants

Enrolled women were pregnant, 18 to 40 years of age, with a measured BMI $\geq$30 kg/m^2 at the screening visit (gestational age, <15 weeks). Obesity was defined as class I: 30$\leq$BMI<35 kg/m^2, class II: 35$\leq$BMI<40 kg/m^2, and class III: BMI$\geq$40 kg/m^2. Women who reported smoking, alcohol, or drug use or had pre-existing hypertension, diabetes (HbA1c $\geq$6.5%), psychological or eating disorders or reported medications/supplements that might affect body weight, planned termination of pregnancy, and bariatric surgery were excluded. Fasting plasma glucose was measured in a venous blood sample, collected after an overnight fast at the research center. Sociodemographic parameters including age, race, parity, family income, education, and employment were obtained from self-report questionnaires. Poverty to income ratio was determined as the ratio of individual income to poverty threshold based on family size.

2.3. Dietary Assessment

Dietary intake was assessed over six days with the SmartIntake® smartphone application, which is a validated food photography method for adult energy intake and diet quality, as assessed by macronutrient intake (kcal from protein, fat, or carbohydrate) and intake of vitamin C, calcium, iron, sodium, or fiber [22]. Prior to analysis, routine data handling procedures were followed and days in which reported caloric intake was <60% of total daily energy expenditure measured by doubly labeled water, were excluded to improve accuracy and eliminate reporting bias by BMI [20]. Total daily energy expenditure was measured for seven days simultaneous to dietary intake [20]. When using SmartIntake®, participants captured images of meals or food items consumed and plate (food) waste. Participants defined the type of meal (breakfast, lunch, dinner, snacks) and every image was automatically time-stamped to allow calculation of eating patterns (first and last meal of a day, eating duration). Images were transmitted automatically in real-time via the phone application and were reviewed as a set by the participant and study staff at the end of the assessment period to document potential missing data. Dietitians determined portion sizes using validated visual comparison procedures [22], and the nutritional characteristics of each food were determined from the United States Department of Agriculture (USDA) Food and Nutrient Database for Dietary Studies 2011–2012 [23] and manufacturers' nutrient information.

Diet quality was defined by macronutrient composition expressed relative to total energy intake (%EI), by the 2015 Healthy Eating Index (HEI) [24] and by macronutrient and micronutrient intake as compared to the intake recommendations by the Institute of Medicine [25,26]. To calculate HEI, foods and beverages were converted into the 37 USDA food pattern components [27] using the Food Patterns Equivalents Database (FPED). The FPED serves as a unique research tool to evaluate food and beverage intakes of Americans with respect to the 2015–2020 Dietary Guidelines for Americans recommendations [28]. The 37 USDA scores were converted into 12 HEI subscores measured as cup equivalents of fruit, vegetables, and dairy; ounce equivalents of grains and protein foods; teaspoon equivalents of added sugars; gram equivalents of solid fats and oils; and the number of alcoholic drinks. The HEI is a composite score of these subscores. The Healthy Eating Index 2015 ranges from 0 to 100, and HEI <51 indicates "Poor", a score between 51 and 80 indicates "Needs Improvement" and a HEI score >80 indicates "Good".

2.4. Nausea and Vomiting of Pregnancy

The Modified-Pregnancy-Unique Quantification of Emesis and Nausea Index (PUQE) questionnaire [29] is a validated instrument that assesses the severity of nausea and vomiting of pregnancy [29,30]. A PUQE Summary Score of ≤6 is considered as having no or mild symptoms of nausea and vomiting of pregnancy, a score between 7 and 12 is considered moderate and a score of ≥13 is defined as severe.

2.5. Eating Inventory

The Eating Inventory (EI), previously known as the Three Factor Eating Questionnaire [31,32], evaluates eating behavior in three factor domains: dietary restraint, disinhibition, and perceived hunger. A low score for dietary restraint, and high scores for disinhibition and perceived hunger, indicate less control over eating behavior and more episodic overeating.

2.6. Food Cravings

Food cravings were evaluated with the Food Craving Inventory (FCI), which measures the frequency of food cravings over the previous month. The FCI measures general cravings as well as cravings for high-fat foods, sweets, carbohydrates/starches, and fast food fats [33]. The version used in this study also included a scale to measure cravings for fruits and vegetables, and cravings for specific foods measured with the FCI have been found to correlate with intake of those foods [34].

2.7. Mindfulness

Mindfulness towards eating was assessed with the Mindful Eating Questionnaire (MEQ) which has been validated in pregnant women [35]. The MEQ explores mindfulness across five subscales, including disinhibition, awareness, external cues, emotional response, and distraction [36]. Mindful eating refers to an unbiased awareness of sensations around eating. Disinhibition measures the inability to stop eating even when full. The awareness subscale measures an individual's awareness of the sensory aspects of eating. Distraction refers to the tendency to think about other things and rush while eating. The external cues subscale refers to eating in response to environmental cues, and emotional response refers to eating in response to negative emotions. The emotional response and distraction subscales are reverse scored, and five questions on the disinhibition are reverse scored. High scores are indicative of mindful eating.

2.8. Statistical Analysis

The sample size was attained from available data of the prospective observational study to assess determinants of gestational weight gain (clinicaltrials.gov: NCT01954342), with energy intake measured by energy intake-balance method [37] as the primary outcome. At the given sample size ($n = 56$), the minimal detectable simple correlation for a power of 80%, at a two-sided significance level of 0.05, was $r = 0.37$. For the regression analysis, we assessed the power (1-β) of independent predictors post-hoc. Relationships between diet quality, eating patterns, and constructs of eating behavior were first evaluated by simple Pearson correlation coefficients. Significant correlations were linear; using power other than 1 did not increase the explained variability (change in $R^2 < 0.01$). To test independent effects of eating behaviors on diet quality adjusted for demographic factors, we performed linear regression with HEI as the dependent variable and significant individual correlates of HEI as independent variables. Frequencies were compared using Chi-Square tests. Comparisons between African-American and White women were performed by independent Student's *t*-test. Statistical analyses were completed using SPSS Inc. software, Version 24 for Windows (IBM Corp, Armonk, NY). Data are presented as mean ± SEM. All tests were performed with significance level $\alpha = 0.05$, and findings were considered significant when $p < \alpha$.

3. Results

Fifty-six women with obesity (36.7 ± 0.7 kg/m^2, 46% White, 50% nulliparous) who collected dietary intake data that satisfied the criteria for inclusion were included in this analysis (Table 1).

Table 1. Subject Characteristics.

	All, *n* = 56	Association with Diet Quality, Healthy Eating Index
	Mean ± SEM	*r*, *p*
Race, *n* (African-American, White, Others)	25, 26, 5	0.11, 0.43
Gestational Age, weeks	11.3 ± 0.3	-
Maternal Age, years	28.3 ± 0.6	0.19, 0.16
Body weight, kg	97.8 ± 2.2	-
Body mass index, kg/m^2	36.7 ± 0.7	0.01, 0.96
Obesity Class, *n* (1, 2, 3)	23, 21, 12	-
Fasting Plasma Glucose, mmol/L (range)	4.9 ± 0.1 (4.2, 6.1)	0.17, 0.20
Education, *n* (1, 2, 3)	6, 39, 11	0.31, 0.02
Employment, *n* (1, 2, 3, 4)	1, 14, 9, 32	0.18, 0.18
Household Income *	3.6 ± 0.3	0.14, 0.30
Parity, *n* (0, 1, ≥2)	28, 16, 12	−0.10, 0.46
Healthy Eating Index	46.7 ± 1.3	-

Education is categorized into High School (1), college (2), postgraduate work (3). Employment into medically disabled (1), unemployed (2), part-time employment (3), and full-time employment (4). * Household income was computed as a percent of federal poverty line ("poverty" < 1.0) according to family size. Parity is defined as number of previous pregnancies of viable infant >20 weeks gestation.

3.1. Dietary Assessment

Participants reported consuming 3.8 ± 0.1 meals per day, of which 2.7 ± 0.05 meals were reported as main meals (breakfast, lunch, or dinner) and 1.1 ± 0.1 meals as snacks. The average reported eating duration (time between first and last photograph of any meal eaten) was 8:28 ± 0:31 h.

The mean reported energy intake was 2165 ± 43 kcal/day, which is equivalent to 84 ± 2% of energy requirements assessed by doubly labeled water during the same period. On average, participants consumed 46 ± 1% of energy as carbohydrates, 38 ± 1% as fat (41% saturated fatty acids, 35% mono-unsaturated fatty acids, 24% poly-unsaturated fatty acids), and 16 ± 1% as protein. The HEI of the diet was 46.7 ± 1.3, which is considered to reflect a "Poor" (<51) diet quality (Table 1). The HEI was positively associated with education level, but was not associated with BMI (as continuous or categorical variable; Class 1: 46.2 ± 1.9, Class 2: 45.9 ± 2.4, Class 3: 49.1 ± 2.6, $p = 0.47$), parity, race, age, income, or employment (Table 1). Breakfast consumption ($p = 0.04$) and an earlier last meal of the day ($p < 0.01$) were associated with a higher HEI.

On an individual level, 71% of women in the cohort ($n = 40$) had a HEI <51 that is "poor", 29% had a HEI between 50 and 80 indicating that diet quality "needs improvement", and none of the participants had a HEI >80 which is "good" diet quality (Supplemental Table S1). Scores of the individual components within the HEI are summarized in Figure 1A and Table S1. Among these, only mean intake of protein foods exceeded 80% of the HEI maximum protein score. Vegetables, dairy, refined grains, and added sugars were between 50% and 80% of the maximum scores within the respective categories, and intake of fruits (total fruits including juices, and whole fruits), greens and beans, whole-grains, seafood, and plant protein, fatty acids and saturated fats, and sodium were below 50%, and thereby "poor".

Macronutrient and fat composition associated significantly with diet quality. HEI associated with intakes of protein (as % of total energy intake, $r = 0.29$, $p = 0.03$), but not carbohydrates. Moreover, HEI was not associated with overall fat intake, but with intakes of saturated fatty acids ($r = -0.37$, $p = 0.005$), mono-unsaturated fatty acids ($r = 0.32$, $p = 0.02$), and the ratio of unsaturated to saturated fatty acids ($r = 0.37$, $p = 0.005$). Macronutrient and micronutrient intakes as compared to the recommendations by the Institute of Medicine are presented in Figure 1B. For majority of nutrients, intakes were close to or exceeding the recommendations, but intakes of fiber (62.5 ± 3.5%), vitamin B12 (41.5 ± 8.0%), vitamin E (69.2 ± 3.8%), and iron (66.0 ± 2.9%) were particularly low.

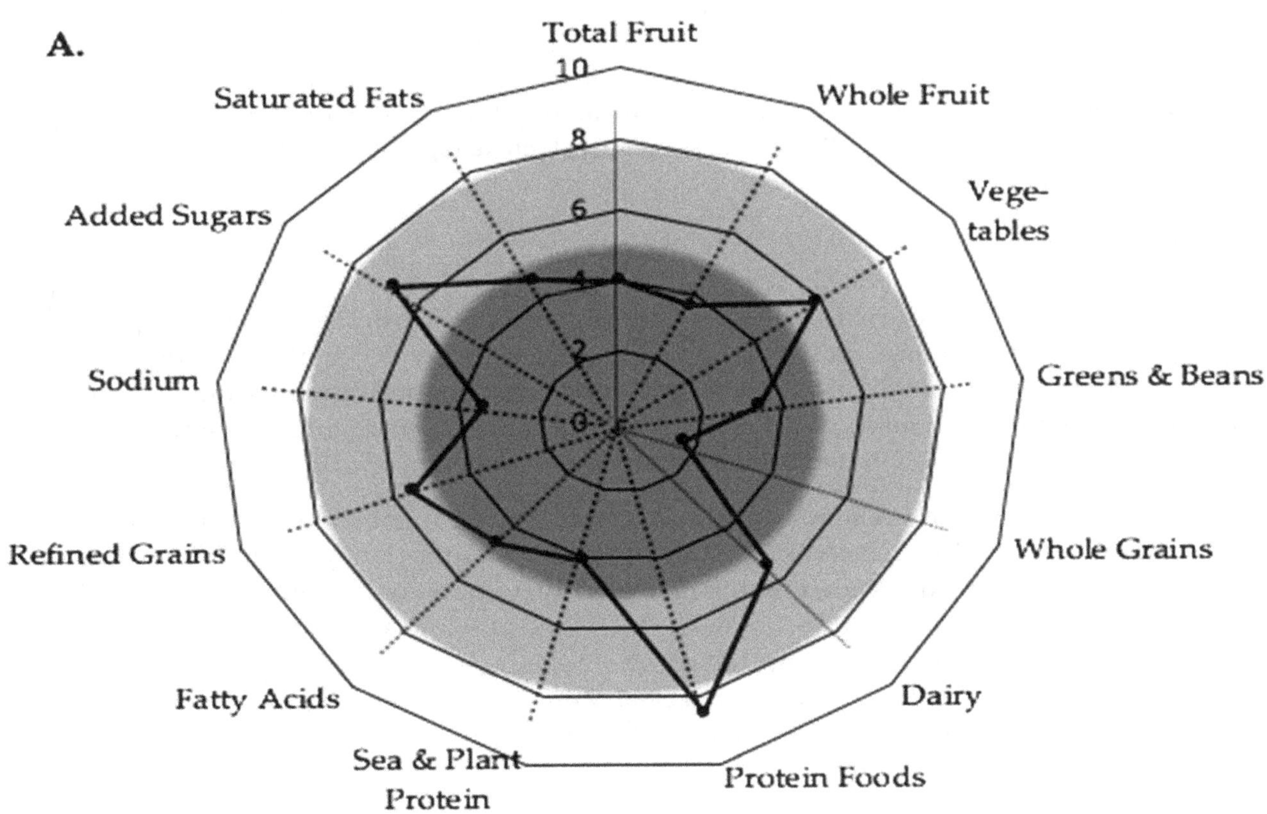

Figure 1. *Cont.*

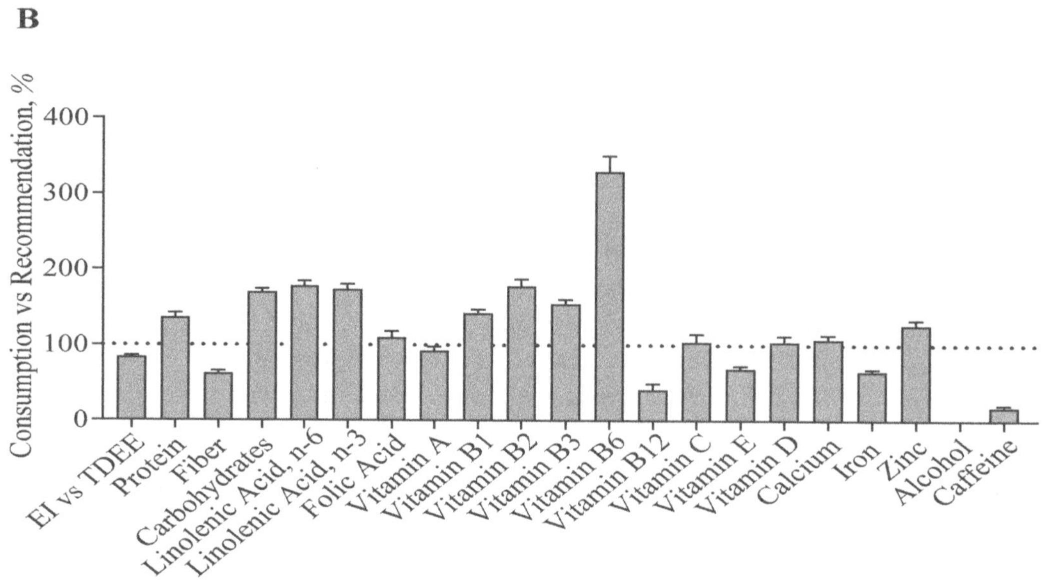

Figure 1. Diet Quality per Healthy Eating Index Components, and Recommendations for Intakes of Macronutrients and Micronutrients. Data are given as mean and mean ± SEM. (**A**) Values in the dark grey area indicate the respective Healthy Eating Index (HEI) food group to be consumed "poorly" (0–5), values in the light grey area as "needs improvement" (5–8) and in the white area as "sufficient" (8–10), according to the HEI guidelines [25]. HEI components scaled from 0–10 are reported as assessed and components scaled 0–5 were multiplied by two to facilitate comparability between factors. (**B**) Values are expressed as intake as compared to the minimal macronutrient and micronutrient intake recommendation by the WHO (maximum intake recommendation for alcohol and caffeine). Macronutrient and Micronutrient intake values are adjusted for the degree of underreporting per individual (−16 ± 2% vs. TDEE, adjusted intake=reported intake/reporting accuracy ["EI vs. TDEE"]).

3.2. Food Cravings

The total food craving score was 2.19 ± 0.07, ranging from 1.09 to 3.33. The most frequent cravings were reported for "fast food fats" and "fruits and vegetables", whereas "high-fat foods" and "sweets" were less frequently craved. In Figure 2, the associations between food cravings and diet quality were reported. Cravings for "high fat foods", "sweets", "carbohydrates and starches", and "fast food fats" associated negatively with HEI, but cravings for "fruit and vegetables" did not associate with HEI.

Cravings for "sweets" correlated significantly with added sugar intake ($r = 0.39$, $p < 0.01$), but were not associated with the reported frequency of snack consumption ($p = 0.65$). Cravings for "fast food fats" were significantly associated with increased consumption of carbohydrate ($r = 0.27$, $p = 0.04$) and less consumption of fats ($r = -0.30$, $p = 0.03$). Increased cravings for both "sweets" and "fast food fats" were associated with poor consumption of whole grains, seafood, and plant proteins ("sweets": $p = 0.02$ and $p = 0.04$, and "fast food fats": $p = 0.04$ and $p = 0.01$, respectively). Cravings for "Fruit and Vegetables" did not correlate with intake of any HEI component.

3.3. Eating Inventory

The average scores from the Eating Inventory were 8.1 ± 0.6 for cognitive restraint, 5.4 ± 0.4 for disinhibition and 3.9 ± 0.3 for hunger. Fourteen (25%) women in the cohort were considered restrained eaters and one (2%) a disinhibited eater (respective subscores >12). The HEI score for diet quality was not associated cognitive restraint ($p = 0.09$), disinhibition ($p = 0.73$), or hunger ($p = 0.43$).

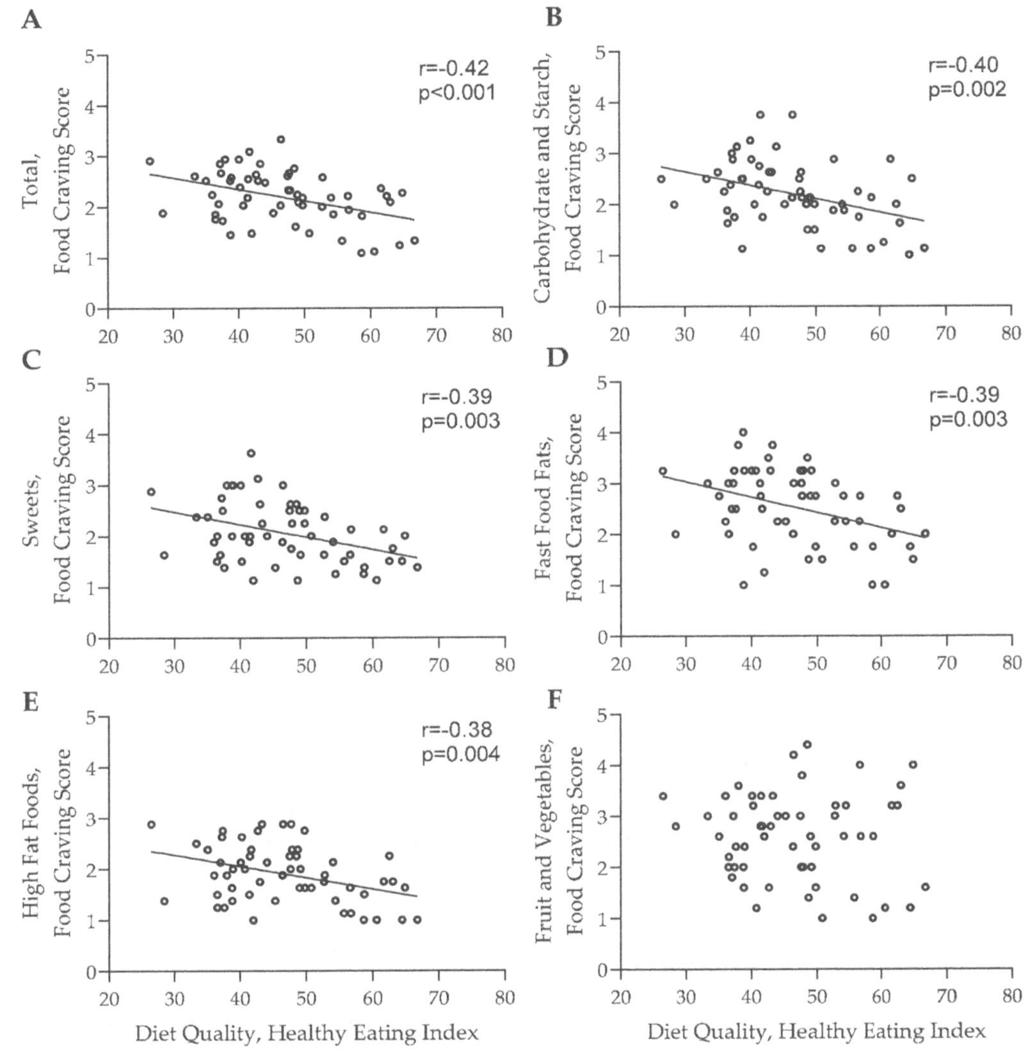

Figure 2. Food Cravings and Diet Quality. Food cravings scores are reported per individual in relation to their respective Healthy Eating Index. Cravings are reported as (**A**) total cravings and as cravings for (**B**) Carbohydrates and Starch, (**C**) Sweets, (**D**) Fast Food Fats, (**E**) High Fat Foods and (**F**) Fruit and Vegetables. Significant associations are indicated by linear regression.

3.4. *Mindful Eating*

The mindful eating summary score was 2.93 ± 0.04. Overall mindfulness as assessed by the summary score was not associated with HEI ($p = 0.22$), meal/snack frequency, or timing. Subscores higher than the overall summary score indicating mindfulness towards these eating behaviors were reported for eating in response to negative emotions ("emotional eating"), inability to stop eating even when full ("disinhibition") and the tendency to think about other things and rush while eating ("distraction"). Of the mindful eating subscores, only awareness correlated with HEI ($r = 0.34$, $p = 0.01$). Awareness associated significantly with consumption of "Greens and Beans" ($r = 0.30$, $p = 0.02$), but not with other HEI components.

3.5. *Nausea and Vomiting and the Influence on Diet Quality*

Forty-six percent of women reported no or only mild symptoms of nausea and vomiting whereas 54% experienced moderate symptoms, and none reported severe symptoms. Nausea and vomiting severity did not correlate with demographic characteristics or HEI but was associated with a lower energy intake ($p = 0.02$), skipping breakfast ($p = 0.02$), eating later in the day ($p < 0.01$), and consuming all meals during a shorter period of time ($p < 0.01$).

3.6. The Influence of Maternal Education on Diet Quality and Eating Behaviors

Education level was positively associated with HEI ($r = 0.31$, $p = 0.02$). Women with higher education consumed more whole grains ($p = 0.03$), greens and beans ($p = 0.02$), and less added sugars ($p = 0.04$). Women with higher education also reported eating more main meals ($r = 0.30$, $p = 0.02$), and increased awareness towards the sensory aspects of eating ($r = 0.33$, $p = 0.01$). Education level was positively associated with disinhibition scores, which indicates that higher educated women had less control over eating behavior ($r = 0.31$, $p = 0.02$). The intent to restrict food intake also was associated with education level (cognitive restraint, $r = 0.29$, $p = 0.03$) and could be in response to the tendency to overeat, as indicated by the association between disinhibition and education level.

3.7. Independent Effects of Awareness, Cravings, and Education

In the linear stepwise regression model with HEI as the dependent variable and significant individual correlates with HEI ($n = 8$) as independent variables, we observed that an early last meal of the day (standardized $\beta = -0.40$, $p < 0.001$, $1-\beta = 0.94$), cravings for sweets (standardized $\beta = -0.35$, $p = 0.004$, $1-\beta = 0.84$), and education (standardized $\beta = 0.27$, $p = 0.02$, $1-\beta = 0.65$) were independent predictors of HEI ($R^2 = 0.38$, $p < 0.001$), but not other cravings, awareness towards eating or breakfast consumption.

3.8. The Influence of Maternal Race on Diet Quality and Eating Behaviors

African-American women reported lower education, less income and higher parity than White women. The HEI was not significantly different between African-American and White women (AA: 45.2 ± 1.8 vs. White: 47.2 ± 1.8, $p = 0.44$). Reported energy intake as compared to energy requirements was also comparable between races. However, eating patterns and eating behaviors differed significantly by maternal race. Compared to White women, African-American women consumed their first meal later in the day (+1:28 ± 0:36 h, $p = 0.03$), and reported eating fewer snacks (African-American vs. White, −0.6 ± 0.2 snacks/day, $p = 0.01$). African-American women reported more cravings for high-fat foods and carbohydrates and starches ($p = 0.02$ and $p = 0.03$, respectively), yet less disinhibition ($p < 0.01$), indicating better control over their eating behavior compared to White women (Table 2).

Table 2. Eating Behavior Assessment.

	African-American, *n* = 26	White, *n* = 25	*p* for Race	Range	High Values Indicative of
Food Cravings					
High Fat	2.12 ± 0.11	1.76 ± 0.10	0.02	1–5	More Craving
Sweets	2.12 ± 0.12	2.04 ± 0.12	0.64	1–5	More Craving
Carbohydrates and Starch	2.42 ± 0.11	2.03 ± 0.13	0.03	1–5	More Craving
Fast Food Fats	2.65 ± 0.12	2.47 ± 0.18	0.41	1–5	More Craving
Fruit and Vegetables	2.79 ± 0.16	2.45 ± 0.18	0.16	1–5	More Craving
Total Score	2.36 ± 0.09	2.08 ± 0.11	0.06	1–5	More Craving
Mindful Eating					
Awareness	2.58 ± 0.12	2.53 ± 0.10	0.77	1–4	Mindfulness
Distraction	3.24 ± 0.10	2.95 ± 0.13	0.09	1–4	Mindfulness
Disinhibition	3.34 ± 0.08	3.00 ± 0.10	0.01	1–4	Mindfulness
Emotional Cues	3.54 ± 0.09	3.32 ± 0.10	0.11	1–4	Mindfulness
External	2.29 ± 0.11	2.69 ± 0.10	0.01	1–4	Mindfulness
Summary Score	2.99 ± 0.06	2.89 ± 0.06	0.24	1–4	Mindfulness
Eating Inventory					
Cognitive Restraint	8.08 ± 1.04	7.69 ± 0.91	0.78	0–21	Greater Control
Disinhibition	4.20 ± 0.47	6.69 ± 0.66	0.004	0–16	Less Control
Hunger	3.52 ± 0.42	4.50 ± 0.40	0.10	0–14	Less Control
PUQE					
Summary Score	6.48 ± 0.43	5.54 ± 0.4	0.12	3–15	Severe Symptoms

PUQE, Modified-Pregnancy-Unique Quantification of Emesis and Nausea Index.

4. Discussion

Improvements in diet quality during pregnancy can prevent poor outcomes in nonobese women [1–9], but dietary interventions have been largely unsuccessful in women with obesity [12,14,16,17,38,39]. We speculate that this may be explained in part by intervention approaches not being specific to the eating patterns and behaviors in women with obesity and thus achieving only small effect sizes on diet quality. Identifying maternal eating patterns that relate to diet quality in women with obesity will help inform the development of future dietary interventions with greater specificity for this group. To this end, we performed an observational cohort study and measured diet quality and eating behavior in 56 healthy women with obesity. In support of our hypothesis, diet quality in early pregnancy was poor, which was related to increased food cravings and less awareness towards eating. Nausea and vomiting severity were not associated with diet quality, but were inversely related to breakfast consumption and energy intake. Lastly, we observed that diet quality and eating behaviors differed by education and race, respectively.

Diet quality in our cohort of pregnant women with obesity was poor (HEI = 47, fat content = 38%) and lower than prior reports of nonpregnancy cohorts in the US (49–64 [40–43]). Interventions in pregnant cohorts with poor diet quality may be more successful in improving maternal and infant outcomes as compared to previous lifestyle intervention studies, because the opportunity for improvement is larger. Diet quality was higher in pregnant women in Australia (HEI = 72 [38]) and the UK (fat content = 31% [15]), and diet quality improved by only 2% [12,38] to 5% [32], as assessed by healthy eating index [38], adherence score to the recommended diet [12], Glycemic Index and Glycemic Load [15].

We observed that poor diet quality is due to poor consumption of all food groups, except for protein intake, and thus appropriate interventions require approaches to target all components of the diet, e.g., Mediterranean diet, DASH diet. Nevertheless, our data also identify specific food groups and behaviors that may affect overall diet quality more than others. For example, strategies to reduce high fat intake, e.g., by reducing fast food intake, will likely reduce saturated fatty acid intake, but may also result in less refined grain consumption. Moreover, increasing fruit and vegetable consumption would likely increase dietary fiber and unsaturated fatty acid intake, thus providing a strategy to improve multiple diet quality components. Increasing fiber intake may not only improve satiety and reduce energy intake [44,45], but also improve gastrointestinal health and glucose homeostasis [46].

Food cravings increase the desire to eat and the satisfaction associated with eating [47]. In the present study, cravings for healthy foods, e.g., fruits and vegetables, were reported more frequently compared to cravings for unhealthy foods, e.g., sweets, fast food, high fat foods. Despite the frequent cravings, fruit was consumed in poor quantities according to the 2015–2020 Dietary Guidelines for Americans [29]. The inability to increase consumption of healthy foods in order to satisfy food cravings for such foods may be due to a lack of availability, perceived cost, or misperception about the health of certain foods [48]. Facilitating indulgence in cravings for healthy foods may also prevent cravings and consumption of unhealthy foods [49].

Conversely to cravings for healthy foods, cravings for foods with poor nutritional value were often indulged in and thereby contributed to poor diet quality, which is consistent with other studies [50]. Specifically, cravings for sweets were linked to intake of added sugar. This data supports and connects evidence for a causal relationship between cravings for sugar [51], consumption of sugar [52] and excess gestational weight gain. We also observed that fast food fats were frequently craved and correlated with poor diet quality, whereas high fat foods were less frequently craved. The fast food fats subscale is comprised solely of pizza, hamburgers, french fries, and potato chips, while the high fat subscale includes eight foods, including bacon, gravy, and sausage. Thus, an important factor distinguishing the two fat subscales is ease of access being that fast food fats are easier to acquire compared to foods on the high fat subscale. Hence, these data support the notion that food accessibility may influence the perception of cravings and the likelihood of eating for indulgence.

Increasing consciousness about diet choices may benefit diet quality [53,54]. We observed that awareness towards eating was associated with better diet quality. This confirms previous reports of mindfulness in pregnant women with overweight and obesity [36,55]. In addition, we show that mindfulness associates specifically with consumption of healthy foods, i.e., 'Greens and Beans', but not with other HEI components. Thus, whereas increasing awareness would likely increase consumption of healthy food items, no direct effect of reducing intake of unhealthy foods would be expected. To our knowledge, only one study has successfully implemented a mindfulness-based intervention in overweight, pregnant women [56,57]; however, the effect of the intervention on diet quality or pregnancy outcomes was not reported.

We hypothesized that diet quality and eating behaviors would be affected by maternal demographic characteristics such as education and race. Diet quality was poor in women with a college degree or postgraduate education (HEI = 49.2) and in women with lower education levels (HEI = 44.4, $p = 0.06$), which confirms similar findings of previous studies [58]. Women with less education were less aware of their eating behavior and had a lower intent to restrict food intake, which may reflect lacking or misguided knowledge on the risks of excess weight gain [59]. Qualitative studies in women enrolled in the Special Supplemental Nutrition Program for Women, Infants, and Children (WIC) program who generally have poor socio-economic status, report that they indeed feel uninformed about weight gain in pregnancy and that receiving more information may increase the intent to restrict food intake to optimize pregnancy outcomes [60]. Women with higher education levels had lower disinhibition scores, indicating poorer self-control. To understand the main independent effects of individual correlates with diet quality, we performed linear regression analysis with HEI as the dependent variable. We identified education, cravings for sweets and an early last meal of the day as independent predictors of diet quality. Awareness towards eating was not a significant predictor in the model, which suggests that the beneficial effect of increased awareness towards eating on diet quality is mediated by eating the last meal of the day earlier, or that education, cravings for sweets, and awareness were low/high in the same women and were thus not independent of each other. Indeed, awareness correlated significantly with both education and cravings for sweets.

We observed significant differences in eating behaviors, but not in diet quality between African-American and White women in the present study, indicating the need for different approaches to improve poor diet quality in all women. African-American women, who reported lower education levels, less income, and higher parity, consumed the first meal later in the day but not the last meal, so eating duration tended to be shorter. The severity of morning sickness was not reported to be different between African-American and White women. The observation that African-American women ate breakfast less frequently, and thus ate later in the day may have contributed to a reduced dietary intake, which we reported previously [21]. In line with these findings, African-American women also reported better control over their eating behavior and reported less snacking despite more cravings.

The strength of this study is the use of food photography. Food photography methods are more accurate in measuring portion sizes and the composition of meals since these are analyzed in an objective manner [22]. Furthermore, the food photography method is performed in real time and is not prone to recall bias as with instruments reliant on recall, yet possibly to "attention bias" for the reporting of snacks [20]. With respect to energy intake, implementation of data quality criteria in the analytical stages minimizes the degree of under-reporting to less than 20% compared to doubly labeled water and eliminates increased reporting bias typically observed with higher energy intake [20]. The major weakness of this study is the lack of prepregnancy data. Thereby, we were unable to determine whether poor diet quality and associated eating behaviors can be targeted prior to pregnancy. Further, the observation period (six days) was relatively short as compared to other instruments such as a food frequency questionnaire which recalls intake over a period of 1 to 12 months. Eating behaviors were assessed by questionnaires and are prone to self-reporting bias. Importantly, all questionnaires were previously validated in pregnancy. In addition, micronutrient, but not macronutrient, intakes may be higher than reported due to prenatal vitamin supplement intake. Lastly, this study did not enroll women without obesity, and therefore we were unable to compare diet quality and eating behaviors between women with normal weight, overweight, or obesity. Early pregnancy diabetes was excluded by HbA1c, but no glucose tolerance test was performed to determine gestational diabetes.

5. Conclusions

The main behavioral determinants of poor diet quality in pregnant women with obesity include the low consumption of fruits and vegetables, the indulgence into cravings for sweets, and eating late in the day. Future intervention strategies developed with a specificity for improving diet quality are therefore to increase the availability of fruits and vegetables rather than sweets or fast foods, which may facilitate indulgence in the observed cravings for healthy foods, and to reduce late-night snacking. In addition, women with lower education levels may benefit from educational interventions on the risks of overeating, whereas women with higher education may benefit from strategies to increase self-control. Future studies are required to show whether strategies to change those behaviors can be successfully implemented and improve pregnancy outcomes in women with obesity.

Author Contributions: Conceptualization, J.M., L.M.R.; methodology, J.M., A.D.A., C.J.R.; software, J.M.; validation, A.D.A., C.J.R. and L.M.R.; formal analysis, J.M., L.M.R.; investigation, J.M., C.J.R., A.D.A., and L.M.R.; resources, L.M.R.; data curation, J.M.; writing—original draft preparation, J.M.; writing—review and editing, J.M., C.J.R., A.D.A., M.S.A. C.K.M. L.M.R.; visualization, J.M.; supervision, L.M.R.; project administration, L.M.R.; funding acquisition, C.K.M. and L.M.R.

Acknowledgments: We are indebted to the participants and clinical/technical support from Porsha Vallo, Elizabeth Sutton, Karissa Elsass, Taylor Ayers and Ray Allen.

References

1. Mijatovic-Vukas, J.; Capling, L.; Cheng, S.; Stamatakis, E.; Louie, J.; Cheung, N.W.; Markovic, T.; Ross, G.; Senior, A.; Brand-Miller, J.C.; et al. Associations of Diet and Physical Activity with Risk for Gestational Diabetes Mellitus: A Systematic Review and Meta-Analysis. *Nutrients* **2018**, *10*, 698. [CrossRef] [PubMed]
2. Schoenaker, D.A.; Soedamah-Muthu, S.S.; Mishra, G.D. Quantifying the mediating effect of body mass index on the relation between a Mediterranean diet and development of maternal pregnancy complications: The Australian Longitudinal Study on Women's Health. *Am. J. Clin. Nutr.* **2016**, *104*, 638–645. [CrossRef] [PubMed]
3. Hillesund, E.R.; Overby, N.C.; Engel, S.M.; Klungsoyr, K.; Harmon, Q.E.; Haugen, M.; Bere, E. Associations of adherence to the New Nordic Diet with risk of preeclampsia and preterm delivery in the Norwegian Mother and Child Cohort Study (MoBa). *Eur. J. Epidemiol.* **2014**, *29*, 753–765. [CrossRef] [PubMed]
4. Zhang, C.; Tobias, D.K.; Chavarro, J.E.; Bao, W.; Wang, D.; Ley, S.H.; Hu, F.B. Adherence to healthy lifestyle and risk of gestational diabetes mellitus: Prospective cohort study. *BMJ* **2014**, *349*, g5450. [CrossRef] [PubMed]
5. Gresham, E.; Collins, C.E.; Mishra, G.D.; Byles, J.E.; Hure, A.J. Diet quality before or during pregnancy and the relationship with pregnancy and birth outcomes: The Australian Longitudinal Study on Women's Health. *Public Health Nutr.* **2016**, *19*, 2975–2983. [CrossRef] [PubMed]
6. Koletzko, B.; Brands, B.; Grote, V.; Kirchberg, F.F.; Prell, C.; Rzehak, P.; Uhl, O.; Weber, M. Early Nutrition Programming Project. Long-Term Health Impact of Early Nutrition: The Power of Programming. *Ann. Nutr. Metab.* **2017**, *70*, 161–169. [CrossRef]
7. Shapiro, A.L.; Kaar, J.L.; Crume, T.L.; Starling, A.P.; Siega-Riz, A.M.; Ringham, B.M.; Glueck, D.H.; Norris, J.M.; Barbour, L.A.; Friedman, J.E.; et al. Maternal diet quality in pregnancy and neonatal adiposity: The Healthy Start Study. *Int. J. Obes.* **2016**, *40*, 1056–1062. [CrossRef]
8. Grandy, M.; Snowden, J.M.; Boone-Heinonen, J.; Purnell, J.Q.; Thornburg, K.L.; Marshall, N.E. Poorer maternal diet quality and increased birth weight. *J. Matern. Fetal Neonatal Med.* **2018**, *31*, 1613–1619. [CrossRef]

9. Brei, C.; Stecher, L.; Meyer, D.M.; Young, V.; Much, D.; Brunner, S.; Hauner, H. Impact of Dietary Macronutrient Intake during Early and Late Gestation on Offspring Body Composition at Birth, 1, 3, and 5 Years of Age. *Nutrients* **2018**, *10*, 579. [CrossRef]
10. Shin, D.; Lee, K.W.; Song, W.O. Pre-Pregnancy Weight Status Is Associated with Diet Quality and Nutritional Biomarkers during Pregnancy. *Nutrients* **2016**, *8*, 162. [CrossRef]
11. Catalano, P.M.; Shankar, K. Obesity and pregnancy: Mechanisms of short term and long term adverse consequences for mother and child. *BMJ* **2017**, *356*, j1. [CrossRef] [PubMed]
12. Koivusalo, S.B.; Rono, K.; Klemetti, M.M.; Roine, R.P.; Lindstrom, J.; Erkkola, M.; Kaaja, R.J.; Poyhonen-Alho, M.; Tiitinen, A.; Huvinen, E.; et al. Gestational Diabetes Mellitus Can Be Prevented by Lifestyle Intervention: The Finnish Gestational Diabetes Prevention Study (RADIEL): A Randomized Controlled Trial. *Diabetes Care* **2016**, *39*, 24–30. [CrossRef] [PubMed]
13. Shieh, C.; Cullen, D.L.; Pike, C.; Pressler, S.J. Intervention strategies for preventing excessive gestational weight gain: Systematic review and meta-analysis. *Obes. Rev.* **2018**. [CrossRef] [PubMed]
14. Dodd, J.M.; McPhee, A.J.; Turnbull, D.; Yelland, L.N.; Deussen, A.R.; Grivell, R.M.; Crowther, C.A.; Wittert, G.; Owens, J.A.; Robinson, J.S.; et al. The effects of antenatal dietary and lifestyle advice for women who are overweight or obese on neonatal health outcomes: The LIMIT randomised trial. *BMC Med.* **2014**, *12*, 163. [CrossRef] [PubMed]
15. Poston, L.; Bell, R.; Croker, H.; Flynn, A.C.; Godfrey, K.M.; Goff, L.; Hayes, L.; Khazaezadeh, N.; Nelson, S.M.; Oteng-Ntim, E.; et al. Effect of a behavioural intervention in obese pregnant women (the UPBEAT study): A multicentre, randomised controlled trial. *Lancet Diabetes Endocrinol.* **2015**, *3*, 767–777. [CrossRef]
16. Simmons, D.; Devlieger, R.; van Assche, A.; Jans, G.; Galjaard, S.; Corcoy, R.; Adelantado, J.M.; Dunne, F.; Desoye, G.; Harreiter, J.; et al. Effect of Physical Activity and/or Healthy Eating on GDM Risk: The DALI Lifestyle Study. *J. Clin. Endocrinol. Metab.* **2017**, *102*, 903–913. [CrossRef]
17. Rono, K.; Grotenfelt, N.E.; Klemetti, M.M.; Stach-Lempinen, B.; Huvinen, E.; Meinila, J.; Valkama, A.; Tiitinen, A.; Roine, R.P.; Poyhonen-Alho, M.; et al. Effect of a lifestyle intervention during pregnancy-findings from the Finnish gestational diabetes prevention trial (RADIEL). *J. Perinatol.* **2018**. [CrossRef]
18. Boswell, R.G.; Kober, H. Food cue reactivity and craving predict eating and weight gain: A meta-analytic review. *Obes. Rev.* **2016**, *17*, 159–177. [CrossRef]
19. Delahanty, L.M.; Meigs, J.B.; Hayden, D.; Williamson, D.A.; Nathan, D.M.; Diabetes Prevenion Program Research Group. Psychological and behavioral correlates of baseline BMI in the diabetes prevention program (DPP). *Diabetes Care* **2002**, *25*, 1992–1998. [CrossRef]
20. Most, J.; Vallo, P.M.; Altazan, A.D.; Gilmore, L.A.; Sutton, E.F.; Cain, L.E.; Burton, J.H.; Martin, C.K.; Redman, L.M. Food Photography Is Not an Accurate Measure of Energy Intake in Obese, Pregnant Women. *J. Nutr.* **2018**, *148*, 658–663. [CrossRef]
21. Most, J.; Gilmore, L.A.; Altazan, A.D.; St Amant, M.; Beyl, R.A.; Ravussin, E.; Redman, L.M. Propensity for adverse pregnancy outcomes in African-American women may be explained by low energy expenditure in early pregnancy. *Am. J. Clin. Nutr.* **2018**, *107*, 957–964. [CrossRef] [PubMed]
22. Martin, C.K.; Correa, J.B.; Han, H.; Allen, H.R.; Rood, J.C.; Champagne, C.M.; Gunturk, B.K.; Bray, G.A. Validity of the Remote Food Photography Method (RFPM) for estimating energy and nutrient intake in near real-time. *Obesity* **2012**, *20*, 891–899. [CrossRef] [PubMed]
23. Martin, C.L.; Montville, J.B.; Steinfeldt, L.C.; Omolewa-Tomobi, G.; Heendeniya, K.Y.; Adler, M.E.; Moshfegh, A.J. *The USDA Food and Nutrient Database for Dietary Studies 2011–2012*; U.S. Department of Agriculture: Beltsville, MD, USA, 2014.
24. The Epidemiology and Genomics Research Program. Overview & Background of the Healthy Eating Index. Available online: https://epi.grants.cancer.gov/hei/ (accessed on 28 May 2019).
25. Mousa, A.; Naqash, A.; Lim, S. Macronutrient and Micronutrient Intake during Pregnancy: An Overview of Recent Evidence. *Nutrients* **2019**, *11*, 443. [CrossRef] [PubMed]
26. Institute of Medicine (US); National Research Council (US) Committee to Reexamine IOM Pregnancy Weight Guidelines. Determining Optimal Weight Gain. In *Weight Gain During Pregnancy: Reexamining the Guidelines*; Rasmussen, K.M., Yaktine, A.L., Eds.; National Academies Press: Washington, DC, USA, 2009. [CrossRef]
27. Bowman, S.A.; Clemens, J.C.; Friday, J.E.; Lynch, K.L.; Moshfegh, A.J. Food Patterns Equivalents Database 2013–2014: Methodology and User Guide. Available online: http://www.ars.usda.gov/nea/bhnrc/fsrg (accessed on 28 May 2019).

28. Millen, B.; Lichtenstein, A.H.; Abrams, S.; Adams-Campbell, L.; Anderson, C.; Brenna, J.T.; Campbell, W.; Clinton, S.; Foster, G.; Hu, F.; et al. 2015–2020 Dietary Guidelines for Americans. Available online: http://health.gov/dietaryguidelines/2015/guidelines/ (accessed on 28 May 2019).
29. Lacasse, A.; Rey, E.; Ferreira, E.; Morin, C.; Berard, A. Validity of a modified Pregnancy-Unique Quantification of Emesis and Nausea (PUQE) scoring index to assess severity of nausea and vomiting of pregnancy. *Am. J. Obstet. Gynecol.* **2008**, *198*, 71.e1–71.e7. [CrossRef] [PubMed]
30. Birkeland, E.; Stokke, G.; Tangvik, R.J.; Torkildsen, E.A.; Boateng, J.; Wollen, A.L.; Albrechtsen, S.; Flaatten, H.; Trovik, J. Norwegian PUQE (Pregnancy-Unique Quantification of Emesis and nausea) identifies patients with hyperemesis gravidarum and poor nutritional intake: A prospective cohort validation study. *PLoS ONE* **2015**, *10*, e0119962. [CrossRef] [PubMed]
31. Stunkard, A.J.; Messick, S. *Eating Inventory Manual*; Harcourt Brace & Company: San Antonio, TX, USA, 1988.
32. Stunkard, A.J.; Waterland, R.A. The Three-Factor Eating Questionnaire-Eating Inventory. In *Obesity Assessment: Tools, Methods, Interpretation*; St Jeor, S.T., Ed.; Chapman and Hall: New York, NY, USA, 1997; pp. 343–370.
33. White, M.A.; Whisenhunt, B.L.; Williamson, D.A.; Greenway, F.L.; Netemeyer, R.G. Development and validation of the food-craving inventory. *Obes. Res.* **2002**, *10*, 107–114. [CrossRef] [PubMed]
34. Martin, C.K.; O'Neil, P.M.; Tollefson, G.; Greenway, F.L.; White, M.A. The association between food cravings and consumption of specific foods in a laboratory taste test. *Appetite* **2008**, *51*, 324–326. [CrossRef]
35. Apolzan, J.W.; Myers, C.A.; Cowley, A.D.; Brady, H.; Hsia, D.S.; Stewart, T.M.; Redman, L.M.; Martin, C.K. Examination of the reliability and validity of the Mindful Eating Questionnaire in pregnant women. *Appetite* **2016**, *100*, 142–151. [CrossRef]
36. Framson, C.; Kristal, A.R.; Schenk, J.M.; Littman, A.J.; Zeliadt, S.; Benitez, D. Development and validation of the mindful eating questionnaire. *J. Am. Diet. Assoc.* **2009**, *109*, 1439–1444. [CrossRef]
37. Thomas, D.M.; Navarro-Barrientos, J.E.; Rivera, D.E.; Heymsfield, S.B.; Bredlau, C.; Redman, L.M.; Martin, C.K.; Lederman, S.A.; L, M.C.; Butte, N.F. Dynamic energy-balance model predicting gestational weight gain. *Am. J. Clin. Nutr.* **2012**, *95*, 115–122. [CrossRef]
38. Dodd, J.M.; Cramp, C.; Sui, Z.; Yelland, L.N.; Deussen, A.R.; Grivell, R.M.; Moran, L.J.; Crowther, C.A.; Turnbull, D.; McPhee, A.J.; et al. The effects of antenatal dietary and lifestyle advice for women who are overweight or obese on maternal diet and physical activity: The LIMIT randomised trial. *BMC Med.* **2014**, *12*, 161. [CrossRef] [PubMed]
39. Dodd, J.M.; Turnbull, D.; McPhee, A.J.; Deussen, A.R.; Grivell, R.M.; Yelland, L.N.; Crowther, C.A.; Wittert, G.; Owens, J.A.; Robinson, J.S.; et al. Antenatal lifestyle advice for women who are overweight or obese: LIMIT randomised trial. *BMJ* **2014**, *348*, g1285. [CrossRef] [PubMed]
40. McCullough, M.L.; Feskanich, D.; Stampfer, M.J.; Rosner, B.A.; Hu, F.B.; Hunter, D.J.; Variyam, J.N.; Colditz, G.A.; Willett, W.C. Adherence to the Dietary Guidelines for Americans and risk of major chronic disease in women. *Am. J. Clin. Nutr.* **2000**, *72*, 1214–1222. [CrossRef] [PubMed]
41. Wilson, M.M.; Reedy, J.; Krebs-Smith, S.M. American Diet Quality: Where It Is, Where It Is Heading, and What It Could Be. *J. Acad. Nutr. Diet.* **2016**, *116*, 302–310. [CrossRef] [PubMed]
42. Gao, S.K.; Beresford, S.A.; Frank, L.L.; Schreiner, P.J.; Burke, G.L.; Fitzpatrick, A.L. Modifications to the Healthy Eating Index and its ability to predict obesity: The Multi-Ethnic Study of Atherosclerosis. *Am. J. Clin. Nutr.* **2008**, *88*, 64–69. [CrossRef] [PubMed]
43. Camhi, S.M.; Whitney Evans, E.; Hayman, L.L.; Lichtenstein, A.H.; Must, A. Healthy eating index and metabolically healthy obesity in U.S. adolescents and adults. *Prev. Med.* **2015**, *77*, 23–27. [CrossRef] [PubMed]
44. Wanders, A.J.; van den Borne, J.J.; de Graaf, C.; Hulshof, T.; Jonathan, M.C.; Kristensen, M.; Mars, M.; Schols, H.A.; Feskens, E.J. Effects of dietary fibre on subjective appetite, energy intake and body weight: A systematic review of randomized controlled trials. *Obes. Rev.* **2011**, *12*, 724–739. [CrossRef] [PubMed]
45. Hervik, A.K.; Svihus, B. The Role of Fiber in Energy Balance. *J. Nutr. Metab.* **2019**, *2019*, 4983657. [CrossRef]
46. Muller, M.; Canfora, E.E.; Blaak, E.E. Gastrointestinal Transit Time, Glucose Homeostasis and Metabolic Health: Modulation by Dietary Fibers. *Nutrients* **2018**, *10*, 275. [CrossRef]
47. Berthoud, H.R. Metabolic and hedonic drives in the neural control of appetite: Who is the boss? *Curr. Opin. Neurobiol.* **2011**, *21*, 888–896. [CrossRef]

48. Reyes, N.R.; Klotz, A.A.; Herring, S.J. A qualitative study of motivators and barriers to healthy eating in pregnancy for low-income, overweight, African-American mothers. *J. Acad. Nutr. Diet.* **2013**, *113*, 1175–1181. [CrossRef]
49. van Kleef, E.; Otten, K.; van Trijp, H.C. Healthy snacks at the checkout counter: A lab and field study on the impact of shelf arrangement and assortment structure on consumer choices. *BMC Public Health* **2012**, *12*, 1072. [CrossRef]
50. Farland, L.V.; Rifas-Shiman, S.L.; Gillman, M.W. Early Pregnancy Cravings, Dietary Intake, and Development of Abnormal Glucose Tolerance. *J. Acad. Nutr. Diet.* **2015**, *115*, 1958–1964. [CrossRef]
51. Orloff, N.C.; Flammer, A.; Hartnett, J.; Liquorman, S.; Samelson, R.; Hormes, J.M. Food cravings in pregnancy: Preliminary evidence for a role in excess gestational weight gain. *Appetite* **2016**, *105*, 259–265. [CrossRef]
52. Renault, K.M.; Carlsen, E.M.; Norgaard, K.; Nilas, L.; Pryds, O.; Secher, N.J.; Olsen, S.F.; Halldorsson, T.I. Intake of Sweets, Snacks and Soft Drinks Predicts Weight Gain in Obese Pregnant Women: Detailed Analysis of the Results of a Randomised Controlled Trial. *PLoS ONE* **2015**, *10*, e0133041. [CrossRef]
53. Warren, J.M.; Smith, N.; Ashwell, M. A structured literature review on the role of mindfulness, mindful eating and intuitive eating in changing eating behaviours: Effectiveness and associated potential mechanisms. *Nutr. Res. Rev.* **2017**, *30*, 272–283. [CrossRef]
54. O'Reilly, G.A.; Cook, L.; Spruijt-Metz, D.; Black, D.S. Mindfulness-based interventions for obesity-related eating behaviours: A literature review. *Obes. Rev.* **2014**, *15*, 453–461. [CrossRef]
55. Hutchinson, A.D.; Charters, M.; Prichard, I.; Fletcher, C.; Wilson, C. Understanding maternal dietary choices during pregnancy: The role of social norms and mindful eating. *Appetite* **2017**, *112*, 227–234. [CrossRef]
56. Vieten, C.; Laraia, B.A.; Kristeller, J.; Adler, N.; Coleman-Phox, K.; Bush, N.R.; Wahbeh, H.; Duncan, L.G.; Epel, E. The mindful moms training: Development of a mindfulness-based intervention to reduce stress and overeating during pregnancy. *BMC Pregnancy Childbirth* **2018**, *18*, 201. [CrossRef]
57. Laraia, B.A.; Adler, N.E.; Coleman-Phox, K.; Vieten, C.; Mellin, L.; Kristeller, J.L.; Thomas, M.; Stotland, N.E.; Lustig, R.H.; Dallman, M.F.; et al. Novel Interventions to Reduce Stress and Overeating in Overweight Pregnant Women: A Feasibility Study. *Matern. Child Health J.* **2018**, *22*, 670–678. [CrossRef]
58. Bodnar, L.M.; Simhan, H.N.; Parker, C.B.; Meier, H.; Mercer, B.M.; Grobman, W.A.; Haas, D.M.; Wing, D.A.; Hoffman, M.K.; Parry, S.; et al. Racial or Ethnic and Socioeconomic Inequalities in Adherence to National Dietary Guidance in a Large Cohort of US Pregnant Women. *J. Acad. Nutr. Diet.* **2017**, *117*, 867–877. [CrossRef]
59. Willcox, J.C.; Ball, K.; Campbell, K.J.; Crawford, D.A.; Wilkinson, S.A. Correlates of pregnant women's gestational weight gain knowledge. *Midwifery* **2017**, *49*, 32–39. [CrossRef]
60. Lindsay, A.C.; Wallington, S.F.; Greaney, M.L.; Tavares Machado, M.M.; De Andrade, G.P. Patient-Provider Communication and Counseling about Gestational Weight Gain and Physical Activity: A Qualitative Study of the Perceptions and Experiences of Latinas Pregnant with their First Child. *Int. J. Environ. Res. Public Health* **2017**, *14*, 1412. [CrossRef]

12

Sialic Acid and Sialylated Oligosaccharide Supplementation during Lactation Improves Learning and Memory in Rats

Elena Oliveros [1,2,*], Enrique Vázquez [1], Alejandro Barranco [1], María Ramírez [1], Agnes Gruart [3], Jose María Delgado-García [3], Rachael Buck [4], Ricardo Rueda [1] and María J. Martín [1]

1 R&D Abbott Nutrition, 18004 Granada, Spain; enrique.vazquez@abbott.com (E.V.); alejandro.barranco@abbott.com (A.B.); maria.ramirez@abbott.com (M.R.); ricardo.rueda@abbott.com (R.R.); maria.j.martin@abbott.com (M.J.M.)

2 Doctoral programme in Biomedicine, School of Health Sciences, University of Granada, 18071 Granada, Spain

3 Division of Neurosciences, Pablo de Olavide University, 41013 Seville, Spain; agrumas@upo.es (A.G.); jmdelgar@upo.es (J.M.D.-G.)

4 R&D Abbott Nutrition, Columbus, OH 43219, USA; rachael.buck@abbott.com

* Correspondence: elena.oliveros@abbott.com

Abstract: Sialic acids (Sia) are postulated to improve cognitive abilities. This study evaluated Sia effects on rat behavior when administered in a free form as N-acetylneuraminic acid (Neu5Ac) or conjugated as 6′-sialyllactose (6′-SL). Rat milk contains Sia, which peaks at Postnatal Day 9 and drops to a minimum by Day 15. To bypass this Sia peak, a cohort of foster mothers was used to raise the experimental pups. A group of pups received a daily oral supplementation of Neu5Ac to mimic the amount naturally present in rat milk, and another group received the same molar amount of Sia as 6′-SL. The control group received water. After weaning, rats were submitted to behavioral evaluation. One year later, behavior was re-evaluated, and in vivo long-term potentiation (LTP) was performed. Brain samples were collected and analyzed at both ages. Adult rats who received Sia performed significantly better in the behavioral assessment and showed an enhanced LTP compared to controls. Within Sia groups, 6′-SL rats showed better scores in some cognitive outcomes compared to Neu5Ac rats. At weaning, an effect on polysialylated-neural cell adhesion molecule (PSA-NCAM) levels in the frontal cortex was only observed in 6′-SL fed rats. Providing Sia during lactation, especially as 6′-SL, improves memory and LTP in adult rats.

Keywords: milk oligosaccharides; infant formula; 6′-sialyllactose; cognitive development; sialic acid

1. Introduction

Breast feeding is associated with multiple health benefits. Infants fed human milk have lower rates of intestinal and autoimmune diseases and food allergies and show higher intellectual quotient (IQ) scores compared to formula-fed infants [1]. The unique composition of human milk plays a key role in optimal development of newborns, and sialic acids (Sia) are considered as one of the components responsible for the multiple benefits. They are present in most mammalian milks, mainly conjugated to proteins and oligosaccharides, but also as free monosaccharides. Within this last group of monosaccharides, there are some key core structures such as N-acetylneuraminic acid (Neu5Ac), N-glycolylneuraminic acid (Neu5Gc) and deaminated neuraminic acid (Kdn), which encompass the so-called Sia molecules [2]. Neu5Ac is the only form of Sia synthesized by humans [2] and is present throughout the body, including brain [3].

Most of the Sia in human milk, approximately 73% [4], are bound to oligosaccharides, generating sialyloligosaccharides, which represent a significant fraction of human milk oligosaccharides (HMOs). Oligosaccharides in human milk are at a higher concentration than in other mammalian milks, ranging from 13.3–23 g/L in colostrum to 3.5–14 g/L in mature milk [4,5], with structural diversity and over 200 different molecules identified so far [6]. Conversely, bovine milk, which is the basis of most infant formula, has an oligosaccharide content over 100-fold [7] lower than human milk. Although goat milk-based infant formula is now available, its use is not as extensive as bovine milk-based infant formulas. Interestingly, goat milk oligosaccharides have significant structural similarities to human milk oligosaccharides [8].

Milk oligosaccharides from any mammal consist of acidic oligosaccharides, predominantly sialylated ones, and neutral oligosaccharides, predominantly fucosylated compounds. There is a significant difference in the distribution of these compounds between human and bovine milk [9]. Sialylated structures represent 70% of bovine milk oligosaccharides compared with 10–20% in human milk [8], while fucosylated glycans are the most abundant form in human milk [10]. Within sialylated compounds, a recent study showed 6′-sialyllactose (6′-SL) is the major representative during the first two months, when it starts to sharply decrease so that 3′-sialyllactose becomes the predominant sialyl-oligosaccharide of human milk beyond the fourth month [11].

Milk oligosaccharides have been linked to different biological functions in the newborn, such as anti-infective activity [12,13], immune system and gastrointestinal development [14,15], modulation of inflammation [16], bifidogenic activity [17], modulation of gut motility and activation of enteric neurons [18] and even enhancement of central nervous system (CNS) functions [19]. Sia has been described as an essential nutrient in the development of infant brain [20], since its highest concentration in milk during early lactation concurs with a rapid increase of brain gangliosides [21]. Furthermore, the content of gangliosides and protein-bound sialic acid is higher in the brain of breast-fed infants in comparison to formula-fed infants [22]. Sia is a key component of brain gangliosides and polysialic acid (polySia) attached to the oligosaccharide chains on neural cell adhesion molecule (NCAM); both brain gangliosides and polysialylated-NCAM (PSA-NCAM) are crucial to ensure synaptic connections and memory formation or neuronal outgrowth [3,20].

HMOs and, by extension, sialyloligosaccharides have been reported as important factors for optimal development and maturation of the immune system [23]. HMOs are also prebiotics favoring the growth of healthy gut microbiota and as pathogen decoys, inhibiting their adhesion to the intestinal mucosa [24–26].

Several studies performed both in rodents [27] and pigs [28] have shown a relationship between Sia and cognitive function. The mechanism of action for the role of Sia on cognitive development has not been proven to date. However, recent research has shown the effects of HMOs on the gut-brain axis (GBA) in rodents [29,30], which compliments their role as prebiotics. The gut-brain axis consists of a bidirectional interaction between the central and the enteric nervous system [31]. The influences of gut microbiota on human health and disease is an important topic in medicine that is believed to occur via gut-brain microbe communication [32]. A recent study demonstrated associations between gut microbiota and cognition in infants [33].

The first two years of life are a critical window for brain development, not only for rapid proliferation and growth of neural cells, but also for increases in synapse connections [34]. Thus, adequate early life nutrition is crucial to ensure optimal cognitive development in infants and children.

The present study was aimed at determining if early Sia supplementation, as a free or conjugated form, plays a role during neural development in rats and whether effects could be detected later in life. For that purpose, rat pups were orally supplemented with Neu5Ac or 6′-SL during the lactation period and were evaluated using behavioral tests and electrophysiological measurements in both young and adult rats.

2. Materials and Methods

2.1. Animals

Pregnant Sprague-Dawley rats (n = 47) in the second week of gestation were purchased from Charles River (Charles River, France) and kept under controlled environmental conditions of temperature (22 °C ± 2), humidity (55% ± 10) and lighting (12 h light/dark cycles). Rats were fed a standard diet ad libitum. Animal experimental protocols were approved by the Ethics Committee of the Estación Experimental del Zaidín-CSIC (Consejo Superior de Investigaciones Científicas, Granada, Spain. Approval number: CBA EEZ-2011/20), and the experiment was performed in accordance with the Spanish and European regulations for the care and use of experimental animals for research.

2.2. Experimental Design

Rodent milk contains sialylated oligosaccharides, in particular 3′-sialyllactose (3′-SL) and 6′-SL [35]. In rat milk, total Sia levels peak at Postnatal Day 9 (PN9), sharply drop until Day 15 and then slightly decrease until the end of lactation [36]. To bypass this peak of Sia, two cohorts of pregnant rats were used with a time lag on the delivery day of 13 days, as shown in the experimental design scheme (see Scheme 1). Animals were maintained on a chow diet for gestation, lactation and growth (2018 Teklad Global 18% Protein Diet) until delivery. The first cohort (n = 20), hereafter called foster mothers, was kept with its respective offspring until PN16. Experimental pups were born from the second cohort of mothers (n = 27) and remained with them until PN3. On that day, 3-day-old pups were removed from their dams, sexed and randomly distributed into 10 pups (5 males and 5 females) groups with balanced weights and litters. Subsequently, they substituted for the 16 day-old pups in foster mother cages. These dams willingly accepted the new litters and took care of them for the rest of the lactation period. Afterwards, foster mothers and their litters were then distributed into 3 experimental groups of 4 dams each.

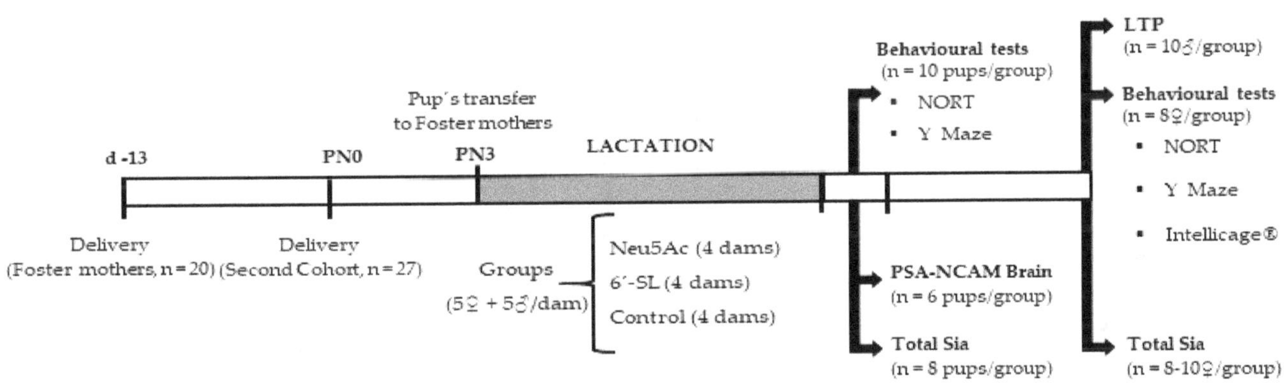

Scheme 1. Experimental design scheme. PN, postnatal day; Neu5Ac, N-acetylneuraminic acid; 6′-SL, 6′-sialyllactose; NORT, Novel Object Recognition Test; PSA-NCAM, polysialylated-neural cell adhesion molecule; LTP, long-term potentiation; Sia, sialic acids; ♀, female; ♂, male.

Since the content of sialic acid in rat milk reaches the lowest values from PN16, all pups raised by foster mothers received less Sia from milk than normally raised rats during early development. To compensate for the deficiency of Sia in milk, one group of pups received an oral supplementation of Neu5Ac from PN3 to weaning, and another group received the same molar amount of Sia given as 6′-SL. The control pups were given water and, therefore, received approximately 5-times less Sia than normally raised rats. In contrast, the 2 experimental groups received the same Sia levels naturally present in rat milk, but from two different sources. Therefore, the model assessed adequate Sia intake during lactation and the influence of the form in which it was provided.

Pups remained undisturbed with the foster rats except for a brief time while they received supplementation (8 times/day; max. 5 min/time). After weaning, all mothers and 2 pups per litter were sacrificed by an intraperitoneal overdose of anesthetic. Brains obtained from the pups were separated into hemispheres. One hemisphere was analyzed to determine Sia content at weaning by high performance liquid chromatography (HPLC), and the other one was used to determine NCAM and PSA-NCAM expression in the frontal cortex by Western blotting. Another set of weaned rats was submitted to classical behavioral tests such as NORT (Novel Object Recognition Test) and Y maze tests. Pups were then maintained for 1 year on a standard chow diet. At that age, males were used for LTP measurements; meanwhile, females were subjected again to psychological tests to evaluate long-term effects on learning and memory. Rats were then sacrificed, and brains were analyzed by HPLC to determine Sia content at adulthood.

2.3. Sialic Acid Doses

Rat milk contains both forms of free Sia, Neu5Ac and Neu5Gc; since Neu5Ac is the most abundant in humans [3] and is present throughout the body including brain, this was the form chosen as a free Sia source to be used in the supplementation.

Rat milk concentration of sialic acid varies through the lactation period having a Sia peak (≈8 mg/mL) at PN9 and dropping to lower levels by Postnatal Day 15 [35] (Figure 1a).

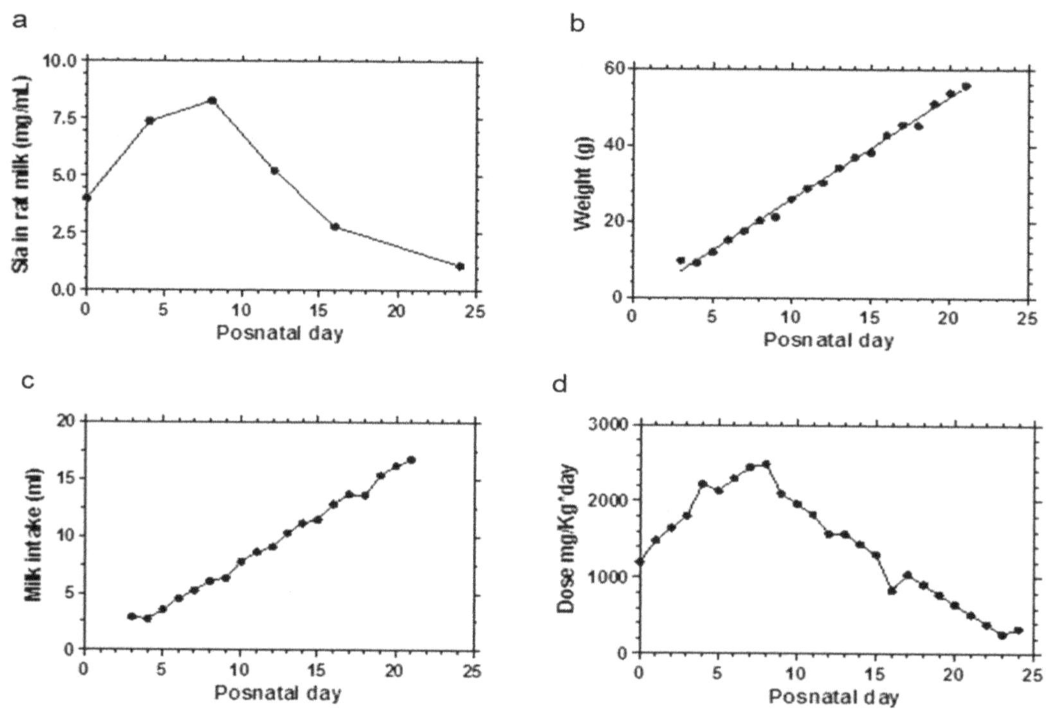

Figure 1. (**a**) Sia concentration (mg/mL) in rat milk throughout the lactation period per the literature [36]. (**b**) Experimental data of rat pups' weight evolution from birth until weaning. (**c**) Estimated data of milk volume intake (mL) in rat pups from birth until weaning per the literature [37]. (**d**) Sialic acid dose (mg/kg/day) that rat pups were receiving from rat milk considering the data shown in graphs (**a**–**c**).

To determine the effects of Sia, a model was designed in which one of the groups received less Sia than that from normal lactation, while the other groups received the same levels of Sia as naturally-nursed pups, either in the free form Neu5Ac or as 6′-SL. The daily dose of Sia was calculated based on Sia content of rat milk, pup body weights and milk intake during lactation according to data found in the literature [36,37] and to internal data from previous experiments (Figure 1b). Figure 1d shows the theoretical Sia dose (mg/kg weight/day) that rat pups would normally receive from rat milk. Equimolar stock solutions with Neu5Ac and 6′-SL were prepared. Variable volumes of these stock solutions were given to the pups per day to adjust the Sia dose, as shown in Figure 1d.

2.4. Analytical Determination of Sialic Acid Content by HPLC

Right hemispheres were analyzed to determine the total amount of sialic acid. After homogenization of the brain, 35 mg were weighed and re-suspended at 0.2 mg/μL in deionized water. Sia were released by mild hydrolysis in 0.2N H_2SO_4 at 80 °C for 1 h. After filtering and centrifuging during 30 min at 10,000 rpm, supernatants were used for derivatization with 5-(difluoromethoxy)-2-mercapto-1H-benzimidazole (DMB) as described by Hara et al. [38] with some modifications. Thus, 50 μL of samples and 50 μL of DMB reagent (8 mM DMB, 1.5 M acetic acid, 14 mM sodium hydrosulfite, 0.8 M 2-mercaptoethanol (Sigma Aldrich, Saint Louis, MO, USA)) were kept for 2.5 h at 50 °C in the dark. A volume of 10 μL of the derivatized solution was injected on an Alliance 2695 HPLC system equipped with a 474-fluorescence detector from Waters (Mildford, MA, USA) as described by Martin et al. [39]. A LiChrosorb RP-18 column (5 μm, 250 mm × 4.6 mm) with a LiChrosorb RP-18 guard cartridge (5 μm), both from Supelco (Bellefonte, PA, USA), was used. DMB derivatives of Sia were isocratically eluted using 7% (*v/v*) methanol, 8% (*v/v*) acetonitrile in water for 40 min at a flow rate of 0.9 mL min^{-1}. All injections were performed at room temperature. The eluent was monitored for fluorescence at 373 nm (excitation wavelength) and 448 nm (emission wavelength). The gain was fixed at 1, and the attenuation at 64 for the 474-fluorescence detector. A set of standards (25–250 ng Neu5Ac) was injected with every set of samples. Data were integrated by the Millennium 4.0 software (Waters, Milford, MA, USA) coupled to the HPLC system. Standard regression and sample quantitation were calculated by Microsoft Excel 2011 and Graph Pad (Prism 4, San Diego, CA, USA).

2.5. Western Blotting

For Western analysis, ≈15–20 mg of frontal cortex samples of pups at weaning (PN22) were homogenized in cold suspension buffer (PBS, 0.1% TritonX100 and protease inhibitor cocktail from Sigma Aldrich, Saint Louis, MO, USA), centrifuged at 10,000 *g* for 15 min, and the supernatant collected. The protein content was determined using the Bradford assay (Bio-Rad, Hercules, CA, USA). Ten micrograms of protein, diluted in phosphate-buffered saline (PBS), were loaded into Criterion XT 4–20% Bis-Tris gels (Bio-Rad). Separation was carried out using MOPS buffer (0.05 M 3-Morpholinopropane-1-sulfonic acid (MOPS), 0.05 M Tris base, 0.003 M SDS, 0.8 mM EDTA) and run at 200 V for 45 min. Separated proteins were transferred onto nitrocellulose membranes for 3.5 h using a Trans-Blot electrophoresis transfer cell. Six samples were run per group. After blocking non-specific binding sites for 1 h with 3% bovine serum albumin (BSA, Sigma Aldrich, Saint Louis, MO, USA) in TBS-TritonX100 (0.025% TritonX100, 20 mM Tris base, 150 mM NaCl, pH 7.6), blots were incubated overnight at 4 °C with one of the following monoclonal antibodies: anti-NCAM (Santa Cruz, CA, USA) at 1:2500; anti-PSA-NCAM (Millipore/Merck, Darmstadt, Germany) at 1:1000. All the antibodies were diluted in TBS containing 1% BSA. After three quick washes in TBS-TritonX100, NCAM blots were incubated for 2 h at room temperature with anti-IgG HRP at 1:5000 (Sigma Aldrich), while PSA-NCAM were incubated with anti-IgG HRP (Bethyl laboratories, Montgomery, TX, USA) at 1:5000 for 2 h. β-actin was used as a control for quantitation and detected with monoclonal antibody (Sigma Aldrich, 1:5000). After five washes in TBS-TritonX100, membranes were developed using Pierce Supersignal West-Pico substrate (Thermo Fisher Scientific, Waltham, MA, USA) and quantified using a Chemidoc XRS system from Bio-Rad (Hercules, CA, USA).

2.6. Long-Term Potentiation Measurement

One-year old male offspring were assigned to this analysis. Animals were anesthetized and implanted with stimulating and recording electrodes in the hippocampus to measure LTP in vivo, as previously described [40]. Based on prior research [41,42], animals were implanted with stimulating electrodes at the Schaffer collateral-commissural pathway of the dorsal hippocampus (3.5 mm lateral and 3.2 mm posterior to Bregma) as per stereotaxic coordinates. Four recording electrodes were also implanted targeting the ipsilateral stratum radiatum beneath the CA1 area (2.5 mm lateral and 3.6 mm posterior to Bregma). Stimulation occurred, and the field excitatory post-synaptic potential (fEPSP) was recorded. After the high-frequency stimulation (HFS) protocols, fEPSPs were recorded for 30 min. Additional 15-min recording sessions were carried out during the following days.

2.7. *Classical Behavioral Tests*

A video tracking system, Sony Camera SSC-G213A (Sony Electronics Inc., Park Ridge, NJ, USA), was used to record all animal trials. Rat performances were then analyzed offline using the analytical software Viewer (Biobserve GmbH, Bonn, Germany) by a technician that was blinded to treatment. An alcohol dilution was used to clean the surface of Y maze and NORT structures after each animal performance to prevent odor cues.

2.7.1. Novel Object Recognition Test

NORT is based on the natural tendency of rodents to explore novel stimuli presented to them; thus, when novel and familiar stimuli are present at the same time, the novel one will be naturally explored for longer [43]. Therefore, this test was run in a black opened plastic chamber (40 × 40 cm), known as the arena. Three objects differing in material, form and color were chosen. After 3 days of habituation to the arena, an acquisition phase took place, and the animals were faced with two different objects (familiar objects) for 10 min. One day later, animals were submitted to a retention test in which a new object (novel object) substituted one of the familiar objects, allowing the animals to explore them for 5 min. Animals were considered as exploring the objects when they approached their whiskers at approximately 1–2 cm or licked them; exploration was never considered when they sat on the objects [44]. The key parameter evaluated in this task was time spent by the rats exploring each object, novel or familiar, during the retention phase.

2.7.2. Y Maze with Blocked Arm Test

The Y maze with blocked arm test measures the ability of rodents to explore new environments and assesses exploratory behavior and memory [45]. The experimental design used was that proposed by Dellu et al. [46] with some modifications. A Y-shape stainless-steeled structure (20 × 10.5 × 50 cm) was used. There are two consecutive phases in the paradigm: an acquisition trial and a retention test. During the acquisition trial, one of the three arms of the maze was blocked (novel arm), and rats could explore the other two arms for 15 min. Four hours later, animals went through the test session in which all arms were open to be explored for 5 min. Novelty was represented by the arm that was not accessible in the acquisition phase. When introduced in the maze after a few hours, animal normal behavior should be to explore first the previously hidden arm; thus, to evaluate animal memory skills, it was analyzed whether animals went first into the novel arm.

2.8. *IntelliCage® Protocol*

The IntelliCage® (NewBehavior AG, Zurich, Switzerland) is a computer-based, fully-automated testing apparatus used to analyze the spontaneous and learning behavior of rodents. This system consists of a cage that presents 4 operant conditioning corners, which can locate one rat at a time. Each corner is equipped with 2 motorized doors, which block or allow access to water bottles placed on both sides of the corner. When a rat tries to access through whichever of the 2 doors (nose poke action), the interruption of a light-beam sensor at either door triggers one or the other doors to open and allow access to a water bottle. Radio frequency identification (RFID) transponders are implanted under the rat skin, allowing for individual recognition; thus, rat entries into the corners are detected through RFID antennas located there. Using this technology, conditioning protocols can be implemented to evaluate the behavioral activities of the rats. Animals were implanted with the RFID-transponders, and 1 day later, they were placed into the IntelliCage® (n = 8 rats/group) and maintained there during

2 weeks for habituation and testing. The habituation process was counted with different stages: 1 day of free exploration with all doors opened; 5 days in which doors were opened only upon a visit to the corner; in the following 2 days, doors opened after a nose poke in the right place; in the last 4 days, one nose poke opened any door only during two drinking sessions of 90 min per night, while the doors remained closed during the rest of the night and day.

Thereafter, a paradigm to measure cognitive outcomes was tested by restricting water access to a specific corner and time periods. During the two-day test, access to water was restricted to one corner (correct corner) only during the two drinking sessions. If the rat nose poked any other corner, water was not available. Each rat was randomly assigned a correct corner. Every visit to this assigned corner was counted as correct, while incorrect visits were those to any other corner. Thus, only rats with adequate cognitive skills could learn which is the correct corner in this place learning paradigm.

2.9. Statistical Analysis

Data are presented as the mean ± SEM. Graph displays and statistical analysis were done using SPSS (SPSS Inc., Chicago, IL, USA) and GraphPad (GraphPad Inc., La Jolla, CA, USA) software. Comparisons between groups were performed by Student's *t*-test and one-way analysis of variance (ANOVA) in NORT and Western blotting. Statistical differences between groups were determined with a two-way repeated measure of the analysis of variance (ANOVA) in LTP measurements. The Y maze test and IntelliCage® paradigm were analyzed through a contingency table analysis using Fisher's test. The significance level was established at $p < 0.05$ for all tests.

3. Results

3.1. Sialic Acid Content in Brain

The content of Neu5Ac in the right brain hemisphere of rats at weaning (PN22) and at 1 year of age is shown in Table 1. Brain concentration of sialic acid (μg NeuAc/mg brain) did not show significant differences among groups at any age.

Table 1. Concentration of Sia (μg Neu5Ac/mg) in brain in weaned and 1-year old rats supplemented with different Sia sources or water during the lactation period. Data are the mean ± SEM.

	Sia Concentration (μg Neu5Ac/mg Brain)			
	Neu5Ac Group	**6′-SL Group**	**Control Group**	**One-Way ANOVA *p*-Value**
Pups rats (n = 8/group)	1.399 ± 0.067	1.405 ± 0.124	1.422 ± 0.058	$p = 0.8336$
1-year old rats (n = 8–10/group)	1.018 ± 0.106	1.067 ± 0.025	0.9745 ± 0.096	$p = 0.2143$

Sia, sialic acids; Neu5Ac, N-acetylneuraminic acid; 6′-SL, 6′-sialyllactose.

3.2. Western Blot

Frontal cortex samples of weaned pups (PN22) were analyzed to determine NCAM and PSA-NCAM expression by Western blotting (6 pups/group). Actin was used as a control for quantitation. The control group was used as the reference group and ratios were calculated between normalized values and the density mean for the control group.

As shown in Figure 2, no differences among groups related to NCAM expression ($p = 0.8819$) were found. However, rats fed 6′-SL in the lactation period expressed significantly more PSA-NCAM in the frontal cortex when compared to rats supplemented with Neu5Ac ($p = 0.012$) or control animals ($p = 0.041$).

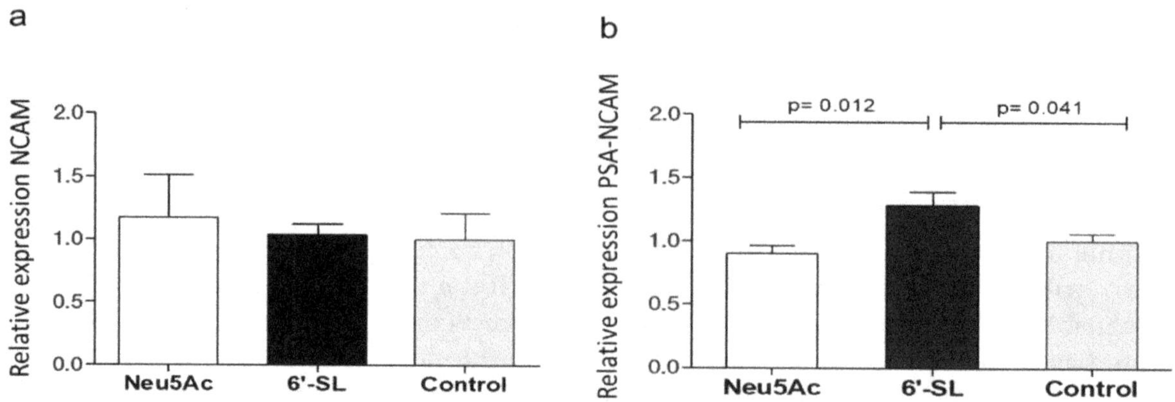

Figure 2. Relative protein expression of NCAM (**a**) and PSA-NCAM (**b**) in frontal cortex samples of rat pups of the three experimental groups at Postnatal Day 22. One-way ANOVA and Student's t-test were used for statistical analysis. Data are expressed as the mean ± SEM (n = 6 rats/group), $p < 0.05$ denotes significant differences. NCAM, neural cell adhesion molecule; PSA-NCAM, polysialylated-neural cell adhesion molecule; Neu5Ac, N-acetylneuraminic acid; 6′-SL, 6′-sialyllactose.

3.3. *In Vivo LTP*

At one-year of age, male rats were submitted to in vivo LTP (10 rats/group). A significant response in LTP was evoked in all the groups following the HFS session (Figure 3). LTP responses were significantly improved in male rats supplemented with 6′-SL during lactation compared to controls. Differences were detectable several days after the stimulation. Neu5Ac group also reached a more intense LTP than the control group, although the difference was not statistically significant.

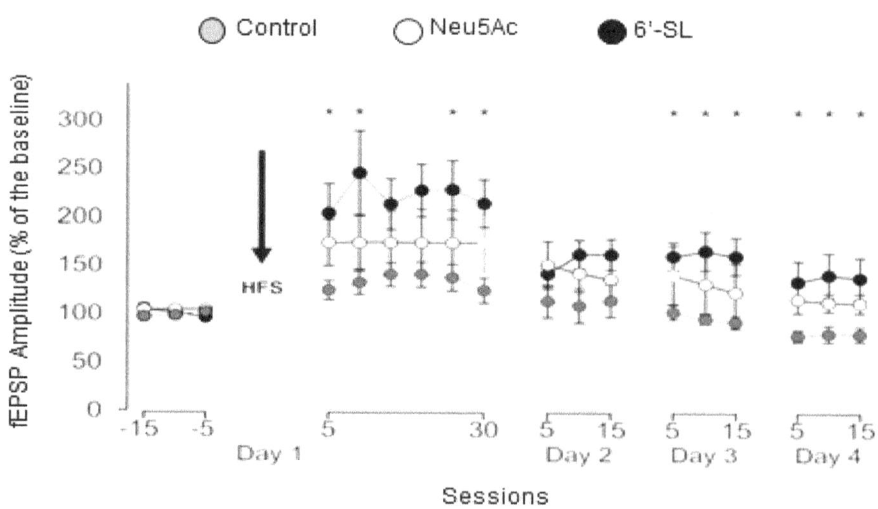

Figure 3. Experimentally-evoked LTP in the groups of animals at one year of age. Data collected from the three groups of animals before and after high-frequency stimulation (HFS) session (indicated by the downward arrow). The HFS was presented after 15 min of baseline recordings. LTP evolution was followed for up to four days. Statistical differences between groups were determined with a two-way repeated measure of the analysis of variance (ANOVA). The three groups of animals presented a significant ($p \leq 0.05$) LTP in relation with baseline values. In addition, field excitatory post-synaptic potential (fEPSP) values evoked after the HFS session were significantly larger (*, $p \leq 0.05$) for the 6′-SL group in comparison with values collected from controls. Data are represented as the mean ± SEM (n = 10 animals/group). Neu5Ac, N-acetylneuraminic acid; 6′-SL, 6′-sialyllactose.

3.4. Classical Behavioral Tests

A behavioral assessment with different paradigms such as NORT and the Y maze test was performed at weaning and when animals were one year old. Results obtained at weaning ($n = 10$ pups/group) did not show any difference in performance of the three groups tested (data not shown). Conversely, data found at adult age ($n = 8$ rats/group) were more conclusive.

3.4.1. NORT

Regarding NORT, the key parameter to study was the time spent exploring the novel object versus the familiar one in the retention phase. Thus, animals with good cognitive abilities tended to explore the novel object for longer. As shown in Figure 4a, rats belonging to the groups that received Sia supplementation, both Neu5Ac and 6′-SL, spent a significantly longer time exploring the novel object than the familiar one. A significant difference in the exploration time of both objects was not found in the control group.

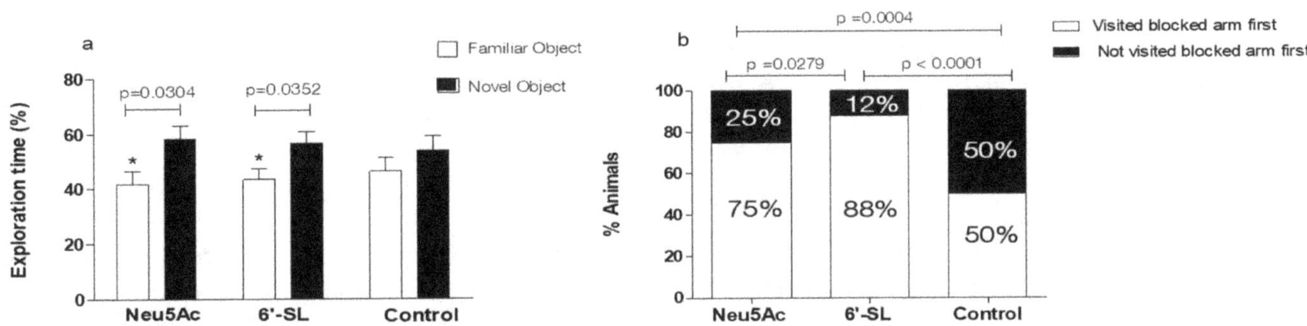

Figure 4. (**a**) Percentage of time spent by the animals exploring a familiar object against a novel object in NORT at one year of age. One-way ANOVA and Student's t-test were applied for statistical analysis; *, $p < 0.05$ denotes significant differences. (**b**) Percentage of animals that chose the novel arm first in the Y maze during the retention test versus those that did not. Fisher's test was applied for statistical analysis; $p < 0.05$ denotes significant differences ($n = 8$ rats/group). Neu5Ac, N-acetylneuraminic acid; 6′-SL, 6′-sialyllactose.

3.4.2. Y Maze with Blocked Arm Test

As for the Y maze task, one-year old rats that received Neu5Ac or 6′-SL during lactation performed significantly better than the control group by clearly identifying the blocked arm. During the retention test, rats with superior cognitive abilities explored the arm first, since it represents novelty. Figure 4b shows the percentage of animals from each group that visited the previously blocked arm first versus the percentage of animals that chose one of the other two arms as their first option. Rats receiving Sia achieved the best score, i.e., 88% of 6′-SL animals visited the novel arm first and 75% of Neu5Ac rats. By contrast, the control group visited the novel arm with the same probability as the other two combined. From a statistical standpoint, the 6′-SL group score was significantly higher, not only when compared to the control group ($p < 0.0001$), but also compared to the Neu5Ac group ($p = 0.0279$). There were also significant differences between Neu5Ac rats and control animals ($p = 0.0004$).

3.5. IntelliCage® Protocol

In the place learning paradigm performed with the IntelliCage® system ($n = 8$ rats/group), results were aligned to the behavior observed in the classical tests. As previously explained, access to water was restricted to the "correct corner" during the two drinking sessions of two consecutive nights. The percentages of visits to the correct corner and visits to incorrect corners were analyzed. Neu5Ac and 6′-SL groups obtained 41% and 39% correct visits, respectively, while the control group reached 25% of visits to the correct corner (Figure 5). Thereby, groups supplemented with Neu5Ac or 6′-SL exhibited a significantly better performance compared to the control group.

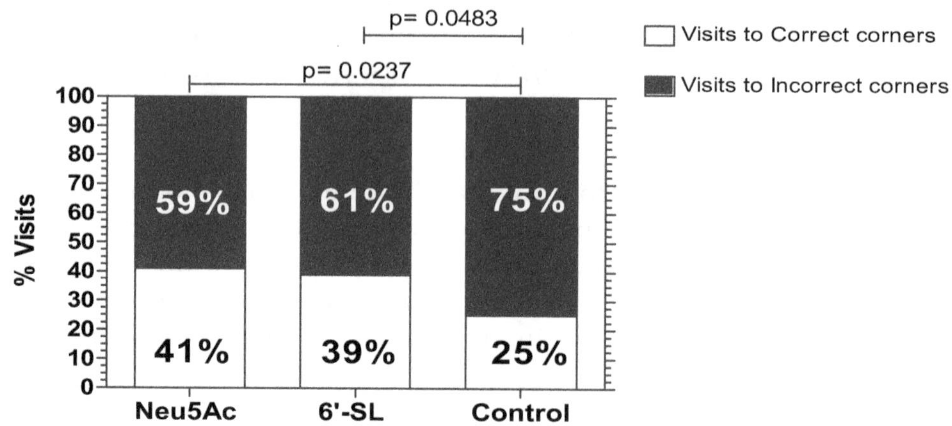

Figure 5. Percentage of total visits to the correct corner versus incorrect corner in the IntelliCage® paradigm for each group of animals during the four drinking sessions of the two days of place learning. Fisher's test was applied for statistical analysis; $p < 0.05$ denotes significant differences; $n = 8$ rats/group; one year of age. Neu5Ac, N-acetylneuraminic acid; 6′-SL, 6′-sialyllactose.

4. Discussion

In the current study, the impact of two forms of sialic acid, either free form or conjugated given during lactation, on cognitive skills later in life was assessed. We evaluated cognitive functions with behavioral and electrophysiological measurements, demonstrating that these sources of Sia given at early stages after birth maintain cognitive function in adulthood when compared to a group that received a lower amount of Sia, and that the provision of Sia as 6′-SL may confer some advantages over the use of the free form.

Pioneering studies in the 1980s showed that exogenous Sia could be incorporated into brain gangliosides and glycoproteins when injected intraperitoneally in rat pups [27]. Wang et al. investigated the metabolic fate of intravenously-administrated ^{14}C-Neu5Ac in piglets, concluding that an exogenous source of sialic acid could cross the blood-brain barrier and be incorporated into various tissues [47]. Carlson and House also demonstrated that Sia given by intraperitoneal injection or orally significantly impacted the concentration of brain gangliosides and glycoproteins [48]. Another study confirmed the impact of orally-administered sialic acid on cortical ganglioside concentration after feeding rat pups a solid diet prepared with different Sia doses from PN17–31. Cortical gangliosides Sia concentration was significantly higher in rats that received a Sia-supplemented diet provided by a protein-bound source of Sia (casein glycomacropeptide) [49].

Considerable research has been carried out to date to elucidate the effects of supplementation with Sia early in life on brain composition and behavior. In a study by Morgan and Winick [27], rat pups were intraperitoneally injected with Neu5Ac or glucose (control group), and an improvement of performance was observed in the Neu5Ac group. A piglet model was used by Wang et al. [28] to evaluate the effect of a sow milk replacer supplemented with several doses of casein glycomacropeptide for 35 days after weaning. Neu5Ac brain concentration, expression of two learning associated genes and learning and memory abilities were positively impacted by the Sia supplementation. However, a research team has recently reported two studies in which supplementation with sialyllactose from PN2–PN22 or PN32 in piglets showed no significant effect on recognition memory [50], but did show a sialic acid increase in hippocampus, prefrontal cortex and corpus callosum [51].

The novelty of the present work is three-fold: (1) the use of a unique foster rat mother model, whereby rat pups were breastfed during the entire lactation period, but received milk with a lower amount of Sia from PN3 until end of lactation; in addition, the animal intervention was performed at an early, developmental stage, which is challenging due to the vulnerability of pups; (2) the timeframe in which Sia content in brain and cognitive outcomes in rats were measured; previous analyses were carried out after weaning, when the Sia supplementation had just finished; herein, brain composition analyses and behavior assessments were performed at the end of Sia supplementation, but also in adult animals that had spent almost one year without receiving additional Sia; and (3) the use of 6′-SL as a source of Sia in comparison to the free form.

Improved cognitive skills reported here were not attributable to an increased Sia content in a brain hemisphere. In fact, Sia content in brain hemispheres samples was the same for the three experimental groups at weaning and in adulthood. According to Wang et al., the ganglioside and glycoprotein sialic acid concentrations in the brain frontal cortex are higher in breastfed infants when compared to formula-fed infants [22]. In a study performed with piglets, it was observed that supplementation with an exogenous source of Sia increased protein-bound sialic acid concentrations in the frontal cortex [28]. Jacobi et al. also demonstrated in piglets that a formula supplemented with dietary 6′-SL and 3′-SL increased the sialic acid bound to gangliosides in several areas of the brain [52]. As described above, Mudd and co-workers have recently published a study in which piglets were fed several diets containing different doses of sialyllactose from PN2–PN32 and showed that dietary sialyllactose increased conjugated Neu5Ac in the prefrontal cortex, among other brain structures [51]. In our study, Neu5Ac determination by HPLC was done in the whole hemisphere instead of in separate structures. Thus, significant differences among groups could have been missed because Neu5Ac may be accumulated in certain brain structures such as frontal cortex. Furthermore, it could be hypothesized that Neu5Ac content in the brain of the different groups was different during an early phase of development, promoting higher rates of axonal growth and enhanced connections between neurons that would support the behavioral differences found in adulthood.

To further explore this, we analyzed NCAM and PSA-NCAM expression levels in the frontal cortex of early weaned pups (PN22). NCAM is a widely-expressed protein involved in the stabilization and modulation of CNS [3]. Polysialic acid (PSA) is a linear homopolymer of α2-8-linked Neu5Ac. PSA is added to NCAM by a regulated post-translational process and varies through development [20]. Polysialylation supports the maintenance of an immature phenotype, allowing the neurites to grow and sprout to connect the complex circuitry of the brain while its graded downregulation enables fine-tuning of NCAM-dependent cell-cell interactions, stabilizing the newly-formed structures. Following the findings of the studies previously cited [28,52], our results in weaned rats showed that PSA-NCAM expression in the frontal cortex was significantly higher in the 6′-SL group when compared to Neu5Ac and the control groups; this result suggests that conjugated Sia such as 6′-SL might be taken up preferentially by the brain, enhancing the sialylation process of proteins highly involved in brain development. The maintenance of PSA-NCAM levels suggests neuroplasticity may be higher in the 6′-SL group.

With regards to cognitive evaluation, several behavioral tests were implemented consisting of two classical tests including the Y Maze with blocked arm and NORT, as well as a novel cognitive paradigm performed in the IntelliCage® system. Y maze and NORT have been used in previous animal studies to evaluate the effects of nutrition on cognition [53,54] and were conducted at both ages in the present work. IntelliCage® paradigm was only performed in adulthood. Data from weaned rats did not show differences among groups in any of the classical tests. In fact, performing cognitive tests at early ages of life entails certain methodological challenges. Leussis and Bolivar [55] pointed out that pre-weanling and weanling rodents normally habituate slower to novel environments, showing low exploratory activity when compared to older animals. It has been suggested that younger animals would perform better in rewarded tasks. Longer periods of exposure or habituation have also been proposed to increase the success of these tests. Based on our experience, the intense physical activity and the lack of focus in very young rodents are the main hurdles found when carrying out cognitive evaluation of weanling animals.

Conversely, significant differences were found in the assessment of cognitive skills in adulthood. In NORT, groups receiving Sia during lactation could distinguish better between novel and familiar objects than the control group. Impairment of the perirhinal cortex, the main brain structure involved in object recognition memory [44,56] has been suggested [57] as the reason why animals are not able to get a good score on memory tasks like NORT. Results obtained from the IntelliCage® paradigm confirmed that animals receiving Sia at early stages performed significantly better than the control group in adulthood. As for the Y maze test, Sia-supplemented animals performed better than the control rats, since they were able to recognize the novel arm easily. An interesting finding to highlight was that, within groups supplemented with Sia, 6′-SL rats had better scores than animals that received Neu5Ac during lactation, suggesting 6′-SL may be a better source of Sia.

An added value of the present study is that animal cognitive assessments were also supported by electrophysiological data based on in vivo LTP measurements. LTP is the basic mechanism for certain types of hippocampal learning [40]. The best results were observed in Sia-supplemented animals, mainly those of the 6′-SL group, while the control group performance was significantly lower than that of 6′-SL rats. These data suggest early supplementation with Sia might enhance processes related to neuronal plasticity.

Remarkably, control animals under-performed in all tests compared to Sia groups. In NORT, there were no differences in exploration time for both objects. In the Y maze, no preference for visiting the blocked arm first was shown. In the IntelliCage®, these animals scored poorly for correct visits, and a low increase in fEPSP amplitude was found in LTP. These results highlighted a certain degree of deficiency in control animals that could be explained by the lower amount of sialic acid and/or other nutrients such as minerals [58] that they received during the lactation period. The data indicate that the exogenous Sia provided by milk is necessary for the establishment of a neuronal network that ensures long-lasting cognitive skills. Lower levels of Sia during this critical timeframe may lead to premature aging of certain brain functions, while an exogenous supply of Sia was shown to be effective in maintaining cognitive skills for a longer duration. This phenomenon agrees with our previous research in which early supplementation during lactation with the HMO 2′-fucosyllactose (2′-FL) induced cognitive benefits in adult animals [42]. This new perspective highlights the concept of early nutrition [59] and the role of sialic acid in brain development.

Although the mechanism of action through which HMOs might exert this positive effect on cognitive outcomes is not yet known, there are several hypotheses. The improved cognitive performance observed in the Sia-supplemented groups could be due to an increase in the polysialylation of NCAM [60] or to an increase of sialylated compounds in brain due to the additional supply of Sia. There is a consistent body of evidence highlighting the potential biological importance of sialylated compounds in brain. Gangliosides are known to be key molecules in many CNS functions such as synaptogenesis, neurite and axonal growth and neural transmission [61–63].

Alternatively, 2′-FL orally given to adult mice also improves cognition and is dependent on gut-brain crosstalk through the vagus nerve [29]. The gut-brain axis (GBA) is a complex bidirectional network that communicates between the brain and gastrointestinal tract and modulates the respective functions [31]. This gut-brain crosstalk is driven by neural pathways and immune and endocrine mechanisms. It is known that one of the main factors able to trigger or modulate GBA is the intestinal microbiota [64] by producing different metabolites, such as short chain fatty acids or neurotransmitters. Several studies have reported how HMOs promote intestinal bacteria such as *Bifidobacterium* and *Lactobacillus* [65,66] based on their prebiotic role. Tarr et al. reported that dietary supplementation with both 6′-SL or 3′-SL effectively altered colonic microbiota communities, as well as diminished stressor-induced alterations in colonic mucosa structure, anxiety-like behavior and immature neuron cell numbers regardless of immune or endocrine functionality [30]. Despite this evidence, the role of 6′-SL as a GBA regulator and the mechanism underlying the reported effects are yet to be explored. Thus, the reported benefits on CNS function could be related either to its prebiotic capability, with its uptake by the brain during the critical neurodevelopment period, inducing long-lasting biochemical changes that ultimately enhance long-term cognitive skills or via GBA regulation.

With regards to the Sia sources used in this study, our results show that free Sia was less effective than 6′-SL, possibly because free Sia is more rapidly eliminated in the urine and, therefore, less bio-available. Nöhle and Schauer [67] suggested that metabolism of sialic acids bound to oligosaccharides might take more time than free Sia, since the former would require hydrolysis. In addition, oral treatment with 6′-SL in a mouse model of symptomatic *GNE* myopathy led to greater restoration of sialylation in muscle and improvement in muscle size and function as compared to the group treated with free Sia [68]. Based on these data, 6′-SL may be a better source of bio-available Sia.

5. Conclusions

In summary, our findings confirm the beneficial effects of supplementation of Neu5Ac or 6′-SL during lactation on long-term cognitive development in rats. Both compounds had positive outcomes; however, the results showed improved scores in behavior and electrophysiological analysis in those animals that received 6′-SL compared to Sia. Further research is needed to delineate the mechanisms of action underlying cognitive benefits and the potential role of intestinal microbiota.

6. Patents

There is one patent resulting from the work reported in this manuscript: the method of achieving memory and learning improvement by the administration of sialic acid. Publication number: WO/2015/085077. International Application Number: PCT/US2014/068582.

Author Contributions: Formal analysis, E.O., A.B., A.G. and J.M.D.-G. Investigation, E.O., A.B., A.G. and J.M.D.-G. Methodology, E.V., M.R. and M.J.M. Supervision, M.J.M. Writing, original draft, E.O. Writing, review and editing, E.V., M.R., R.B., R.R. and M.J.M. The results described in this manuscript are part of the doctoral thesis project of E.O. within the doctoral programme in Biomedicine of the University of Granada.

Acknowledgments: The authors would like to thank the technical staff for their assistance.

References

1. Anderson, J.W.; Johnstone, B.M.; Remley, D.T. Breast-feeding and cognitive development: A meta-analysis. *Am. J. Clin. Nutr.* **1999**, *70*, 525–535. [CrossRef] [PubMed]
2. Varki, A.; Schauer, R. Sialic acids. In *Essentials of Glycobiology*, 2nd ed.; Varki, A., Cummings, R.D., Esko, J.D., Freeze, H.H., Stanley, P., Bertozzi, C.R., Hart, G.W., Etzler, M.E., Eds.; Cold Spring Harbor Laboratory Press: Cold Spring Harbor, NY, USA, 2009.
3. Wang, B. Sialic acid is an essential nutrient for brain development and cognition. *Annu. Rev. Nutr.* **2009**, *29*, 177–222. [CrossRef] [PubMed]
4. Ten Bruggencate, S.J.; Bovee-Oudenhoven, I.M.; Feitsma, A.L.; van Hoffen, E.; Schoterman, M.H. Functional role and mechanisms of sialyllactose and other sialylated milk oligosaccharides. *Nutr. Rev.* **2014**, *72*, 377–389. [CrossRef] [PubMed]
5. Coppa, G.V.; Pierani, P.; Zampini, L.; Carloni, I.; Carlucci, A.; Gabrielli, O. Oligosaccharides in human milk during different phases of lactation. *Acta Paediatr. Suppl.* **1999**, *88*, 89–94. [CrossRef] [PubMed]
6. Ninonuevo, M.R.; Park, Y.; Yin, H.; Zhang, J.; Ward, R.E.; Clowers, B.H.; German, J.B.; Freeman, S.L.; Killeen, K.; Grimm, R.; et al. A strategy for annotating the human milk glycome. *J. Agric. Food Chem.* **2006**, *54*, 7471–7480. [CrossRef] [PubMed]
7. Jantscher-Krenn, E.; Bode, L. Human milk oligosaccharides and their potential benefits for the breast-fed neonate. *Minerva Pediatr.* **2012**, *64*, 83–99. [PubMed]
8. Kiskini, A.; Difilippo, E. Oligosaccharides in goat milk: Structure, health effects and isolation. *Cell. Mol. Biol.* **2013**, *59*, 25–30. [PubMed]
9. Martin-Sosa, S.; Martin, M.J.; Garcia-Pardo, L.A.; Hueso, P. Sialyloligosaccharides in human and bovine milk and in infant formulas: Variations with the progression of lactation. *J. Dairy Sci.* **2003**, *86*, 52–59. [CrossRef]

10. Peterson, R.; Cheah, W.Y.; Grinyer, J.; Packer, N. Glycoconjugates in human milk: Protecting infants from disease. *Glycobiology* **2013**, *23*, 1425–1438. [CrossRef] [PubMed]
11. Austin, S.; De Castro, C.A.; Bénet, T.; Hou, Y.; Sun, H.; Thakkar, S.K.; Vinyes-Pares, G.; Zhang, Y.; Wang, P. Temporal Change of the Content of 10 Oligosaccharides in the Milk of Chinese Urban Mothers. *Nutrients* **2016**, *8*, 346. [CrossRef] [PubMed]
12. Weichert, S.; Jennewein, S.; Hufner, E.; Weiss, C.; Borkowski, J.; Putze, J.; Schroten, H. Bioengineered 2′-fucosyllactose and 3-fucosyllactose inhibit the adhesion of pseudomonas aeruginosa and enteric pathogens to human intestinal and respiratory cell lines. *Nutr. Res.* **2013**, *33*, 831–838. [CrossRef] [PubMed]
13. Weichert, S.; Koromyslova, A.; Singh, B.K.; Hansman, S.; Jennewein, S.; Schroten, H.; Hansman, G.S. Structural basis for norovirus inhibition by human milk oligosaccharides. *J. Virol.* **2016**, *90*, 4843–4848. [CrossRef] [PubMed]
14. Goehring, K.C.; Marriage, B.J.; Oliver, J.S.; Wilder, J.A.; Barrett, E.G.; Buck, R.H. Similar to those who are breastfed, infants fed a formula containing 2′-fucosyllactose have lower inflammatory cytokines in a randomized controlled trial. *J. Nutr.* **2016**, *146*, 2559–2566. [CrossRef] [PubMed]
15. Donovan, S.M.; Comstock, S.S. Human milk oligosaccharides influence neonatal mucosal and systemic immunity. *Ann. Nutr. Metab.* **2016**, *69*, 42–51. [CrossRef] [PubMed]
16. He, Y.; Liu, S.; Kling, D.E.; Leone, S.; Lawlor, N.T.; Huang, Y.; Feinberg, S.B.; Hill, D.R.; Newburg, D.S. The human milk oligosaccharide 2′-fucosyllactose modulates cd14 expression in human enterocytes, thereby attenuating lps-induced inflammation. *Gut* **2016**, *65*, 33–46. [CrossRef] [PubMed]
17. Jost, T.; Lacroix, C.; Braegger, C.; Chassard, C. Impact of human milk bacteria and oligosaccharides on neonatal gut microbiota establishment and gut health. *Nutr. Rev.* **2015**, *73*, 426–437. [CrossRef] [PubMed]
18. Bienenstock, J.; Buck, R.H.; Linke, H.; Forsythe, P.; Stanisz, A.M.; Kunze, W.A. Fucosylated but not sialylated milk oligosaccharides diminish colon motor contractions. *PLoS ONE* **2013**, *8*, e76236. [CrossRef] [PubMed]
19. Nakano, T.; Sugawara, M.; Kawakami, H. Sialic acid in human milk: Composition and functions. *Acta Paediatr. Taiwan* **2001**, *42*, 11–17. [PubMed]
20. Wang, B. Molecular mechanism underlying sialic acid as an essential nutrient for brain development and cognition. *Adv. Nutr. Int. Rev. J.* **2012**, *3*, 465S–472S. [CrossRef] [PubMed]
21. Asakuma, S.; Akahori, M.; Kimura, K.; Watanabe, Y.; Nakamura, T.; Tsunemi, M.; Arai, I.; Sanai, Y.; Urashima, T. Sialyl oligosaccharides of human colostrum: Changes in concentration during the first three days of lactation. *Biosci. Biotechnol. Biochem.* **2007**, *71*, 1447–1451. [CrossRef] [PubMed]
22. Wang, B.; McVeagh, P.; Petocz, P.; Brand-Miller, J. Brain ganglioside and glycoprotein sialic acid in breastfed compared with formula-fed infants. *Am. J. Clin. Nutr.* **2003**, *78*, 1024–1029. [CrossRef] [PubMed]
23. Chichlowski, M.; German, J.B.; Lebrilla, C.; Mills, D.A. The influence of milk oligosaccharides on microbiota of infants: Opportunities for formulas. *Annu. Rev. Food Sci. Technol.* **2011**, *2*, 331–351. [CrossRef] [PubMed]
24. German, J.B.; Freeman, S.L.; Lebrilla, C.B.; Mills, D.A. Human milk oligosaccharides: Evolution, structures and bioselectivity as substrates for intestinal bacteria. *Nestle Nutr. Workshop Ser. Pediatr. Program.* **2008**, *62*, 205–218. [PubMed]
25. Jantscher-Krenn, E.; Marx, C.; Bode, L. Human milk oligosaccharides are differentially metabolised in neonatal rats. *Br. J. Nutr.* **2013**, *110*, 640–650. [CrossRef] [PubMed]
26. Bode, L. Human milk oligosaccharides: Every baby needs a sugar mama. *Glycobiology* **2012**, *22*, 1147–1162. [CrossRef] [PubMed]
27. Morgan, B.L.; Winick, M. Effects of administration of n-acetylneuraminic acid (nana) on brain nana content and behavior. *J. Nutr.* **1980**, *110*, 416–424. [CrossRef] [PubMed]
28. Wang, B.; Yu, B.; Karim, M.; Hu, H.; Sun, Y.; McGreevy, P.; Petocz, P.; Held, S.; Brand-Miller, J. Dietary sialic acid supplementation improves learning and memory in piglets. *Am. J. Clin. Nutr.* **2007**, *85*, 561–569. [CrossRef] [PubMed]
29. Vazquez, E.; Barranco, A.; Ramirez, M.; Gruart, A.; Delgado-Garcia, J.M.; Jimenez, M.L.; Buck, R.; Rueda, R. Dietary 2′-fucosyllactose enhances operant conditioning and long-term potentiation via gut-brain communication through the vagus nerve in rodents. *PLoS ONE* **2016**, *11*. [CrossRef] [PubMed]
30. Tarr, A.J.; Galley, J.D.; Fisher, S.E.; Chichlowski, M.; Berg, B.M.; Bailey, M.T. The prebiotics 3′sialyllactose and 6′sialyllactose diminish stressor-induced anxiety-like behavior and colonic microbiota alterations: Evidence for effects on the gut-brain axis. *Brain Behav. Immun.* **2015**, *50*, 166–177. [CrossRef] [PubMed]

31. Carabotti, M.; Scirocco, A.; Maselli, M.A.; Severi, C. The gut-brain axis: Interactions between enteric microbiota, central and enteric nervous systems. *Ann. Gastroenterol.* **2015**, *28*, 203–209. [PubMed]
32. Dinan, T.G.; Cryan, J.F. Gut instincts: Microbiota as a key regulator of brain development, ageing and neurodegeneration. *J. Physiol.* **2017**, *595*, 489–503. [CrossRef] [PubMed]
33. Carlson, A.L.; Xia, K.; Azcarate-Peril, M.A.; Goldman, B.D.; Ahn, M.; Styner, M.A.; Thompson, A.L.; Geng, X.; Gilmore, J.H.; Knickmeyer, R.C. Infant gut microbiome associated with cognitive development. *Biol. Psychiatry* **2018**, *83*, 148–159. [CrossRef] [PubMed]
34. Benton, D.; ILSI Europe a.i.s.b.l. The influence of children's diet on their cognition and behavior. *Eur. J. Nutr.* **2008**, *47* (Suppl. 3), 25–37. [CrossRef]
35. Sprenger, N.; Duncan, P.I. Sialic acid utilization. *Adv. Nutr.* **2012**, *3*, 392S–397S. [CrossRef] [PubMed]
36. Dickson, J.J.; Messer, M. Intestinal neuraminidase activity of suckling rats and other mammals. Relationship to the sialic acid content of milk. *Biochem. J.* **1978**, *170*, 407–413. [CrossRef] [PubMed]
37. Dominguez, H.D.; Thomas, J.D. Artificial Rearing. In *Alcohol: Methods and Protocols*; Nagy, L.E., Ed.; Humana Press: Totowa, NJ, USA, 2008; Volume 447, pp. 85–100.
38. Hara, S.; Takemori, Y.; Yamaguchi, M.; Nakamura, M.; Ohkura, Y. Fluorometric high-performance liquid chromatography of N-acetyl- and N-glycolylneuraminic acids and its application to their microdetermination in human and animal sera, glycoproteins, and glycolipids. *Anal. Biochem.* **1987**, *164*, 138–145. [CrossRef]
39. Martin, M.J.; Vazquez, E.; Rueda, R. Application of a sensitive fluorometric HPLC assay to determine the sialic acid content of infant formulas. *Anal. Bioanal. Chem.* **2007**, *387*, 2943–2949. [CrossRef] [PubMed]
40. Gruart, A.; Munoz, M.D.; Delgado-Garcia, J.M. Involvement of the ca3-ca1 synapse in the acquisition of associative learning in behaving mice. *J. Neurosci.* **2006**, *26*, 1077–1087. [CrossRef] [PubMed]
41. Vazquez, E.; Barranco, A.; Ramirez, M.; Gruart, A.; Delgado-García, J.M.; Martinez-Lara, E.; Blanco, S.; Martin, M.J.; Castanys-Muñoz, E.; Buck, R.H.; et al. Effects of a human milk oligosacharide, 2′-fucosyllactose, on hippocampal long term potentiation and learning capabilities in rodents. *JNB* **2015**, *26*, 455–465. [PubMed]
42. Oliveros, E.; Ramirez, M.; Vazquez, E.; Barranco, A.; Gruart, A.; Delgado-Garcia, J.M.; Buck, R.; Rueda, R.; Martin, M.J. Oral supplementation of 2′-fucosyllactose during lactation improves memory and learning in rats. *J. Nutr. Biochem.* **2016**, *31*, 20–27. [CrossRef] [PubMed]
43. Antunes, M.; Biala, G. The novel object recognition memory: Neurobiology, test procedure, and its modifications. *Cogn. Process.* **2012**, *13*, 93–110. [CrossRef] [PubMed]
44. Ennaceur, A.; Delacour, J. A new one-trial test for neurobiological studies of memory in rats. 1: Behavioral data. *Behav. Brain Res.* **1988**, *31*, 47–59. [CrossRef]
45. Wolf, A.; Bauer, B.; Abner, E.L.; Ashkenazy-Frolinger, T.; Hartz, A.M. A comprehensive behavioral test battery to assess learning and memory in 129s6/tg2576 mice. *PLoS ONE* **2016**, *11*. [CrossRef] [PubMed]
46. Dellu, F.; Mayo, W.; Cherkaoui, J.; Le Moal, M.; Simon, H. A two-trial memory task with automated recording: Study in young and aged rats. *Brain Res.* **1992**, *588*, 132–139. [CrossRef]
47. Wang, B.; Downing, J.A.; Petocz, P.; Brand-Miller, J.; Bryden, W.L. Metabolic fate of intravenously administered n-acetylneuraminic acid-6-14c in newborn piglets. *Asia Pac. J. Clin. Nutr.* **2007**, *16*, 110–115. [PubMed]
48. Carlson, S.E.; House, S.G. Oral and intraperitoneal administration of n-acetylneuraminic acid: Effect on rat cerebral and cerebellar n-acetylneuraminic acid. *J. Nutr.* **1986**, *116*, 881–886. [CrossRef] [PubMed]
49. Scholtz, S.A.; Gottipati, B.S.; Gajewski, B.J.; Carlson, S.E. Dietary sialic acid and cholesterol influence cortical composition in developing rats. *J. Nutr.* **2013**, *143*, 132–135. [CrossRef] [PubMed]
50. Fleming, S.A.; Chichlowski, M.; Berg, B.M.; Donovan, S.M.; Dilger, R.N. Dietary sialyllactose does not influence measures of recognition memory or diurnal activity in the young pig. *Nutrients* **2018**, *10*, 395. [CrossRef] [PubMed]
51. Mudd, A.T.; Fleming, S.A.; Labhart, B.; Chichlowski, M.; Berg, B.M.; Donovan, S.M.; Dilger, R.N. Dietary sialyllactose influences sialic acid concentrations in the prefrontal cortex and magnetic resonance imaging measures in corpus callosum of young pigs. *Nutrients* **2017**, *12*, 1297. [CrossRef] [PubMed]
52. Jacobi, S.K.; Yatsunenko, T.; Li, D.; Dasgupta, S.; Yu, R.K.; Berg, B.M.; Chichlowski, M.; Odle, J. Dietary isomers of sialyllactose increase ganglioside sialic acid concentrations in the corpus callosum and cerebellum and modulate the colonic microbiota of formula-fed piglets. *J. Nutr.* **2016**, *146*, 200–208. [CrossRef] [PubMed]
53. Cutuli, D.; De Bartolo, P.; Caporali, P.; Laricchiuta, D.; Foti, F.; Ronci, M.; Rossi, C.; Neri, C.; Spalletta, G.;

Caltagirone, C.; et al. N-3 polyunsaturated fatty acids supplementation enhances hippocampal functionality in aged mice. *Front. Aging Neurosci.* **2014**, *6*, 220. [CrossRef] [PubMed]
54. Hiratsuka, S.; Honma, H.; Saitoh, Y.; Yasuda, Y.; Yokogoshi, H. Effects of dietary sialic acid in n-3 fatty acid-deficient dams during pregnancy and lactation on the learning abilities of their pups after weaning. *J. Nutr. Sci. Vitaminol. (Tokyo)* **2013**, *59*, 136–143. [CrossRef] [PubMed]
55. Leussis, M.P.; Bolivar, V.J. Habituation in rodents: A review of behavior, neurobiology, and genetics. *Neurosci. Biobehav. Rev.* **2006**, *30*, 1045–1064. [CrossRef] [PubMed]
56. Aggleton, J.P.; Albasser, M.M.; Aggleton, D.J.; Poirier, G.L.; Pearce, J.M. Lesions of the rat perirhinal cortex spare the acquisition of a complex configural visual discrimination yet impair object recognition. *Behav. Neurosci.* **2010**, *124*, 55–68. [CrossRef] [PubMed]
57. Albasser, M.M.; Davies, M.; Futter, J.E.; Aggleton, J.P. Magnitude of the object recognition deficit associated with perirhinal cortex damage in rats: Effects of varying the lesion extent and the duration of the sample period. *Behav. Neurosci.* **2009**, *123*, 115–124. [CrossRef] [PubMed]
58. Keen, C.L.; Lönnerdal, B.; Clegg, M.; Hurley, L.S. Developmental changes in composition of rat milk: Trace elements, minerals, protein, carbohydrate and fat. *J. Nutr.* **1981**, *111*, 226–236. [CrossRef] [PubMed]
59. Anjos, T.; Altmae, S.; Emmett, P.; Tiemeier, H.; Closa-Monasterolo, R.; Luque, V.; Wiseman, S.; Perez-Garcia, M.; Lattka, E.; Demmelmair, H.; et al. Nutrition and neurodevelopment in children: Focus on nutrimenthe project. *Eur. J. Nutr.* **2013**, *52*, 1825–1842. [CrossRef] [PubMed]
60. Becker, C.G.; Artola, A.; Gerardy-Schahn, R.; Becker, T.; Welzl, H.; Schachner, M. The polysialic acid modification of the neural cell adhesion molecule is involved in spatial learning and hippocampal long-term potentiation. *J. Neurosci. Res.* **1996**, *45*, 143–152. [CrossRef]
61. Schnaar, R.L.; Gerardy-Schahn, R.; Hildebrandt, H. Sialic acids in the brain: Gangliosides and polysialic acid in nervous system development, stability, disease, and regeneration. *Physiol. Rev.* **2014**, *94*, 461–518. [CrossRef] [PubMed]
62. Hwang, H.M.; Wang, J.T.; Chiu, T.H. Effects of exogenous gm1 ganglioside on ltp in rat hippocampal slices perfused with different concentrations of calcium. *Neurosci. Lett.* **1992**, *141*, 227–230. [CrossRef]
63. Ledeen, R.W.; Wu, G.; Lu, Z.H.; Kozireski-Chuback, D.; Fang, Y. The role of gm1 and other gangliosides in neuronal differentiation. Overview and new finding. *Ann. N. Y. Acad. Sci.* **1998**, *845*, 161–175. [CrossRef] [PubMed]
64. Burokas, A.; Moloney, R.D.; Dinan, T.G.; Cryan, J.F. Microbiota regulation of the mammalian gut-brain axis. *Adv. Appl. Microbiol.* **2015**, *91*, 1–62. [PubMed]
65. Coppa, G.V.; Zampini, L.; Galeazzi, T.; Facinelli, B.; Ferrante, L.; Capretti, R.; Orazio, G. Human milk oligosaccharides inhibit the adhesion to caco-2 cells of diarrheal pathogens: *Escherichia coli*, vibrio cholerae, and salmonella fyris. *Pediatr. Res.* **2006**, *59*, 377–382. [CrossRef] [PubMed]
66. Bindels, L.B.; Delzenne, N.M.; Cani, P.D.; Walter, J. Towards a more comprehensive concept for prebiotics. *Nat. Rev. Gastroenterol. Hepatol.* **2015**, *12*, 303–310. [CrossRef] [PubMed]
67. Nöhle, U.; Schauer, R. Metabolism of sialic acids from exogenously administered sialyllactose and mucin in mouse and rat. *Hoppe Seylers Z. Physiol. Chem.* **1984**, *365*, 1457–1467. [CrossRef] [PubMed]
68. Yonekawa, T.; Malicdan, M.C.; Cho, A.; Hayashi, Y.K.; Nonaka, I.; Mine, T.; Yamamoto, T.; Nishino, I.; Noguchi, S. Sialyllactose ameliorates myopathic phenotypes in symptomatic gne myopathy model mice. *Brain* **2014**, *137*, 2670–2679. [CrossRef] [PubMed]

13

The Impact of Mediterranean Dietary Patterns During Pregnancy on Maternal and Offspring Health

Federica Amati *, Sondus Hassounah and Alexandra Swaka

Department of Primary Care and Public Health, Imperial College London, London W6 8RP, UK; s.hassounah@imperial.ac.uk (S.H.); a.swaka@imperial.ac.uk (A.S.)
* Correspondence: f.amati@imperial.ac.uk

Abstract: (1) Background: Pregnancy outcomes for both mother and child are affected by many environmental factors. The importance of pregnancy for 'early life programming' is well established and maternal nutrition is an important factor contributing to a favourable environment for developing offspring. We aim to assess whether following a Mediterranean Diet during pregnancy is beneficial for maternal and offspring outcomes; (2) Methods: a systematic review was performed using standardized reporting guidelines with the National Heart Lung and Blood Iinstitute quality assessment tool for selection and extraction; (3) Results: results show that being on a Mediterranean Diet during pregnancy is associated with favourable outcomes for both maternal and offspring health, particularly for gestational diabetes in mothers and congenital defects in offspring (4) Conclusions: Following a Mediterranean dietary pattern during gestation is beneficial for the health of both the mother and offspring. Pregnant women and those trying to conceive should be advised to follow a Mediterranean Diet to potentially decrease, for example, the likelihood of atopy (OR 0.55) in the offspring and Gestational Diabetes Mellitus in the mother (OR 0.73).

Keywords: maternal nutrition; Mediterranean diet; offspring health

---

1. Introduction

The maternal diet before conception and during pregnancy has long-term implications for maternal and offspring health, from placental development [1], risk of developing gestational diabetes [2], birth complications [3], birth weight [4] and risk of developing allergies in childhood [5–8]. Exposure to an unfavourable environment in early pregnancy is known to significantly increase the risk of diseases in adult life; this is known as 'early life programming' and one of the most important factors is the maternal diet [9]. Pregnancy presents an opportune time window for healthcare professionals' intervention to improve health for both the mother and child, making the evidence surrounding maternal diet an important tool for the healthcare practice.

Maternal diet is a blueprint for the diet which children are likely to follow into adolescence. This is due to the fact that, typically, mothers are responsible for feeding their children. Without intervention, pregnant women who do not follow a healthy diet or lifestyle choices are unlikely to change their patterns of behaviour. Sometimes obstacles to changes in behaviour can present themselves even for well-known harmful habits such as smoking during pregnancy, but as a unique window of opportunity, focusing health service efforts to impact the behaviour of pregnant women is crucial.

The Mediterranean Diet (MD) and Mediterranean Diet Adherence (MDA) is characterized by a high intake of fruits, vegetables, whole grain cereals, legumes, fish and nuts; low-to-moderate consumption of dairy products and limited amounts of red meat and red wine. It is low in saturated fats and high in antioxidants, fibre and mono and polyunsaturated fatty acids mainly derived from extra virgin olive oil (evoo) (MUFAs) and oily fish (n-3 PUFAs). The MD is known to have many beneficial effects for longevity and disease prevention, demonstrated in numerous high-quality studies, reviews and meta-analyses, making it the most widely studied and evidence-based dietary approach to healthy eating and disease prevention [10–13]. The unique synergy of various health benefitting nutrients makes MD an effective approach to improving health [11].

Recording dietary patterns through food diaries and food frequency questionnaires (FFQs) is a valuable tool to analyse eating behaviours and better understand which foods and food groups are consumed. Individual foods, such as extra virgin olive oil (evoo), as well as food groups, such as pulses, provide an insight to the nutrients consumed in the recorded foods, such as monounsaturated fatty acids (MUFAs) and fibre, respectively. Asking an individual to recount specific nutrient amounts is more complex than recounting what foods were consumed as part of the daily diet, making dietary pattern analysis more attainable for patients and crucial for research.

Evidence on the impact of diet during pregnancy on health outcomes focusses on either individual nutrients, such as folic acid, or the Mediterranean Diet for their impact on specific disease outcomes such as neural tube defects [14] or leukaemia [15]. The degree of evidence available for the impact of specific nutrients in pregnancy on outcomes for offspring health is more powerful than that for dietary patterns. For instance, the necessity for appropriate levels of folic acid during gestation is well-documented in the prevention of neural tube defects, and the mechanism by which folic acid prevents neural tube defects is well understood and documented. Whereas supplements are the quicker and easier way to address certain nutritional deficiencies of individual nutrients [11], dietary patterns are a useful way of studying the effects of dietary exposure, in turn, making recommended diets a potential health improvement intervention alongside appropriate and necessary supplementation in pregnancy.

The Mediterranean Diet is well established as beneficial in the literature [16]. Previous reviews of the evidence where several dietary patterns have been evaluated highlight that maternal dietary patterns are important factors in early life programming. Maternal dietary patterns which reflect the MD showed consistent associations with a lower risk for allergic disease in children [17], appropriate infant birthweight [18], and lower risk of pre-eclampsia and preterm birth [19]. This Review investigates and presents current evidence exclusively on the Mediterranean Diet's multifactorial impact on overall health outcomes for both the mother and offspring, as the sole dietary pattern of interest.

Our results indicate that the Mediterranean Diet has a significantly positive impact on maternal and offspring health, strengthening the evidence base to encourage its adoption as a preventive measure against diseases throughout the life course and especially in pregnancy when the outcome of two or more individuals can be positively impacted.

2. Materials and Methods

2.1. Data Sources and Search Strategy

This systematic review was performed using a predetermined, unpublished protocol and in accordance with standardized reporting guidelines [20]. Search terms identification and classification were guided by previous comprehensive relevant reviews [21]. One reviewer (FA) performed searches in the following online electronic databases (Medline, Embase, Web of Science, Scopus, Maternity & infant care and Cochrane). The search of online databases is up to date to February 2019. The search was not restricted by language or date.

The search was broken down into four main categories. To identify the relevant population, the first Boolean search was done using the term "OR" to explode (search by subject heading) and map (search by keyword) the following MeSH headings "child health" or "offspring" or "newborn" or "neonate" or "child" or "baby" or "gestation" or "pregnancy" or "pregnant woman" or "perinatal period" or "prenatal exposure" or "prenatal". To identify relevant interventions the second Boolean search used the term "OR" to explode and map "Mediterranean diet" or "fruit" or "vegetable" or "legume" or "nut" or "olive oil" or "evoo" or "oily fish" or "seafood" or "tomato". The third category of

MeSH headings was also related to the intervention and included ((low or little or medium or moderate or less or decrease or reduce or restrict) (intake or consumption or consume or eat or amount)) AND ("dairy product" or "red meat" or "processed meat" or "red wine"). Finally, the fourth group of key terms was used to identify the study design whereby a Boolean search using the term "OR" was used to explode and map the keywords "randomized controlled trial" or "controlled clinical trial" or "placebo" or "Retrospective Studies" or "Cohort Studies". The four search categories were then combined using the Boolean operator "AND". The hand searching of results in the Maternity & infant care database for a Mediterranean diet highlighted that using the terminology of 'child health' was not capturing some relevant papers, thus, the papers which were the result of searching for a Mediterranean diet in this database were hand-searched instead. For a full list of the search terms in each database please see Appendix A.

2.2. *Study Selection*

Three reviewers (FA, AS and SH) independently evaluated articles for eligibility in a three-stage procedure. In stage one, all identified titles and abstracts were reviewed. In stage two, a full-text review was performed on all the articles that met the predefined inclusion criteria as well as all articles for which there was uncertainty as to eligibility. In stage three, full texts were re-evaluated for data extraction.

2.3. *Inclusion/Exclusion Criteria*

Studies, publications or reports in the English-language describing an association between the Mediterranean diet during pregnancy and infant development were eligible for inclusion. Studies, publications or reports were included for analysis if they included the following:

1. Exposure: Comprehensive dietary assessment: Food frequency questionnaire (FFQ), 24 h diet recall, food record, diet history, Use of a priori dietary score or index;
2. Outcome: Clinical neonatal outcome, disorders assessed by study staff, medical records or clinician diagnosed (for example, Foetal growth restriction (FGR) and preterm delivery (PTD)), developmental issues assessed by validated scale/questionnaire;
3. Design: Observational studies (cross-sectional, cohort, case-control), Interventional studies (clinical trials);
4. Population: Pregnant women (at any gestational age).

Articles were excluded if they investigated pregnant women with other dietary complications (non-gestational diabetes, obesity, anorexia, malnourishment) and/or if they explored a specific nutrient impact as opposed to a dietary pattern (e.g., Omega-3 supplementation as a feature of the Med Diet.)

2.4. *Data Extraction and Quality Assessment*

Two reviewers (FA and AS) independently extracted data from all studies that satisfied the inclusion criteria. Any disagreement in data extraction and/or study inclusion was resolved through discussion between the two reviewers and, when necessary, a third reviewer (SH).

The primary outcome was the impact on maternal and offspring health. A number of other study characteristics were also extracted including geographic location, description of the study population, primary outcomes, description of intervention and control, and results. Furthermore, data pertaining to sample size, number, and features of the intervention were also extracted.

2.5. *Quality Assessment*

The methodological quality of studies was assessed and scored independently by two reviewers (FA and AS) using the validated National Heart, Lung, and Blood Institute (NHLBI) study Quality Assessment Tool [22] (see Appendix B Table A1). Disagreements were resolved through discussion. The summary score for each study was calculated (minimum: 1, maximum: 10) and categorised into three categories. Studies with a score of 8 or above were considered of high-quality, studies with a score of 5–7 were considered of fair quality and studies with a score of 4 or below were considered of poor quality. These categories were used to evaluate whether outcomes significantly varied according to study quality and to determine which weight studies should be given in the synthesis of the findings.

2.6. Data Synthesis and Presentation

Since exploring heterogeneity is one of the main aims of an SLR/MA, a descriptive synthesis approach was used instead of meta-analytic procedures. Our review includes studies with diverse designs and all shared comprehensive dietary assessment tools to measure MD adherence, with neonatal and maternal clinical markers as outcomes. The results of the quality assessment are presented in Table 1. As the narrative synthesis was used to analyse and present the findings, the results of data abstraction are summarized in Table 2, which outlines the type, objective and target of intervention, and measurement of effect for each intervention. Study results are summarized in Table 3 according to categories/themes and whether the MD was found to have a Protective, Null or Negative effect on outcomes.

3. Results

3.1. Literature Selection

Our initial database search is outlined in Figure 1, showing that a total of 125 articles were initially identified based on our search criteria, 14 duplicates were removed, leaving 111 articles for title and abstract screening, of which 67 were excluded for the title (25 were the wrong type of article for this review, 19 targetted the non-objective population, 8 were studies that included dietary complications or risk factors, and 15 focused on a specific nutrient impact); 16 at abstract following the inclusion/exclusion criteria (9 were the wrong type of article for this review, 3 targetted a non-objective population, 3 for studies that included dietary complications or risk factors, and 2 focused on specific nutrient impact); and 6 after full text screening, included in the Appendix C (2 were the wrong type of article for this review, 3 targetted a non-objective population, and 1 focused on specific nutrient impact), for a total of 22 articles reviewed and included in this paper.

The studies included all used a comprehensive dietary assessment tool to measure MD adherence, with neonatal and maternal clinical markers as outcomes. The selected studies included observational, interventional studies, randomized trials, and all studies included a population of pregnant women at any gestational age with neonatal or child follow-ups. Table 1 shows our quality assessment results and Appendix C Figure A1 shows papers excluded after full text review.

Table 1. The quality assessment score values: <4 = Low, 4–7 = Medium, 8–10 = High.

Author	Design	Score (1–10)	Quality Assessment
Assaf-Balut, C; Garcia de la Torre, N; A Duran et al. [23]	Prospective randomized interventional study	8	High
Assaf-Balut, Carla; Garcia de la Torre, et al. [24]	Prospective randomized controlled trial (The St Carlos GDM prevention study)	9	High
Botto, Lorenzo D.; Krikov, Sergey; et al. [25]	Multicentre population-based case-control study	9	High
Chatzi, L.; Rifas-Shiman, S.; [26]	Prospective Cohort study (Project Viva + Rhea Study)	9	High
Chatzi L.; Torrent, M.; et al. [27]	Prospective Cohort study	7	High
Chatzi, L.; Garcia, R.; et. al. [28]	Cohort study (INMA and Rhea Study)	9	High
E, Parlapani; et al. [29]	Cohort study	7	Medium
Fernandez-Barres, S.; et al. [30]	Birth Cohort study (INMA)	8	High
Gesteiro, E.; Rodriguez B., et al. [31]	Cohort study	7	Medium
Gesteiro, E.; Bastida S., et al. [32]	Cross-sectional study	7	Medium
Gonzalez-Nahm, S. et al. [33]	Cohort study	8	High
Haugen, M.; et al. [34]	Prospective Cohort study (MoBa)	8	High
House, J.; et al. [35]	Prospective Cohort study	9	High
Castro-Rodriguez, J.; et al. [36]	Cohort study	7	Medium

Table 1. *Cont.*

Author	Design	Score (1–10)	Quality Assessment
Lange, N. [37]	Longitudinal pre-birth cohort study	9	High
Mantzoros, C.; et al. [38]	Prospective cohort study (Project Viva)	8	High
Monteagudo, C.; et al. [39]	Cohort study	8	High
Peraita-Costa, I. et al. [40]	Retrospective cross-sectional population-based study	7	Medium
Saunders, L.; et al. [41]	Cohort study (TIMOUN)	8	High
Steenweg-de Graaff, J.; et al. [42]	Population-based cohort (The Generation R Study)	9	High
Vujkovic, M.; et al. [43]	Case-control study	7	Medium
Smith, L.; et al. [44]	Population-based cohort study	7	Medium

GDM = gestational diabetes mellitus, INMA = INfancia y Medio Ambiente study, TIMOUN= French Caribeean Mother Child cohort study.

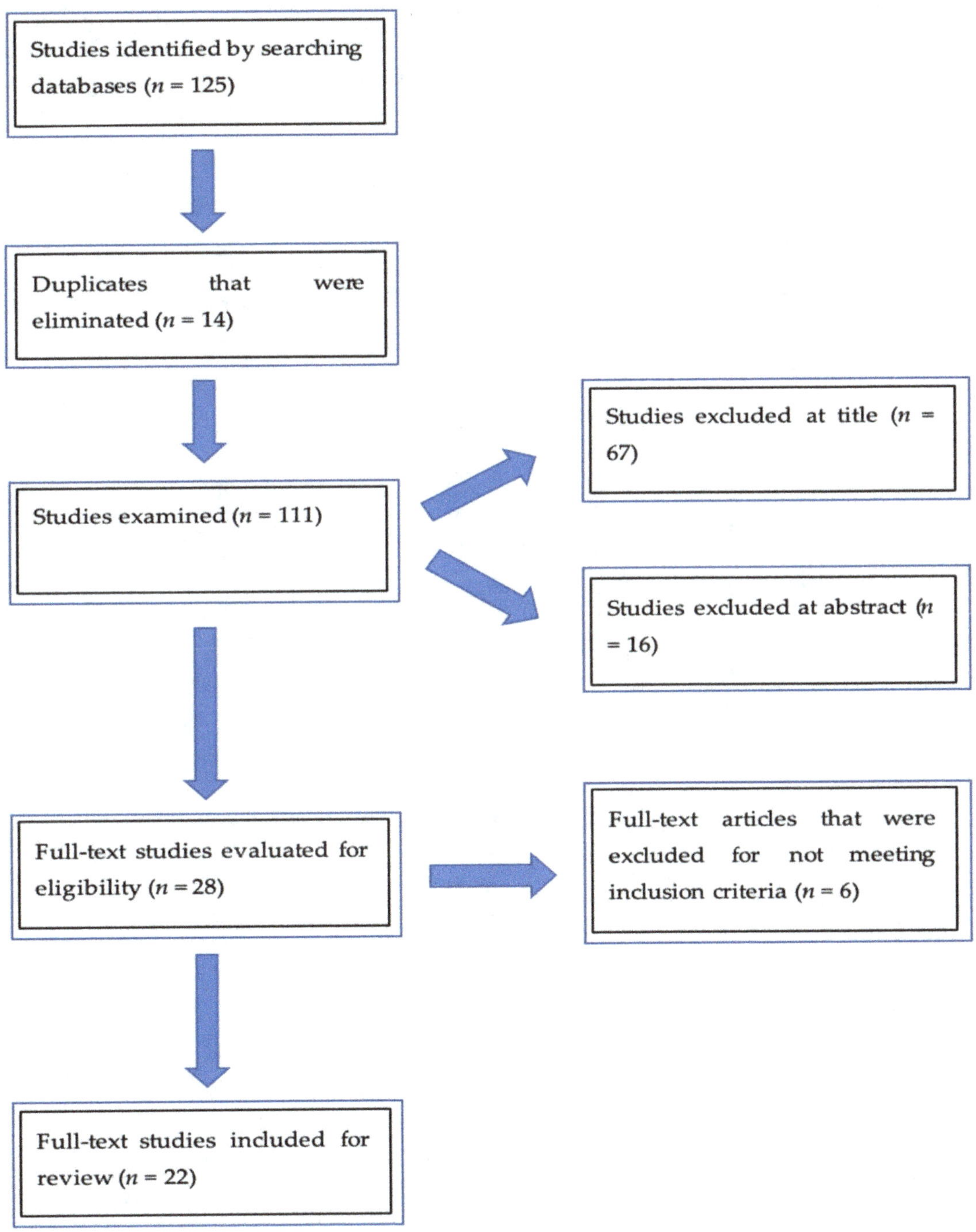

Figure 1. The flow diagram of the process for study selection.

Table 2. The outcomes and effect estimates for the included studies.

Authors	Design and Cohort	Included Participants and Gestational Age	Intervention Type and Comparator	Results
Assaf-Balut, C; Garcia de la Torre, N; A Duran et al. [23] Spain	Prospective randomized interventional study	874; First Trimester	MD nutritional therapy	As an early nutritional intervention, MD reduces the incidence of GDM. Comparison of HbA_{1c} levels at 24–28 weeks in women with GDM and normal glucose tolerance: $p = 0.001$. Values became similar at 36–38 gestational weeks with intervention.
Assaf-Balut, Carla; Garcia de la Torre, et al. [24] Spain	Prospective randomized controlled trial	874; intervention group (IG), $n = 434$ control group (CG), $n = 440$; 8–12 gestational weeks (First Trimester)	MD nutritional therapy with additional evoo and pistachios	Supplemented MD reduces the incidence of GDM as an early nutritional intervention. IG showed reduced rates of insulin-treated GDM: $p = < 0.05$
Botto, Lorenzo D.; Krikov, Sergey; et al. [25] USA	Multicentre population-based case-control study	Mothers of babies with major non-syndromic congenital heart defects ($n = 9885$); mothers with unaffected babies ($n = 9468$); maternal diet assessed in the year before pregnancy	A priori defined MDS with Quartiles 1–4 (worst to best)	Better diet quality is associated with a reduced occurrence of some conotruncal and septal heart defects Overall conotruncal defects: OR 0.63, 95% CI 0.49 to 0.80 Overall tetralogy of Fallot: OR 0.76, 95% CI 0.64 to 0.91 Overall septal defects: OR 0.77, 95% CI 0.63 to 0.94 Overall atrial septal defects: OR 0.86, 95% CI 0.75 to 1.00
Chatzi, L.; Rifas-Shiman, S.; [26] USA, Greece	Cohort study; Project Viva	Mother-child pairs from USA: 997 Greece: 569 MDA measured during pregnancy with follow-up at median 4.2 and 7.7 years	MDA with a priori defined MDS through FFQ	Greater adherence to MD during pregnancy may protect against excess offspring cardiometabolic risk. For each 3-point increase in MDS, offspring BMI decreased by 0.14 units (95% confidence interval, −0.15 to −0.13)
Chatzi L.; Torrent, M.; et al. [27] Spain	Cohort study	507 mothers during the gestational period; 460 children at 6.5 years post-gestational follow-up	Impact of MDA during pregnancy on asthma and atopy in childhood using a priori defined MDS	Adherence to Med Diet during pregnancy support protective effect against asthma-like symptoms and atopy in childhood Persistent wheeze: OR 0.22; 95% CI 0.08 to 0.90 Atopic wheeze: OR 0.30; 95% CI 0.10 to 0.90 Atopy: (OR 0.55; 95% CI 0.31 to 0.97
Chatzi, L.; Garcia, R.; et al. [28] Spain, Greece	Cohort study; INMA (Spain) RHEA (Greece)	During pregnancy with follow-up within 1 year post-gestational; 1771 mother-newborn pairs (Spain); 745 pairs (Greece)	MDA calculated through completed FFQ	High meat intake during pregnancy may increase the risk of a wheeze in the first year of life; high dairy intake may decrease it RR 0.83, 95% CI 0.72, 0.96
E, Parlapani; et al. [29] Greece	Cohort study	82 women delivering preterm singletons ≤34 weeks	FFQ and MDA	High adherence to MD, may favourably affect intrauterine growth (IUGR), premature birth and maternal hypertension (HTN); Low-MDA neonates group had a higher rate of IUGR: OR 3.3 Low-MDA mothers had a higher rate of prematurity: OR 1.6 Low-MDA mothers had a higher gestational HTN: OR 3.8
Fernandez-Barres, S.; et al. [30] Spain	Cohort study; INMA	1827 mother-child pairs, assessed during pregnancy	FFQ and MDA	Adherence to MD during pregnancy not associated with a risk of childhood obesity, but is linked to a lower waist circumference; p-value for trend = 0.009

Table 2. *Cont.*

Authors	Design and Cohort	Included Participants and Gestational Age	Intervention Type and Comparator	Results
Gesteiro, E.; Rodriguez, B., et al. [31] Spain	Cohort study	35 women with 'adequate' or 'inadequate' diets according to HEI (healthy eating index) and MDA score; 1st trimester	13 point MDA score via FFQ	Maternal diets during the 1st trimester with low HEIs or adherence to MD have a negative effect on insulin markers at birth; Low MDA-score diets had low-fasting glycaemia: $p = 0.025$ and delivered infants with high insulinaemia: $p = 0.049$
Gesteiro, E.; Sanchez-Muiz FJ, et al. [32] Spain	Cross-sectional study	53 mother-neonate pairs; GDM screening at 24–28 gestational weeks	Maternal MDA and offspring lipoprotein profile	Neonates of mothers who consumed low adherence of MD during pregnancy presented impaired lipoprotein and higher homocysteine levels; Mothers' diet in the nAA + AT x mTT group (neonates carrying FTO rs9939609 T allele x Mothers homozygous for FTO rs9939609 T allele) had a significantly lower MDA score: $p = 0.05$
Gonzalez-Nahm, S. et al. [33] USA	Cohort study	390 women whose infants had DNA methylation cord blood data available; FFQ at preconception or 1st trimester	MDA via FFQ	Suggests that maternal diet can have a sex-specific impact on infant DNA methylation at specific imprinted DMRs; OR = 7.40, 95% CI = 1.88–20.09
Haugen, M.; et al. [34] Norway	Cohort study; MoBa	MD criteria met: 569 women; 1–4 criteria met: 25,397 women; 0 MD criteria met: 159 women; 18–24 gestational weeks	MDA via FFQ	Women who adhered to the MD criteria did not have a reduced risk of preterm birth compared to women who met none of the criteria; OR: 0.73, 95% CI: 0.32, 1.68 Intake of fish twice a week or more associated with lower preterm birth; OR: 0.84; 95% CI: 0.74, 0.95
House, J.; et al. [35] USA	Cohort study; NEST	325 mother-infant pairs; 1st trimester; follow-up at 2 years post-gestation	MDA via FFQ	Offspring of women with high MDA less likely to exhibit neurobehavioural effects: Depression; OR = 0.28 Anxiety; OR = 0.42 Social relatedness; OR = 2.38
Castro-Rodriguez, J.; et al. [36] Spain, Chile	Cohort study	Gestational period; follow-up in 1000 preschoolers (at 1.5 yrs and 4 yrs)	MDA via FFQ	Low fruit and high meat consumption by the child had a negative effect on allergic responses (wheezing, rhinitis, or dermatitis); as did the high consumption of pasta and potatoes by the mother
Lange, N. [37] USA	Longitudinal prebirth cohort study; Project Viva	1376 mother-infant pairs; 1st and 2nd trimesters with follow-up at 3 years post-gestation	MDA via FFQ	Dietary pattern during pregnancy not associated with recurrent wheeze; OR per 1-point increase in MD: 0.98, 95% CI, 0.98–1.08
Mantzoros, C.; et al. [38] USA	Prospective cohort study; Project Viva	780 women; 1st and 2nd trimesters; post-gestational cord blood	MDA	Adherence to MD during pregnancy not associated with cord blood leptin or adiponectin; *p*-value = 0.38
Monteagudo, C.; et al. [39] Spain	Cohort study	320 umbilical cord serum samples	MDS-p (med diet score adapted to pregnancy)	Adherence to the MD and folic acid supplementation during pregnancy may indicate being overweight in newborns; OR = 3.33 ($p = 0.019$)

Table 2. *Cont.*

Authors	Design and Cohort	Included Participants and Gestational Age	Intervention Type and Comparator	Results
Peraita-Costa, I. et al. [40] Spain	Retrospective cross-sectional population-based study	492 mother-child pairs; immediately post-delivery and for 6 months thereafter	MDA with two groups identified: low and high adherence	Low adherence to an MD was not associated with a higher risk of a low birthweight newborn; aOR = 1.68; 95% CI 1.02–5.46
Saunders, L.; et al. [41] French West Indies	Cohort study; TIMOUN	728 pregnant women who delivered liveborn singletons with no malformations	Semi-quantitative FFQ analysed for MDA	Results suggest that adherence to a Caribbean diet may include benefits of MD, contributing to a reduction in preterm delivery in overweight women; A OR: 0.7, 95% CI 0.6, 0.9
Steenweg-de Graaff, J.; et al. [42] The Netherlands	Population-based cohort; Generation R Study	During pregnancy at median 13.5 weeks; Post-gestation in 3104 children at 1.5, 3, and 6 years of age	MDA via FFQ	High adherence to traditional Dutch diet and low adherence to MD are linked to an increased risk of child externalizing problems; OR per SD in MDS: 0.90, 95% CI: 0.83–0.97 OR per SD in Traditionally Dutch Score: 1.11, 95% CI: 1.03–1.21
Vujkovic, M.; et al. [43] The Netherlands	Case-control study	50 mothers of children with Spinal Bifida; 81 control mothers post-gestation	Dietary assessment via FFQ	MD seems to show an association with reducing the risk of offspring being affected by SB; Weak MDA; OR: 2.7 (95% CI 1.2–6.1) High MDA; OR: 3.5 (95% CI 1.5–7.9)
Smith, L.; et al. [44] United Kingdom	Population-based cohort study	922 LMPT; 965 term births; 32–36 weeks gestation (3rd Trimester)	Maternal interview for dietary factors: MDA, low fruit and vegetable intake, use of folic acid supplements	Women with 0 adherence to MD were nearly twice as likely to deliver LMPT; RR 1.81 (1.04 to 3.14) Smokers and low consumption of fruit and vegetables had a particularly high risk; RR 1.81 (1.29 to 2.55)

MD = Mediterranean Diet, MDS = Mediterranean Diet Score, MDA = Mediterranean Diet Adherance, FFQ = Food Frequency Questionnaire, HEI = Healthy Eating Index.

3.2. *Study Characteristics*

The studies included ($n = 22$) were published between 2008 and 2018 and were conducted in 8 countries, which included Spain, USA, Greece, Holland, Norway, Chile, French West Indies, and the United Kingdom. The common dietary measurements used were the adherence to the Mediterranean Diet Score (MDS) and an adapted MDS for pregnancy (MDS-p).

The MDS is an a priori defined score developed to measure compliance to a high intake of Mediterranean Diet foods with a score ranging from 0 to 9, where 9 indicates greater adherence to the diet [13]. The MDS-p is a scoring system that was designed by Montegaudo et al. [45] for pregnant women to better quantify the micronutrients in their diets such as calcium, folic acid, and iron, which are especially relevant in pregnancy [39].

Of the included studies, 16 were cohort studies, 1 was a randomized interventional study, 1 was a randomized controlled trial, 2 were case-control studies, and 2 were cross-sectional studies. All studies were conducted during the gestational period with follow-ups after birth. Table 2 shows the summarized characteristics of the studies including design, measures used, and results reported. The total number of participants for all of the studies is 63,336.

3.3. *MAIN RESULTS*

3.3.1. Allergic Disorders

Four studies focused on the relationship between maternal adherence to a Mediterranean Diet during pregnancy and neonatal or childhood outcomes of asthma and atopy. A cohort study by Chatzi, L; Torrent, M.; et al. [27] found that adherence to the MD during pregnancy supports a protective effect against asthma-like symptoms and atopy in childhood at 6.5 years old. Chatzi, L.; Garcia, R.; et al. [28] found that while adherence to the MD was not associated with the risk of wheeze and eczema in any cohort, high meat intake during pregnancy might increase the risk of wheeze during the first year of life. Through questionnaires of epidemiological factors, maternal diet during pregnancy, and childhood diet, Castro-Rodriguez, J.; M. Ramirez-Hernandez et al. [36], found that wheezing, rhinitis or dermatitis were negatively affected by high potato and pasta consumption by the mother and subsequent low fruit and high meat consumption by the child. Lange, N. et al. [37] however, examined 1376 mother-infant pairs and found that the dietary pattern is not associated with recurrent wheeze.

3.3.2. Premature Birth, Birth Weight, Childhood Obesity

Six studies examined the implications of the diet on premature birth, gestational diabetes (please see Table 3), birth weight, and/or childhood obesity. Parlapani, E. et al. [29] found that neonates of mothers with low adherence to the MD had significantly higher intrauterine growth restriction and lower birth weights. Haugen, M. et al. [34] investigated the association between women who met the MD adherence criteria and those who did not. The study showed that those who met the MD criteria of fish $\geq$2 times a week, fruit and vegetables $\geq$5 times a day, use of olive/canola oil, red meat intake $\leq$2 times a week, and $\leq$2 cups of coffee a day, did not have a lower risk of preterm birth compared to women who met none of the criteria. A population-based cohort study involving 922 late and moderate preterm births (LMPT) by Smith, L. et al. [44], identified that women who did not include any aspects of the MD during pregnancy were nearly twice as likely to have LMPT in comparison to higher adherence mothers. Fernandez-Barres, et al. [30] evaluated associates between adherence to the MD during pregnancy, but found no risk to childhood obesity, however, it was associated with a lower waist circumference, which is related to abdominal obesity and is an important health marker. Peraita-Costa et al. [40] administered the "Kidmed" questionnaire to collect dietary information from mothers on adherence to the MD. Of the 492 women, 40.2% showed low adherence to the MD, but this study did not directly correlate the results to low birth weight due to potentially confounding factors including smoking, low education levels, and low dairy intake. Saunders, L. et al. [41] found that low adherence to the MD could implicate a positive correlation between maternal diet and small birth weight.

Table 3. A summary of findings from our review of the evidence.

Health Outcomes	Impact of Maternal MD		
Outcome Variable	**Protective**	**Negative**	**Inconclusive**
Allergic Disorders	3 (27,28,36)		1 (37)
Premature birth, birth weight, childhood obesity	5 (29,30,39,41,44)		2 (30,36)
Cardiometabolic and congenital defects	3 (25,26,43)		
Gestational diabetes & pre-eclampsia	2 (23,24,29)		
DNA Methylation	2 (33,35)		
Biomarkers	2 (31,32)		1(38)
Behavioural development	1 (42)		

3.3.3. Cardiometabolic and Congenital Defects

Three studies examined the link between better maternal diet quality with congenital heart defects or metabolic factors. Chatzi, L.; Rifas-Shiman, S.; et al. [26] studied 997 mother-child pairs, finding that improved adherence to the MD during pregnancy showed lower systolic and diastolic blood pressures and may protect offspring against cardiometabolic risk. Botto, L. [25] et al. found, in a high-quality study, that diet quality was a factor of reduced conotruncal and atrial septal heart defects. Vujkovic, M. et al. [43] found that because of the higher levels of serum and RBC folate, Vitamin B12 and lower plasma homocysteine contained in the MD, offspring have a reduced risk of spina bifida.

3.3.4. Gestational Diabetes and Pre-Eclampsia

Two studies found that gestational nutrition based on the MD reduces the incidence of Gestational Diabetes (GDM). In a prospective randomized interventional study by A Duran, [24] 177 women out of 874 were diagnosed with GDM and found that with early intervention using the MD, gestational outcomes were improved. Likewise, the results of a randomized controlled trial conducted by Assaf-Balut, C. et al. [24] show that the incidence of GDM was reduced by early dietary intervention with a diet rich in EVOO and pistachios. Parlapani et al. [29] found that MDA was an independent predictor of gestational hypertension and pre-eclampsia.

3.3.5. DNA Methylation

Two studies examined the association between maternal adherence to the MD and DNA methylation in infants. One study conducted by Gonzalez-Nahm et al. [33] showed evidence that maternal diet of low MD adherence had an increased risk of female sex-linked hypo-methylation at the MEG3-IG differentially methylated region. House, J. et al. [35] also found an association between maternal adherence to the MD and female sex-linked methylation at MEG3, IGF2, and SGCE/PEG10 DMRs, and identified an association between MD and favourable neurobehavioral outcomes in early childhood.

3.3.6. Biomarkers

Four studies were associated with adherence to the MD and subsequent repercussions on biomarkers and implications of the pregnancy and on the newborn. Gesteiro, E. et al. [31] aimed to determine the relationship between diet within the first trimester and biomarkers of insulin resistance at birth. They found that women consuming low MD adherence diets had low-fasting glycaemia and delivered infants with high insulinaemia. A follow up cross-sectional study by Gasteiro, E., Bastida, S. et al. [32] aiming to identify the relationship between diet quality during pregnancy and serum lipid, arylesterase and homocysteine values at birth identified that neonates whose mothers had low adherence to the MD presented impaired levels of the referenced biomarkers. In a cohort study by Mantzoros et al. [38], multivariable linear regression was used to analyse the correlation between maternal diet during the 1st and 2nd trimesters and cord blood levels of leptin and adiponectin. High adherence to the MD was not found to be associated with these levels. Conversely, a study by Monteagudo et al. [39] on the exposure to organochlorine pesticides and maternal diet indicated that higher folic acid supplementation and greater exposure to the endocrine-disrupting residues were related to higher newborn weight.

3.3.7. Behavioural Development

One cohort study by Steenweg-de Graaff et al. [42], examining the pregnancies and follow-up of the 3104 children born, found that the MD was not associated with internalizing problems such as anxiety or depression, while low adherence to the MD was positively associated with increased child externalizing problems, such as aggression or inattention.

Of the 22 studies included, 18 found that adherence to the Mediterranean Diet during pregnancy had protective factors on the health of the newborn and 4 of the studies were inconclusive or showed no correlation. None of the studies showed a negative association between the MD and the outcomes.

4. Discussion

The mechanisms by which the MD exerts its effect on fetal development and maternal health are complex and need further research. By reviewing the available literature focusing specifically on MD interventions/exposure, as opposed to all dietary patterns as in previous reviews, we have a good overview of how the MD pattern effects mothers and their offspring on a variety of outcomes. Particularly interesting insights can be gleaned from the numerical values associated with some of the risk factors. The studies in this review are of good quality and represent a combined study population >63,000.

The observed heterogeneity of interventions, study populations and outcomes measured, allows for a big picture view of how the MD diet exerts its effects at all gestational ages and in the early years of life. For instance, when looking at behavioural outcomes, this review concluded that adherence to the MD in pregnancy has a statistically significant impact on decreasing the likelihood of offspring exhibiting depressive behaviours (OR 0.28) [35] in an ethnically diverse cohort, and another study added to this with a reduced OR of 0.90 [42] for developing externalising behaviours (such as aggression) for offspring of mothers with a high MDA.

Though some of the outcome categories we have identified only have 2 or 3 studies, they give a good starting point for future research to build on the current knowledge. Berti et al.'s comprehensive literature review of early life nutritional exposures on life-long health splits its findings into 'sections' [46] which, again, give a big picture overview on the vast impact that maternal, early life and even pre-conceptional nutrition can have. Unlike some more focused reviews, investigating the impact of maternal diet on allergic diseases [47], for instance, we hope that our review's heterogeneity contributes to a wider understanding of maternal dietary impact.

This review brings together some ideas of how the MD may be contributing to in-utero development through specific mechanistic pathways. The methylation of specific sites in two of the studies (see Table 3) present results on how the MD, as opposed to specific nutrients, contribute to this very time-sensitive window of change of DNA methylation during fetal development.

The results on atopy, asthma and eczema highlight that whilst the MD is not always protective, it is associated with a reduced likelihood of allergic disorders as a result of maternal MD diet adherence and compounded further by offspring MD adherence. This type of follow up warrants attention; further investigation into the impacts which MD adherence for offspring of mothers who had high adherence to the MD during pregnancy and lactation, compared to non-MD adherent mother-child pairs would allow for dietary recommendations to be evidence-based through the course of pregnancy and early life as a one-time course. Intuitively, this would be a good way to approach dietary recommendations for improving health, as most children adopt their mother's dietary choices as the main provider of food in early life.

With regards to premature birth, low birth weight and childhood obesity, the evidence is more mixed. The studies that found no association between the MD and decreased likelihood of premature birth were of high quality. Some of the uncertainty is due to the limitations of the studies, some not controlling for confounders of specific outcomes like intrauterine growth, such as smoking. Despite this, the studies that were inconclusive on the impact of the MD on their primary chosen outcome, for instance the INMA birth cohort study for childhood obesity [30] and Parlapani et al.'s work [29] on birth complications and prematurity, still found statistically significant positive associations between MD adherence and other health outcomes in their results, such as waist circumference and likelihood of pre-eclampsia and necrotizing enterocolitis for each study, respectively.

A strong case for the positive impact of the MD can be seen in the results of the studies focusing on cardiometabolic and congenital defects, GDM and DNA methylation. Though these studies investigated hugely different markers and outcomes, it is clear that the MD has a protective effect on them all. The evidence presented here regarding DNA methylation and biomarkers reflects a novel way to measure the impact of dietary changes and contributes to the understanding of the mechanisms behind the long-term impacts which 'early-life programming' has. The nature of DNA methylation in the fetal development time-course makes it possible to observe the impact which specific intra-uterine exposures have on offspring DNA methylations 20, 30 or 40 years later. For example, studies on the impact of intra-uterine exposure to famine showed that lower methylation of 5 CpG dinucleotides within the insulin-like growth factor-II differentially methylated region (DMR) [48] was detected in affected offspring decades later. Thus, the potential for future research on the impact of the MD on methylation sites of interest is vast, as dietary exposure has such a large impact.

The pattern of MD that may influence the reduction of adverse effects most appears to be one where there is purposefully added evoo and nuts. As seen in the present literature, increased vegetables and oily fish and decreased processed foods delivered positive results, and the effects are seen both in metabolically healthy and compromised gestation, indicating that the MD could be a diet with beneficial outcomes for GDM and metabolically healthy pregnancies.

The results of this review add to the growing body of evidence that the Mediterranean Diet is a beneficial dietary recommendation throughout the life course. By collating the evidence on outcomes of the MD for the mother and child, we highlight the broad range of effects this dietary intervention has. The limitations of this work are the small number of studies per outcome group, with the biggest group here being 'premature birth and birth weight' at only 7 studies total. Regular updates of this review are important as research around the topic is growing, and with an expanding evidence base, the possibility of meta-analysis for each category is likely. The biggest strength of this review is that, even with small numbers of studies, it highlights the impact which MDA in pregnancy and early childhood can have on several different health outcomes. The implications for clinical practice are great, as prescribing an MD pattern to women of reproductive age is a simple intervention, with important clinical potential for both the mother and offspring.

5. Conclusions

The Mediterranean Diet in pregnancy and early infancy is safe and beneficial for a wide range of maternal and offspring outcomes. Further research to ascertain the relationship and mechanisms maternal MD has with health outcomes of interest in different populations is needed to position it as a public health intervention for all populations.

Acknowledgments: This article presents independent research commissioned by the National Institute for Health Research (NIHR) under the Collaborations for Leadership in Applied Health Research and Care (CLAHRC) programme for North West London. The views expressed in this publication are those of the authors and not necessarily those of the NHS, NIHR or the Department of Health.

Appendix A Search Strategy

Database: MEDLINE <1946 to February 04, 2019>:

1. exp Fruit/ or Fruit.mp. (131831)
2. edible grain/ or exp vegetables/ (42391)
3. Leguminosae.mp. or exp Fabaceae/ (69062)
4. nut.mp. or Nuts/ (6941)
5. exp Olive Oil/ or evoo.mp. (4609)
6. extra virgin olive oil.mp. (931)
7. monounsaturated fatty acids.mp. or exp Fatty Acids, Monounsaturated/ (45287)
8. Fishes/ or oily fish.mp. or Fatty Acids, Omega-3/ or Seafood/ (75289)
9. Lycopersicon esculentum/ or tomato*.mp. (23549)
10. ((high or more or increase* or elevat* or much or rais*) adj6 (intake or consumption or consume or eat* or amount*)).tw. (179734)
11. 1 or 2 or 3 or 4 or 5 or 6 or 7 or 8 or 9 (348823)
12. 10 and 11 (14459)
13. Milk/ or exp Dairy Products/ or dairy.mp. (120218)
14. red meat.mp. or exp Red Meat/ (4259)
15. Meat Products/ or processed meat.mp. (7285)
16. Wine/ or red wine.mp. (11501)
17. 13 or 14 or 15 or 16 (141175)
18. ((low or little or medium or moderate or less or decrease* or reduc* or restrict*) adj6 (intake or consumption or consume or eat* or amount*)).tw. (177151)
19. 17 and 18 (6736)
20. Mediterranean Diet.mp. or exp Diet, Mediterranean/ (4636)
21. exp Pregnancy/ or pregnan*.mp. (966432)
22. maternal diet.mp. (1885)
23. prenatal.mp. or Prenatal Nutritional Physiological Phenomena/ or Prenatal Exposure Delayed Effects/ (161569)
24. 21 or 22 or 23 (994947)
25. child health.mp. or Child/ or Child Health/ (1617258)
26. newborn.mp. or exp Infant, Newborn/ (717150)
27. 25 or 26 (2178391)
28. exp animals/ not humans.sh. (4543138)
29. randomized controlled trial.mp. or Randomized Controlled Trial/ (498499)
30. controlled clinical trial.mp. or Controlled Clinical Trial/ (105353)
31. placebo.de. (0)
32. trial.mp. (1103671)
33. Retrospective Studies/ or Cohort Studies/ or cohort stud*.mp. (994814)
34. 29 or 30 or 31 or 32 or 33 (2049754)
35. 34 not 28 (1998518)
36. ((12 and 19) or 20) and 24 and 27 and 35 (22)

Database: Embase Classic+Embase <1947 to 2019 February 04>:

1. exp Fruit/ (127584)
2. fruit.mp. (110586)

3. vegetable*.mp. or leafy vegetable/ or vegetable/ (128062)
4. exp legume/ or legume.mp. (79855)
5. exp nut/ or nut*.mp. (670576)
6. extra virgin olive oil/ or olive oil/ or evoo.mp. (12921)
7. monounsaturated fatty acids.mp. or exp monounsaturated fatty acid/ (8992)
8. exp fish/ or oily fish.mp. or omega 3 fatty acid/ (240566)
9. sea food/ (9239)
10. tomato*.mp. or tomato/ (24952)
11. ((high or more or increase* or elevat* or much or rais*) adj6 (intake or consumption or consume or eat* or amount*)).tw. (242744)
12. 1 or 2 or 3 or 4 or 5 or 6 or 7 or 8 or 9 or 10 (1171930)
13. 11 and 12 (49587)
14. exp dairy product/ (111325)
15. red meat/ or red meat.mp. (5486)
16. processed meat.mp. or exp processed meat/ (2238)
17. red wine.mp. or exp red wine/ (5583)
18. 14 or 15 or 16 or 17 (122438)
19. ((low or little or medium or moderate or less or decrease* or reduc* or restrict*) adj6 (intake or consumption or consume or eat* or amount*)).tw. (234104)
20. 18 and 19 (7553)
21. Mediterranean Diet.mp. or exp Mediterranean diet/ (7990)
22. gestation*.mp. (314747)
23. maternal diet.mp. or maternal nutrition/ (11842)
24. pregnancy/ or pregnant woman/ or pregnant.mp. or pregnancy.mp. (1002075)
25. perinatal.mp. or perinatal period/ (133359)
26. prenatal period/ or prenatal exposure/ or prenatal.mp. (242919)
27. 22 or 23 or 24 or 25 or 26 (1257012)
28. child health.mp. or child health/ (76176)
29. offspring.mp. or progeny/ (100561)
30. newborn.mp. or newborn/ (696375)
31. neonat*.mp. (351653)
32. child/ (1815590)
33. baby.mp. or exp baby/ (71511)
34. 28 or 29 or 30 or 31 or 32 or 33 (2643576)
35. (exp animal/ or nonhuman/) not exp human/ (6800562)
36. clinical trial.de. (974978)
37. randomized controlled trial.de. (537435)
38. randomization.de. (81390)
39. single blind procedure.de. (33905)
40. double blind procedure.de. (160469)
41. crossover procedure.de. (58496)
42. placebo.de. (340801)
43. prospective study.de. (502412)
44. (randomi?ed controlled adj1 trial*).mp. [mp=title, abstract, heading word, drug trade name, original title, device manufacturer, drug manufacturer, device trade name, keyword, floating subheading word, candidate term word] (744347)
45. rct.mp. (32969)

46. (random* adj1 allocat*).mp. [mp=title, abstract, heading word, drug trade name, original title, device manufacturer, drug manufacturer, device trade name, keyword, floating subheading word, candidate term word] (37316)
47. (single adj1 blind*).mp. [mp=title, abstract, heading word, drug trade name, original title, device manufacturer, drug manufacturer, device trade name, keyword, floating subheading word, candidate term word] (45468)
48. (double adj1 blind*).mp. [mp=title, abstract, heading word, drug trade name, original title, device manufacturer, drug manufacturer, device trade name, keyword, floating subheading word, candidate term word] (245874)
49. ((treble or triple) adj1 (blind* or placebo*)).mp. [mp=title, abstract, heading word, drug trade name, original title, device manufacturer, drug manufacturer, device trade name, keyword, floating subheading word, candidate term word] (1080)
50. 36 or 37 or 38 or 39 or 40 or 41 or 42 or 43 or 44 or 45 or 46 or 47 or 48 or 49 (2093989)
51. (exp animal/ or nonhuman/) not exp human/ (6800562)
52. ((13 and 20) or 21) and 27 and 34 and 50 (26)
53. 52 not 51 (26)

Database: Web of Science to February 04, 2019

1. (fruit*) (263,892)
2. (vegetable*) (112,459)
3. (legume*) (36,972)
4. (nut or nuts) (23,002)
5. ("olive oil*") (20,491)
6. (evoo) (626)
7. (oily fish) (417)
8. (seafood or "sea food") (11,311)
9. (tomato*) (71,792)
10. 9 or 8 or 7 or 6 or 5 or 4 or 3 or 2 or 1 (461,691)
11. ((high*or more or increase* or elevat* or raise*) Near/2 (intake* or consumption or cosume* or eat* or amount)) (263,946)
12. 11 and 10 (21,325)
13. (dairy) (120,668)
14. ("red meat*") (3894)
15. ("processed meat*") (2493)
16. ("red wine*") (12,350)
17. 16 or 15 or 14 or 13 (138,033)
18. ((low* or little or moderate or less or decrease* or reduc* or restric*) Near/2 (intake of consumption of consume or eat* or amount*)) (278,089)
19. 18 and 17
20. 19 and 12 (960)
21. (Mediterranean Near/2 diet*) (7.892)
22. 21 or 20 (8715)
23. (pregnancy or pregnant) (448,186)
24. (gestation) (97,107)
25. (maternal near/2 nutrition*) (3839)
26. (maternal near/2 diet*) (4936)
27. (perinatal) (65,900)
28. 27 or 26 or 25 or 24 or 23 (529,985)

29. (child* near/2 health*) (73,055)
30. (offspring) (84,383)
31. (baby or babies) (62,022)
32. (newborn*) (139,175)
33. (f?etus*) (6686)
34. 33 or 32 or 31 or 30 or 29 (347,022)
35. 34 and 28 (76,415)
36. 35 and 22 (76)

Cochrane: <xx to February 04, 2019>:

TITLE-ABS-KEY ("Mediterranean Diet" AND (pregnan* OR prenatal OR perinatal OR pregnan* OR maternal) AND (offspring OR baby OR child AND health OR newborn))

Appendix B

Table A1. The based on National Institutes of Health (NIH) study quality assessment tools for controlled trials [1].

Criteria	Yes	No	Other
Cohort/cross-sectional studies			(CD, NR, NA) *
1. Was the research question or objective in this paper clearly stated?			
2. Was the study population clearly specified and defined?			
3. Was the participation rate of eligible persons at least 50%?			
4. Were all the subjects selected or recruited from the same or similar populations (including the same time period)? Were inclusion and exclusion criteria for being in the study prespecified and applied uniformly to all participants?			
5. Was a sample size justification, power description, or variance and effect estimates provided?			
6. For the analyses in this paper, were the exposure(s) of interest measured prior to the outcome(s) being measured?			
7. Was the timeframe sufficient so that one could reasonably expect to see an association between exposure and outcome if it existed?			
8. For exposures that can vary in amount or level, did the study examine different levels of the exposure as related to the outcome (e.g., categories of exposure, or exposure measured as continuous variable)?			
9. Were the exposure measures (independent variables) clearly defined, valid, reliable, and implemented consistently across all study participants?			
10. Was the exposure(s) assessed more than once over time?			
11. Were the outcome measures (dependent variables) clearly defined, valid, reliable, and implemented consistently across all study participants?			
12. Were the outcome assessors blinded to the exposure status of participants?			
13. Was loss to follow-up after baseline 20% or less?			
14. Were key potential confounding variables measured and adjusted statistically for their impact on the relationship between exposure(s) and outcome(s)?			
Quality Rating (Good, Fair, or Poor)			
Rater #1 FA:			
Rater #2 AS:			
Additional Comments (If POOR, please state why):			
Randomized Control Trials			
1. Was the study described as randomized, a randomized trial, a randomized clinical trial, or an RCT?			
2. Was the method of randomization adequate (i.e., use of randomly generated assignment)?			
3. Was the treatment allocation concealed (so that assignments could not be predicted)?			
4. Were study participants and providers blinded to the treatment group assignment?			
5. Were the people assessing the outcomes blinded to the participants' group assignments?			
6. Were the groups similar at baseline on important characteristics that could affect outcomes (e.g., demographics, risk factors, co-morbid conditions)?			
7. Was the overall drop-out rate from the study at endpoint 20% or lower of the number allocated to treatment?			
8. Was the differential drop-out rate (between treatment groups) at the endpoint 15 percentage points or lower?			
9. Was there high adherence to the intervention protocols for each treatment group?			
10. Were other interventions avoided or similar in the groups (e.g., similar background treatments)?			
11. Were outcomes assessed using valid and reliable measures, implemented consistently across all study participants?			
12. Did the authors report that the sample size was sufficiently large to be able to detect a difference in the main outcome between groups with at least 80% power?			
13. Were outcomes reported or subgroups analyzed prespecified (i.e., identified before analyses were conducted)?			

Table A1. *Cont.*

Criteria	Yes	No	Other
14. Were all randomized participants analyzed in the group to which they were originally assigned, i.e., did they use an intention-to-treat analysis?			
Quality Rating (Good, Fair, or Poor)			
Rater #1 initials:			
Rater #2 initials:			
Additional Comments (If POOR, please state why):			

* CD, cannot determine; NA, not applicable; NR, not reported; [1] National Heart, Lung, and Blood Institute (NHLBI). Study Quality Assessment Tools. NHLBI. Available at: https://www.nhlbi.nih.gov/health-topics/study-quality-assessment-tools.

Appendix C

The studies excluded after full text screening:

Schulpis, Kleopatra H.; Gavrili, Stavroula; Vlachos, George; Karikas, George A.; Michalakakou, Kelly; Demetriou, Elisabeth; Papassotiriou, Ioannis	2006	The effect of nutritional habits on maternal-neonatal lipid and lipoprotein serum levels in three different ethnic groups	Annals of Nutrition and Metabolism
Rasmussen, Morten Arendt; Maslova, Ekaterina; Halldorsson, Thorhallur Ingi; Olsen, Sjurdur Frodi	2014	Characterization of Dietary Patterns in the Danish National Birth Cohort in Relation to Preterm Birth	Plos One
Cuervo, Marta; Sayon-Orea, Carmen; Santiago, Susana; Alfredo Martinez, Jose	2014	Dietary and Health Profiles of Spanish Women in Preconception, Pregnancy and Lactation	Nutrients
Balci, Yasemin Isik; Ergin, Ahmet; Karabulut, Aysun; Polat, Aziz; Dogan, Mustafa; Kucuktasci, Kazim	2014	Serum Vitamin B12 and Folate Concentrations and the Effect of the Mediterranean Diet on Vulnerable Populations	Pediatric Hematology and Oncology
Andrusaityte, Sandra; Grazuleviciene, Regina; Petraviciene, Inga	2017	Effect of diet and maternal education on allergies among preschool children: A case-control study	Environmental Research
Haggarty, Paul; Campbell, Doris M.; Duthie, Susan; Andrews, Katherine; Hoad, Gwen; Piyathilake, Chandrika; McNeill, Geraldine	2009	Diet and deprivation in pregnancy	British Journal of Nutrition

Figure A1. The papers excluded after full-text screening.

References

1. Reijnders, I.F.; Mulders, A.G.M.G.J.; van der Windt, M.; Steegers, E.A.P.; Steegers-Theunissen, R.P.M. The impact of periconceptional maternal lifestyle on clinical features and biomarkers of placental development and function: A systematic review. *Hum. Reprod. Update* **2019**, *25*, 72–94. [CrossRef] [PubMed]
2. Kampmann, U.; Madsen, L.R.; Skajaa, G.O.; Iversen, D.S.; Moeller, N.; Ovesen, P. Gestational diabetes: A clinical update. *World J. Diabetes* **2015**, *6*, 1065–1072. [CrossRef] [PubMed]
3. Kind, K.L.; Moore, V.M.; Davies, M.J. Diet around conception and during pregnancy – effects on fetal and neonatal outcomes. *Reprod. Biomed. Online* **2006**, *12*, 532–541. [CrossRef]

4. Zerfu, T.A.; Pinto, E.; Baye, K. Consumption of dairy, fruits and dark green leafy vegetables is associated with lower risk of adverse pregnancy outcomes (APO): A prospective cohort study in rural Ethiopia. *Nutr. Diabetes* **2018**, *8*, 52. [CrossRef] [PubMed]
5. Sewell, D.A.; Hammersley, V.S.; Devereux, G.; Robertson, A.; Stoddart, A.; Weir, C.; Worth, A.; Sheikh, A. Investigating the effectiveness of the Mediterranean diet in pregnant women for the primary prevention of asthma and allergy in high-risk infants: Protocol for a pilot randomised controlled trial. *Trials Electron. Resour.* **2013**, *14*, 173. [CrossRef] [PubMed]
6. Seyedrezazadeh, E.; Moghaddam, M.P.; Ansarin, K.; Vafa, M.R.; Sharma, S.; Kolahdooz, F. Fruit and vegetable intake and risk of wheezing and asthma: A systematic review and meta-analysis. *Nutr. Rev.* **2014**, *72*, 411–428. [CrossRef]
7. Nurmatov, U.; Devereux, G.; Sheikh, A. Nutrients and foods for the primary prevention of asthma and allergy: Systematic review and meta-analysis. *J. Allergy Clin. Immunol.* **2011**, *127*, 724–733. [CrossRef]
8. Venter, C.; Brown, K.R.; Maslin, K.; Palmer, D.J. Maternal dietary intake in pregnancy and lactation and allergic disease outcomes in offspring. *Pediatr. Allergy Immunol.* **2017**, *28*, 135–143. [CrossRef] [PubMed]
9. Moody, L.; Chen, H.; Pan, Y.-X. Early-Life Nutritional Programming of Cognition—The Fundamental Role of Epigenetic Mechanisms in Mediating the Relation between Early-Life Environment and Learning and Memory Process12. *Adv. Nutr.* **2017**, *8*, 337–350. [CrossRef] [PubMed]
10. Estruch, R.; Martínez-González, M.A.; Corella, D.; Salas-Salvadó, J.; Ruiz-Gutiérrez, V.; Covas, M.I.; Fiol, M.; Gómez-Gracia, E.; López-Sabater, M.C.; Vinyoles, E.; et al. Effects of a Mediterranean-style diet on cardiovascular risk factors: A randomized trial. *Ann. Int. Med.* **2006**, *145*, 1–11. [CrossRef]
11. Jacobs, D.R.; Gross, M.D.; Tapsell, L.C. Food synergy: An operational concept for understanding nutrition. *Am. J. Clin. Nutr.* **2009**, *89*, 1543S–1548S. [CrossRef] [PubMed]
12. Reduction in the Incidence of Type 2 Diabetes with the Mediterranean Diet | Diabetes Care. Available online: http://care.diabetesjournals.org/content/34/1/14.short (accessed on 6 March 2019).
13. Widmer, R.J.; Flammer, A.J.; Lerman, L.O.; Lerman, A. The Mediterranean Diet, its Components, and Cardiovascular Disease. *Am. J. Med.* **2015**, *128*, 229–238. [CrossRef]
14. Fischer, M.; Stronati, M.; Lanari, M. Mediterranean diet, folic acid, and neural tube defects. *J. Pediatr.* **2017**, *43*, 74. [CrossRef] [PubMed]
15. Dessypris, N.; Karalexi, M.A.; Ntouvelis, E.; Diamantaras, A.-A.; Papadakis, V.; Baka, M.; Polychronopoulou, S.; Sidi, V.; Stiakaki, E.; Petridou, E.T. Association of maternal and index child's diet with subsequent leukemia risk: A systematic review and meta analysis. *Cancer Epidemiol.* **2017**, *47*, 64–75. [CrossRef]
16. Sofi, F.; Abbate, R.; Gensini, G.F.; Casini, A. Accruing evidence on benefits of adherence to the Mediterranean diet on health: An updated systematic review and meta-analysis. *Am. J. Clin. Nutr.* **2010**, *92*, 1189–1196. [CrossRef] [PubMed]
17. Netting, M.J.; Middleton, P.F.; Makrides, M. Does maternal diet during pregnancy and lactation affect outcomes in offspring? A systematic review of food-based approaches. *Nutrition* **2014**, *30*, 1225–1241. [CrossRef]
18. Grieger, J.A.; Clifton, V.L. A Review of the Impact of Dietary Intakes in Human Pregnancy on Infant Birthweight. *Nutrients* **2014**, *7*, 153–178. [CrossRef] [PubMed]
19. Chen, X.; Zhao, D.; Mao, X.; Xia, Y.; Baker, P.N.; Zhang, H. Maternal Dietary Patterns and Pregnancy Outcome. *Nutrients* **2016**, *8*, 351. [CrossRef]
20. Liberati, A.; Altman, D.G.; Tetzlaff, J.; Mulrow, C.; Gøtzsche, P.C.; Ioannidis, J.P.A.; Clarke, M.; Devereaux, P.J.; Kleijnen, J.; Moher, D. The PRISMA Statement for Reporting Systematic Reviews and Meta-Analyses of Studies That Evaluate Health Care Interventions: Explanation and Elaboration. *PLoS Med.* **2009**, *6*, e1000100. [CrossRef] [PubMed]
21. Rees, K.; Hartley, L.; Flowers, N.; Clarke, A.; Hooper, L.; Thorogood, M.; Stranges, S. "Mediterranean" dietary pattern for the primary prevention of cardiovascular disease. *Cochrane Database Syst. Rev.* **2013**, *12*, CD009825. [CrossRef]
22. National Heart, Lung, and Blood Institute (NHLBI). Study Quality Assessment Tools. Available online: https://www.nhlbi.nih.gov/health-topics/study-quality-assessment-tools (accessed on 23 March 2019).

23. Assaf-Balut, C.; Garcia de la Torre, N.; Durán, A.; Fuentes, M.; Bordiú, E.; del Valle, L.; Valerio, J.; Familiar, C.; Jiménez, I.; Herraiz, M.A.; et al. Medical nutrition therapy for gestational diabetes mellitus based on Mediterranean Diet principles: A subanalysis of the St Carlos GDM Prevention Study. *BMJ Open Diabetes Res. Care* **2018**, *6*, e000550. [CrossRef] [PubMed]
24. Assaf-Balut, C.; Garcia de la Torre, N.; Duran, A.; Fuentes, M.; Bordiu, E.; Del Valle, L.; Familiar, C.; Ortolá, A.; Jiménez, I.; Herraiz, M.A.; et al. A Mediterranean diet with additional extra virgin olive oil and pistachios reduces the incidence of gestational diabetes mellitus (GDM): A randomized controlled trial: The St. Carlos GDM prevention study. *PLoS ONE* **2017**, *12*, e0185873. [CrossRef] [PubMed]
25. Botto, L.D.; Krikov, S.; Carmichael, S.L.; Munger, R.G.; Shaw, G.M.; Feldkamp, M.L. Lower rate of selected congenital heart defects with better maternal diet quality: A population-based study. *Arch. Dis. Child. Fetal Neonatal Ed.* **2016**, *101*, 43–49. [CrossRef] [PubMed]
26. Chatzi, L.; Rifas-Shiman, S.L.; Georgiou, V.; Joung, K.E.; Koinaki, S.; Chalkiadaki, G.; Margioris, A.; Sarri, K.; Vassilaki, M.; Vafeiadi, M.; et al. Adherence to the Mediterranean diet during pregnancy and offspring adiposity and cardiometabolic traits in childhood. *Pediatr. Obes.* **2017**, *12*, 47–56. [CrossRef] [PubMed]
27. Chatzi, L.; Torrent, M.; Romieu, I.; Garcia-Esteban, R.; Ferrer, C.; Vioque, J.; Kogevinas, M.; Sunyer, J. Mediterranean diet in pregnancy is protective for wheeze and atopy in childhood. *Thorax* **2008**, *63*, 507–513. [CrossRef] [PubMed]
28. Chatzi, L.; Kogevinas, M. Prenatal and childhood Mediterranean diet and the development of asthma and allergies in children. *Public Health Nutr.* **2009**, *12*, 1629–1634. [CrossRef] [PubMed]
29. Parlapani, E.; Agakidis, C.; Karagiozoglou-Lampoudi, T.; Sarafidis, K.; Agakidou, E.; Athanasiadis, A.; Diamanti, E. The Mediterranean diet adherence by pregnant women delivering prematurely: Association with size at birth and complications of prematurity. *J. Mater. Fetal Neonatal Med.* **2017**, *13*, 1–8. [CrossRef]
30. Fernandez-Barres, S.; Romaguera, D.; Valvi, D.; Martinez, D.; Vioque, J.; Navarrete-Munoz, E.M.; Amiano, P.; Gonzalez-Palacios, S.; Guxens, M.; Pereda, E.; et al. Mediterranean dietary pattern in pregnant women and offspring risk of overweight and abdominal obesity in early childhood: The INMA birth cohort study. *Pediatr. Obes.* **2016**, *11*, 491–499. [CrossRef] [PubMed]
31. Gesteiro, E.; Rodriguez Bernal, B.; Bastida, S.; Sanchez-Muniz, F.J. Maternal diets with low healthy eating index or Mediterranean diet adherence scores are associated with high cord-blood insulin levels and insulin resistance markers at birth. *J. Clin. Nutr.* **2012**, *66*, 1008–1015. [CrossRef]
32. Gesteiro, E.; Sanchez-Muniz, F.J.; Ortega-Azorin, C.; Guillen, M.; Corella, D.; Bastida, S. Maternal and neonatal FTO rs9939609 polymorphism affect insulin sensitivity markers and lipoprotein profile at birth in appropriate-for-gestational-age term neonates. *J. Physiol.* **2016**, *72*, 169–181. [CrossRef]
33. Gonzalez-Nahm, S.; Mendez, M.; Robinson, W.; Murphy, S.K.; Hoyo, C.; Hogan, V.; Diane, R. Low maternal adherence to a Mediterranean diet is associated with increase in methylation at the MEG3-IG differentially methylated region in female infants. *Environ. Epigenetics* **2017**, *3*. [CrossRef]
34. Haugen, M.; Meltzer, H.M.; Brantsaeter, A.L.; Mikkelsen, T.; Osterdal, M.L.; Alexander, J.; Olsen, S.F.; Bakketeig, L. Mediterranean-type diet and risk of preterm birth among women in the Norwegian Mother and Child Cohort Study (MoBa): A prospective cohort study. *Acta Obstet. Gynecol. Scand.* **2008**, *87*, 319–324. [CrossRef]
35. House, J.S.; Mendez, M.; Maguire, R.L.; Gonzalez-Nahm, S.; Huang, Z.; Daniels, J.; Susan KMurphy, B.; Fuemmeler, F.A.; Wright, C.H. Periconceptional Maternal Mediterranean Diet Is Associated with Favorable Offspring Behaviors and Altered CpG Methylation of Imprinted Genes. *Front. Cell Dev. Biol.* **2018**, *6*. [CrossRef]
36. Castro-Rodriguez, J.A.; Ramirez-Hernandez, M.; Padilla, O.; Pacheco-Gonzalez, R.M.; Pérez-Fernández, V.; Garcia-Marcos, L. Effect of foods and Mediterranean diet during pregnancy and first years of life on wheezing, rhinitis and dermatitis in preschoolers. *Allergol. Immunopathol. (Madr)* **2016**, *44*, 400–409. [CrossRef]
37. Lange, N.E.; Rifas-Shiman, S.L.; Camargo, C.A.; Gold, D.R.; Gillman, M.W.; Litonjua, A.A. Maternal dietary pattern during pregnancy is not associated with recurrent wheeze in children. *J. Allergy Clin. Immunol.* **2010**, *126*, 250–255. [CrossRef]
38. Mantzoros, C.S.; Sweeney, L.; Williams, C.J.; Oken, E.; Kelesidis, T.; Rifas-Shiman, S.L.; Gillman, M.W. Maternal diet and cord blood leptin and adiponectin concentrations at birth. *Clin. Nutr.* **2010**, *29*, 622–626. [CrossRef]

39. Monteagudo, C.; Mariscal-Arcas, M.; Heras-Gonzalez, L.; Ibanez-Peinado, D.; Rivas, A.; Olea-Serrano, F. Effects of maternal diet and environmental exposure to organochlorine pesticides on newborn weight in Southern Spain. *Chemosphere* **2016**, *1*, 135–142. [CrossRef]
40. Peraita-Costa, I.; Llopis-Gonzalez, A.; Perales-Marin, A.; Sanz, F.; Llopis-Morales, A.; Morales-Suarez-Varela, M. A Retrospective Cross-Sectional Population-Based Study on Prenatal Levels of Adherence to the Mediterranean Diet: Maternal Profile and Effects on the Newborn. *J. Environ. Res.* **2018**, *15*, 1530. [CrossRef]
41. Saunders, L.; Guldner, L.; Costet, N.; Kadhel, P.; Rouget, F.; Monfort, C.; Thomé, J.P.; Multigner, L. Cordier S.Effect of a Mediterranean diet during pregnancy on fetal growth and preterm delivery: Results from a French Caribbean Mother-Child Cohort Study (TIMOUN). *Paediatr. Perinat. Epidemiol.* **2014**, *28*, 235–244. [CrossRef]
42. Steenweg-de Graaff, J.; Tiemeier, H.; Steegers-Theunissen, R.P.M.; Hofman, A.; Jaddoe, V.W.V.; Verhulst, F.C.; Roza, S.J. Maternal dietary patterns during pregnancy and child internalising and externalising problems. The Generation R Study. *Clin. Nutr.* **2014**, *33*, 115–121. [CrossRef]
43. Vujkovic, M.; Steegers, E.A.; Looman, C.W.; Ocké, M.C.; Spek, P.; van der Steegers-Theunissen, R.P. The maternal Mediterranean dietary pattern is associated with a reduced risk of spina bifida in the offspring. *BJOG Int. J. Obstet. Gynaecol.* **2009**, *116*, 408–415. [CrossRef]
44. Smith, L.K.; Draper, E.S.; Evans, T.A.; Field, D.J.; Johnson, S.J.; Manktelow, B.N.; Seaton, S.E.; Marlow, N.; Petrou, S.; Boyle, E.M. Associations between late and moderately preterm birth and smoking, alcohol, drug use and diet: A population-based case-cohort study. *Arch. Dis. Child. Fetal Neonatal Ed.* **2015**, *100*, F486–F491. [CrossRef]
45. Mariscal-Arcas, M.; Rivas, A.; Monteagudo, C.; Granada, A.; Cerrillo, I.; Olea-Serrano, F. Proposal of a Mediterranean diet index for pregnant women. *J. Nutr.* **2009**, *102*, 744–749. [CrossRef]
46. Berti, C.; Agostoni, C.; Davanzo, R.; Hyppönen, E.; Isolauri, E.; Meltzer, H.M.; Steegers-Theunissen, R.P.; Cetin, I. Early-life nutritional exposures and lifelong health: Immediate and long-lasting impacts of probiotics, vitamin D, and breastfeeding. *Nutr. Rev.* **2017**, *75*, 83–97. [CrossRef]
47. Beckhaus, A.A.; Garcia-Marcos, L.; Forno, E.; Pacheco-Gonzalez, R.M.; Celedón, J.C.; Castro-Rodriguez, J.A. Maternal nutrition during pregnancy and risk of asthma, wheeze, and atopic diseases during childhood: A systematic review and meta-analysis. *Allergy* **2015**, *70*, 1588–1604. [CrossRef]
48. Heijmans, B.T.; Tobi, E.W.; Stein, A.D.; Putter, H.; Blauw, G.J.; Susser, E.S.; Slagboom, P.E.; Lumey, L.H. Persistent epigenetic differences associated with prenatal exposure to famine in humans. *Proc. Natl. Acad. Sci. USA* **2008**, *105*, 17046–17049. [CrossRef]

Permissions

All chapters in this book were first published by MDPI; hereby published with permission under the Creative Commons Attribution License or equivalent. Every chapter published in this book has been scrutinized by our experts. Their significance has been extensively debated. The topics covered herein carry significant findings which will fuel the growth of the discipline. They may even be implemented as practical applications or may be referred to as a beginning point for another development.

The contributors of this book come from diverse backgrounds, making this book a truly international effort. This book will bring forth new frontiers with its revolutionizing research information and detailed analysis of the nascent developments around the world.

We would like to thank all the contributing authors for lending their expertise to make the book truly unique. They have played a crucial role in the development of this book. Without their invaluable contributions this book wouldn't have been possible. They have made vital efforts to compile up to date information on the varied aspects of this subject to make this book a valuable addition to the collection of many professionals and students.

This book was conceptualized with the vision of imparting up-to-date information and advanced data in this field. To ensure the same, a matchless editorial board was set up. Every individual on the board went through rigorous rounds of assessment to prove their worth. After which they invested a large part of their time researching and compiling the most relevant data for our readers.

The editorial board has been involved in producing this book since its inception. They have spent rigorous hours researching and exploring the diverse topics which have resulted in the successful publishing of this book. They have passed on their knowledge of decades through this book. To expedite this challenging task, the publisher supported the team at every step. A small team of assistant editors was also appointed to further simplify the editing procedure and attain best results for the readers.

Apart from the editorial board, the designing team has also invested a significant amount of their time in understanding the subject and creating the most relevant covers. They scrutinized every image to scout for the most suitable representation of the subject and create an appropriate cover for the book.

The publishing team has been an ardent support to the editorial, designing and production team. Their endless efforts to recruit the best for this project, has resulted in the accomplishment of this book. They are a veteran in the field of academics and their pool of knowledge is as vast as their experience in printing. Their expertise and guidance has proved useful at every step. Their uncompromising quality standards have made this book an exceptional effort. Their encouragement from time to time has been an inspiration for everyone.

The publisher and the editorial board hope that this book will prove to be a valuable piece of knowledge for researchers, students, practitioners and scholars across the globe.

List of Contributors

Prasad P. Devarshi, Ryan W. Grant, Chioma J. Ikonte and Susan Hazels Mitmesser
Science and Technology, Pharmavite, LLC,West Hills, CA 91304, USA

Annica F. Dörsam, Sophia B. Lörcher, Stephan Zipfel and Katrin E. Giel
Department of Psychosomatic Medicine and Psychotherapy, Medical University Hospital Tübingen, 72076 Tübingen, Germany

Hubert Preißl
Institute for Diabetes Research and Metabolic Diseases of the Helmholtz Center Munich at the University of Tübingen; fMEG Center; German Center for Diabetes Research (DZD), 72076 Tübingen, Germany

Nadia Micali
Department of Psychiatry, Faculty of Medicine, University of Geneva, 1205 Geneva, Switzerland

Giorgia Sebastiani, Ana Herranz Barbero, Cristina Borrás-Novell, Miguel Alsina Casanova, Victoria Aldecoa-Bilbao, Mireia Pascual Tutusaus and Oscar García-Algar
Neonatology Unit, Hospital Clinic-Maternitat, ICGON, BCNatal, 08028 Barcelona, Spain

Vicente Andreu-Fernández
Grup de Recerca Infancia i Entorn (GRIE), Institut d'investigacions Biomèdiques August Pi I Sunyer (IDIBAPS), 08028 Barcelona, Spain

Silvia Ferrero Martínez and María Dolores Gómez Roig
BCNatal | Barcelona Center for Maternal Fetal and Neonatal Medicine Hospital Sant Joan de Déu, 08028 Barcelona, Spain

Aneta Lewicka
Laboratory of Epidemiology, Military Institute of Hygiene and Epidemiology, Kozielska 4, 01-163 Warsaw, Poland

Łukasz Szymański
Department of Microwave Safety, Military Institute of Hygiene and Epidemiology, Kozielska 4, 01-163 Warsaw, Poland

Kamila Rusiecka, Anna Kucza, Robert Zdanowski and Sławomir Lewicki
Department of Regenerative Medicine and Cell Biology, Military Institute of Hygiene and Epidemiology, Kozielska 4, 01-163 Warsaw, Poland

Anna Jakubczyk
Department of Biochemistry and Food Chemistry, University of Life Sciences, Skromna 8, 20-704 Lublin, Poland

Jasper Most and Leanne M Redman
Pennington Biomedical Research Center, Baton Rouge, LA 70808, USA

Sheila Dervis, Francois Haman and Kristi B Adamo
School of Human Kinetics, University of Ottawa, Ottawa, ON K1N 6N5, Canada

Ingibjorg Gunnarsdottir and Bryndis Eva Birgisdottir
Unit for Nutrition Research, Landspitali University Hospital and Faculty of Food Science and Nutrition, University of Iceland, Eiríksgata 29 101 Reykjavik, Iceland

Laufey Hrolfsdottir
Unit for Nutrition Research, Landspitali University Hospital and Faculty of Food Science and Nutrition, University of Iceland, Eiríksgata 29 101 Reykjavik, Iceland
Institution of Health Science Research, University of Akureyri and Akureyri Hospital, Eyrarlandsvegi, 600 Akureyri, Iceland

Alexander Kr. Smarason
Institution of Health Science Research, University of Akureyri and Akureyri Hospital, Eyrarlandsvegi, 600 Akureyri, Iceland

Ingibjorg Th Hreidarsdottir
Department of Obstetrics and Gynecology, Landspitali University Hospital, Hringbraut, 101 Reykjavík, Iceland

Hildur Hardardottir
Department of Obstetrics and Gynecology, Landspitali University Hospital, Hringbraut, 101 Reykjavík, Iceland
Faculty of Medicine, University of Iceland, Vatnsmýrarvegi 16, 101 Reykjavík, Iceland

Thorhallur I. Halldorsson
Unit for Nutrition Research, Landspitali University Hospital and Faculty of Food Science and Nutrition, University of Iceland, Eiríksgata 29 101 Reykjavik, Iceland
Centre for Fetal Programming, Department of Epidemiology Research, Statens Serum Institut, Artillerivej 5, 2300 Copenhagen, Denmark

Suzanne Phelan
Department of Kinesiology & Public Health, California Polytechnic State University, 1 Grand Ave, San Luis Obispo, CA 93407, USA

Barbara Abrams
Division of Epidemiology, University of California at Berkeley School of Public Health, 2121 Berkeley Way #5302, Berkeley, CA 94720-7360, USA

Rena R. Wing
Warren Alpert Medical School at Brown University Department of Psychiatry and Human Behavior, 197 Richmond Street, Providence, RI 02906, USA

Tinu M. Samuel, Olga Sakwinska and Kimmo Makinen
Nestlé Research, 1000 Lausanne, Switzerland

Graham C. Burdge
School of Human Development and Health, Faculty of Medicine, University of Southampton, Southampton SO16 6YD, UK

Keith M. Godfrey
MRC Lifecourse Epidemiology Unit and NIHR Southampton Biomedical Research Centre, University of Southampton & University Hospital Southampton NHS Foundation Trust, Southampton SO16 6YD, UK

Irma Silva-Zolezzi
Nestlé Research, Singapore 618802, Singapore

Emily E. Hohman
Center for Childhood Obesity Research, The Pennsylvania State University, University Park, State College, PA 16802, USA

Jennifer S. Savage and Katherine M. McNitt
Center for Childhood Obesity Research, The Pennsylvania State University, University Park, State College, PA 16802, USA
Department of Nutritional Sciences, The Pennsylvania State University, University Park, State College, PA 16802, USA

Alison D. Gernand
Department of Nutritional Sciences, The Pennsylvania State University, University Park, State College, PA 16802, USA

Abigail M. Pauley and Krista S. Leonard
Exercise Psychology Laboratory, Department of Kinesiology, The Pennsylvania State University, University Park, State College, PA 16802, USA

Tricia Turner
Diagnostic Medical Sonography, South Hills School of Business and Technology, State College, PA 16801, USA

Danielle Symons Downs
Exercise Psychology Laboratory, Department of Kinesiology, The Pennsylvania State University, University Park, State College, PA 16802, USA
Department of Obstetrics and Gynecology, Penn State College of Medicine, Hershey, PA 17033, USA

Jaimey M. Pauli
Department of Obstetrics and Gynecology, Penn State College of Medicine, Hershey, PA 17033, USA
Department of Maternal & Fetal Medicine, Penn State College of Medicine, Hershey, PA 17033, USA

Daniel E. Rivera
Control Systems Engineering Laboratory, School for Engineering of Matter, Transport, and Energy, Arizona State University, Tempe, AZ 85287, USA

Yu-Chin Lien and David E Condon
Center for Research on Reproduction and Women's Health, Perelman School of Medicine, The University of Pennsylvania, Philadelphia, PA 19104, USA

Michael K Georgieff and Phu V Tran
Department of Pediatrics, University of Minnesota School of Medicine, Minneapolis, MN 55455, USA

Rebecca A Simmons
Center for Research on Reproduction and Women's Health, Perelman School of Medicine, The University of Pennsylvania, Philadelphia, PA 19104, USA
Children's Hospital of Philadelphia, Philadelphia, PA 19104, USA

Jasper Most, Abby D. Altazan and Leanne M. Redman
Reproductive Endocrinology and Women's Health, Pennington Biomedical Research Center, Baton Rouge, LA 70817, USA

Candida J. Rebello
Clinical Trials Unit, Pennington Biomedical Research Center, Baton Rouge, LA 70817, USA

Corby K. Martin
Ingestive Behavior, Weight Management, and Health Promotion Laboratory, Pennington Biomedical Research Center, Baton Rouge, LA 70817, USA

Marshall St Amant
Woman's Hospital, 100 Woman's Way, Baton Rouge, LA 70817, USA

Enrique Vázquez, Alejandro Barranco, María Ramírez, Ricardo Rueda and María J. Martín
R&D Abbott Nutrition, 18004 Granada, Spain

Elena Oliveros
R&D Abbott Nutrition, 18004 Granada, Spain
Doctoral programme in Biomedicine, School of Health Sciences, University of Granada, 18071 Granada, Spain

Rachael Buck
R&D Abbott Nutrition, Columbus, OH 43219, USA

Agnes Gruart and Jose María Delgado-García
Division of Neurosciences, Pablo de Olavide University, 41013 Seville, Spain

Federica Amati, Sondus Hassounah and Alexandra Swaka
Department of Primary Care and Public Health, Imperial College London, London W6 8RP, UK

Index